Computed Tomography

Physical Principles, Clinical Applications,
and Quality Control

Second Edition

COMPUTED TOMOGRAPHY

Physical Principles, Clinical Applications, and Quality Control

Second Edition

Euclid Seeram, RT (R), BSc, MSc, FCAMRT
Medical Imaging, Advanced Studies
British Columbia Institute of Technology
Burnaby, British Columbia, Canada

W.B. SAUNDERS COMPANY

A Harcourt Health Sciences Company
Philadelphia   London   New York   St. Louis   Sydney   Toronto

W.B. SAUNDERS COMPANY
A Harcourt Health Sciences Company

The Curtis Center
Independence Square West
Philadelphia, Pennsylvania 19106-3399

Executive Editor: Jeanne Wilke
Developmental Editor: Jennifer Genett
Project Manager: Linda McKinley
Production Editor: Ellen Forest
Book Design Manager: Judi Lang
Cover Design: Liz Rudder

Library of Congress Cataloging-in-Publication Data

Seeram, Euclid.
    Computed tomography : physical principles, clinical applications, & quality control /
Euclid Seeram.
        p. cm.
    Includes bibliographical references and index.
    ISBN 0-7216-8173-5 (alk. paper)
        1. Tomography.   I. Title.

RC78.7.T6 S36 2000
616.07'57—dc21   00-063497

Cover photograph courtesy of Marconi.

COMPUTED TOMOGRAPHY: PHYSICAL PRINCIPLES, CLINICAL APPLICATIONS,   ISBN 0-7216-8173-5
AND QUALITY CONTROL
SECOND EDITION

Printed in the United States of America.

Last digit is the print number: 9   8   7   6   5   4   3   2   1

Contributors

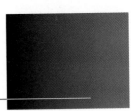

Robert Cacak, PhD
Director of Medical Physics
Salem Hospital
Salem, Oregon

Lois Doody, RT (R), AC
Instructor, British Columbia Institute of Technology;
Burnaby, British Columbia, Canada

Borys Flak, MD
Associate Professor, Department of Radiology
University of British Columbia
Vancouver, British Columbia, Canada

Donna Keobke, RT (R)
CT and MRI Technologist
Radiology Department
Vancouver General Hospital
Vancouver, British Columbia, Canada

David KB Li, MD, FRCPA
Professor, Department of Radiology
University of British Columbia;
Associate Head, Department of Radiology
Vancouver General Hospital and University of
British Columbia Hospitals
Vancouver, British Columbia, Canada

Jeremy Lysne, RT(R)(CT)
Department of Radiology
Denver Children's Hospital
Denver, Colorado

Robert Nugent, MD
Associate Professor, Department of Radiology
University of British Columbia;
Staff Neuroradiologist, Department of Radiology
Vancouver General Hospital
Vancouver, British Columbia, Canada

Bryan Westerman, PhD
Clinical Sciences Manager
Toshiba America Medical Systems
Tustin, California

Reviewers

Joseph R. Bittengle, M Ed, RT(R)(ARRT)
Chairman and Assistant Professor
Department of Radiologic Technology
University of Arkansas for Medical Sciences
Little Rock, Arkansas

Deborah L. Durham, MA, RT(R)(MR)(CT)
Department Chair, CT/MR Curricula
Forsyth Technical Community College
Winston-Salem, North Carolina

This book is affectionately
dedicated
to
my brothers and sisters,

Lolita, *Robin*, *Virgil*, *Sabrina*, and *Nirvani*

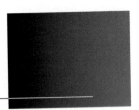

Preface to the Second Edition

The publication of the first edition of *Computed Tomography: Physical Principles, Clinical Applications & Quality Control* resulted in the only in-depth text dedicated solely to computed tomography and its clinical uses. Topics included the physical principles of computed tomography; digital image processing; image reconstruction, quality, and manipulation; instrumentation; radiation dose; and quality control. The text also focused on the clinical applications of CT, including pediatric CT.

The evolution of CT physical principles, instrumentation, and clinical applications continue at a steady pace and have led to a number of recent significant developments. The most significant of these is multislice volume CT scanning, which was announced and demonstrated in 1998 at the meeting of the Radiological Society of North America in Chicago. Multislice CT has revolutionized CT scanning and resulted in the wide range of new clinical applications that are examined in this book. This expansion of CT technology and its applications has resulted in a new, expanded edition of *Computed Tomography: Physical Principles, Clinical Applications, and Quality Control* that reflects the current state of CT technology.

PURPOSE

Although the second edition has grown by six chapters to accommodate all the recent advances in CT, the text remains dedicated to its original manifold purposes: to provide comprehensive coverage of the physical principles of CT and its clinical applications for both adults and children; to lay the foundation necessary for the practice of CT scanning; to enhance communication between the CT technologist and other medical personnel; and to promote an understanding of sectional anatomic images as they relate to CT.

CONTENT AND ORGANIZATION

Chapter 1 lays the foundations of computed tomography by reviewing its history, including the introduction of the CT scanner as a diagnostic medical imaging tool. Because the digital computer is central to the CT scanner, Chapter 2 takes a closer look at the concepts of computer technology. This chapter begins with an overview of computer systems and concludes with computer applications in radiology, including picture archiving and communication systems and three-dimensional (3D) imaging. Chapter 3 examines the topic of image processing and representation and explores the relevancy of CT to the technology of digital image processing.

Chapter 4 begins a more in-depth examination of the physical principles of CT, including the meaning of CT numbers and the concept of windowing. Chapter 5 addresses the concepts of data acquisition, the first step in image production. Chapter 6 focuses on what the CT technologist needs to know to understand the process of image reconstruction. Chapter 7 is devoted to CT instrumentation. The discussion of image manipulation continues in Chapter 8, which includes an introduction to multiplanar reconstruction and 3D imaging. Chapter 9 describes Electron Beam CT used to overcome the difficulties of imaging moving internal organs, and Chapter 10 describes mobile CT. The focus on physical principles and instrumentation concludes with Chapters 11 and 12, which examine image quality and patient dose, respectively.

Chapters 13–16 are devoted to the physical concepts of volume CT scanning: Chapter 13 details the fundamentals of single-slice spiral/helical CT (also called *volume CT*), and Chapter 14 outlines the major advances in volume scanning. Chapter 15 furthers the discussion of volume scanning by examining multislice spiral/helical CT, and Chapter 16 examines in depth one of the major advances in volume scanning, continuous imaging, also called *real-time CT fluoroscopy*.

Because the advances in spiral/helical CT have resulted in an increased use of 3D display of sectional anatomy, Chapters 17-19 examine 3D CT imaging. Chapter 17 examines the fundamental concepts of 3D CT. Chapters 18 and 19 explore two applications of 3D CT: CT angiography and virtual endoscopy.

The next three chapters include updated and expanded coverage of the clinical applications of CT: Chapter 20, "CT of the Head, Neck, and Spine"; Chapter 21, "CT of the Body"; and Chapter 22, "Pediatric CT." The final chapter, Chapter 23, presents updated information on CT quality control. Four appendices summarize the historical and technical developments in CT and list specifications for three modern CT scanners.

NEW TO THIS EDITION

The second edition keeps up with the latest advances in CT imaging with six new chapters that provide full coverage of the latest in multislice spiral/helical CT and its clinical applications. Chapter 14 outlines the most recent advances in volume scanning and their clinical applications, most notably continuous, or real-time, imaging, subsecond scanning, and multislice detectors and image reconstruction. Chapter 15, reviews the development of multislice CT, describes the physical principles of data acquisition and image reconstruction, and explains the equipment components used in multislice spiral CT. Chapter 16 elaborates on the principles and technology of real-time CT fluoroscopy by examining imaging principles, equipment components, and performance considerations such as image quality and radiation dose. Chapter 17 gives technologists the tools needed to enhance their interaction with 3-D imaging systems by outlining the fundamental concepts of 3D imaging in CT. This chapter concludes with an overview of the clinical applications of 3D imaging in CT and MRI and looks toward the future of 3D imaging in radiology. Chapter 18 elaborates on the technical requirements of computed tomography angiography through a discussion of patient preparation, acquisition parameters, and contrast media administration. The chapter also develops an outline of several 3D visualization tools for use in CTA. Finally, Chapter 19 examines the ideas of virtual CT imaging and the future of virtual endoscopy in radiology.

In addition, each chapter from the previous edition has been expanded and updated to include state-of-the-art technology and the most up-to-date information on physical principles, instrumentation, and quality control.

The addition of 130 new images demonstrates the achievements of these technologic advances. New line drawings provide a better representation of important concepts in the text, and a new page layout makes it easier to locate information.

USE AND SCOPE

This comprehensive text is written to meet the wide and varied requirements of its users, students, and instructors alike, and it can meet many different educational and program needs. *Computed Tomography: Physical Principles, Clinical Applications, and Quality Control* can be used as the primary text for introductory CT courses at the diploma, associate, and baccalaureate degree levels; it serves as a resource for continuing education programs; it functions as a reference text for the CT technologist and other imaging personnel; and it provides the necessary overview of the physical and clinical aspects of CT, which is a prerequisite for graduate-level courses in CT.

The content is intended to meet the educational requirements of various radiologic technology professional associations including the American Society of Radiologic Technologists, the American Registry for Radiologic Technologists, the Canadian Association of Medical Radiation Technologists, the College of Radiographers in the United Kingdom, as well as those in Africa, Asia, Australia, and continental Europe.

CT has become an integral part of the education of radiologic technologists who play a significant role in the care and management of patients undergoing sophisticated imaging procedures.

Read on, learn, and enjoy. Your patients will benefit from your wisdom.

Euclid Seeram, RT(R), BSc, MSc, FCAMRT
British Columbia, Canada

Acknowledgments

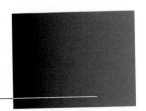

It is indeed a pleasure to express sincere thanks to several individuals whose time and efforts have contributed tremendously to this second edition. First and foremost, I must thank all my contributors—three radiologists, two physicists, and three technologists extraordinnaire—who gave their time and expertise to write selected chapters in this book. They are listed on a separate page. In particular, I am indebted to Dr. Robert Cacak, PhD from whom I have learned much about radiation dose in CT.

The content of this book is built around the works and expertise of several noted physicists, radiologists, computer scientists, and biomedical engineers employed in universities, hospitals, and the manufacturing industry. In essence, they are the tacit authors of this text, and I am truly grateful to all of them. In this regard, I owe a good deal of thanks to Dr. Godfrey Hounsfield and Dr. Allan Cormack, both of whom shared the Nobel Prize for Medicine and Physiology for their work in the invention and development of the CT scanner. I have been in personal communication with Dr. Hounsfield and he has graciously provided me with details of his biography and his original experiments. I am also grateful to Dr. Robert Ledley, inventor of the first whole-body CT scanner, and the current president of the National Biomedical Research Foundation at Georgetown University Medical Center, and to Professor Dr. Willi Kalender, PhD, of the Institute of Medical Physics in Germany, for providing me with details of their biographies and photographs. One individual who provided me with a photograph of Allan Cormack is Professor Robert Gonsalves, chairman of the Department of Electrical Engineering and Computing Science, Tufts University. Thanks for your time and efforts in locating this important photograph.

Additionally, I am appreciative of the efforts of Dr. Hui Hu, PhD, a physicist at General Electric Medical Systems and "Ken" Katsuyuki Taguchi of Toshiba Medical Systems in Japan for reading, critiquing, and offering constructive comments on my description of image reconstruction in multislice CT. I also appreciate the efforts of Dr. Hui He, PhD, and Dr. Jiang Hsieh, PhD, both physicists at General Electric Medical Systems, for feedback on some technical details on multislice CT and for providing several CT image artifacts, respectively.

In addition, I must acknowledge the efforts of all the individuals from CT manufacturers who have assisted me generously with technical details and photographs of their CT scanners for use in the book. In particular, I am grateful to Fredric Friedberg (senior Vice President and general counsel), Dr. Bryan Westerman, PhD, Carol Malin, and Philip Moore of Toshiba Medical Systems; Rick Boone, Mike Sims (who explained quite a bit on Picker's approach to multislice CT scanning), Paula Newell, and Mary Beth Zadel of Picker International; Sandy Clark of General Electric Medical Systems; Irene Jemczyk and Bob Carter of Philips Medical Systems; Kimberly Cooper of Siemens Medical Systems; and Hiromichi Kawachi of Shimadzu Medical Systems. Additionally, I would like to thank Elscint for permission to use selected photographs from its CT brochures.

Equally important are three other individuals who provided me with several CT images for use in the text. They are John C Posh, RT, (R) (MR), Chief MRI Technologist at Muhlenberg Hospital Center; Ryan Hennen of Vital Images in Minneapolis, Minnesota; and Martin Ratner of Nuclear Associates, Carle Place, New York.

In this book I have used several illustrations from original papers published in the professional literature and I an indeed thankful to all the publishers and especially to the authors who have done the original work.

Three individuals who deserve special mention are Jayaram Udupa, PhD, and Gabor Herman, PhD, of the Medical Image Processing Group at the University of Pennsylvania; and Michael Vannier, MD, FACR of the Mallinckrodt Institute of Radiology, Washington University School of Medicine in St. Louis, for their work on 3D imaging and its applications in CT.

Additionally, I must acknowledge the work of the two reviewers of this book, Joseph Bittengle and Deborah Durham, who offered constructive comments to help improve the quality of the chapters. Their efforts are very much appreciated.

The people at Mosby and W.B. Saunders, Harcourt Health Sciences Companies, deserve special thanks for their hard work, encouragement and support of this project. They are Andrew Allen, PhD, Editor-in-Chief; Jeanne Wilke, Executive Editor; Jennifer Genett, Developmental Editor; and Michelle Robinson, Editorial Assistant. Thanks, Jennifer, for keeping me on track. I must also thank the individuals in the production department at Mosby for doing a wonderful job on the manuscript to bring it to its final form. In particular, I am grateful to Ellen Forest, Production Editor, who has worked exceptionally hard during the production of this book, especially in the page-proof stage.

Finally, my family deserves special mention for their love, support, and encouragement while I worked into the evenings on the manuscript. I appreciate the efforts of my lovely wife, Trish, a special person in my life, and my son, David, a very wise and special young man. Thanks for everything, especially for thinking that I am the greatest husband and dad. I would also like to acknowledge here the love, support, and encouragement of both my parents, Betty and Samuel (thanks for having me) and my in-laws, Joan and Edward Penner.

Last but not least, I must thank the thousands of students who have diligently completed my CT Physics course. Thanks for all the stimulating and challenging questions. Keep on learning and enjoy the pages that follow.

Contents

Computed Tomography

Physical Principles, Clinical Applications,
and Quality Control

Second Edition

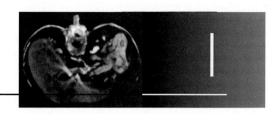

Computed Tomography

Medical imaging has experienced significant changes in both the technologic and clinical arenas. Innovations have become common in the radiology department, and today the introduction of new ideas and methods and refinements in existing techniques are apparent. The goal of these developments is the acquisition of optimal diagnostic information while the quality of care afforded to patients is improved. One such development that is a revolutionary tool of medicine, particularly in medical imaging, is computed tomography (CT). This chapter explores the meaning of CT through a brief description of its fundamental principles and historical perspectives. In addition, it summarizes the growth of CT from its introduction in the 1970s to today's technology.

MEANING

The word *tomography* is not new. It can be traced back to the early 1920s, when a number of investigators were developing methods to image a specific layer or section of the body. At that time, terms such as "body section radiography" and "stratigraphy" (from *stratum*, meaning "layer") were used to describe the technique. In 1935 Grossman refined the technique and labeled it *tomography* (from the Greek *tomos*, meaning "section"). A conventional tomogram is an image of a section of the patient that is oriented parallel to the film.

In 1937, Watson developed another tomographic technique in which the sections were transverse sections (cross-sections); this technique was referred to as *transverse axial tomography*. However, these images lacked enough detail and clarity to be useful in diagnostic radiology, preventing the technique from being fully realized as a clinical tool.

Image Reconstruction from Projections

CT overcomes limitations in detail and clarity by using image reconstruction from projections to produce sharp, clear images of cross-sectional anatomy. Image reconstruction from projections had its theoretic roots in 1917 when the Austrian mathematician Radon proved it possible to reconstruct or build up an image of a two- or three-dimensional object from a large number of its projections from different directions. This procedure has been used in a number of fields, ranging from astronomy to electron microscopy. For example, in

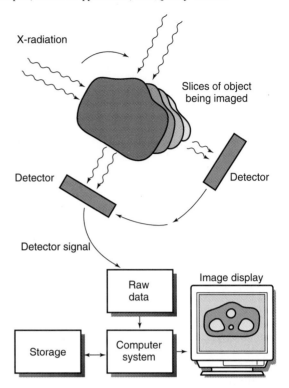

FIG. 1-1. Image reconstruction from projections. From many different directions, radiation passes through each slice or cross-section of the object being imaged. This radiation is projected onto a detector that sends signals to a computer for processing into an image that reveals the internal structure of the object.

astronomy, images of the sun have been reconstructed, and in microscopy, images of the molecular structure of bacteria can be reconstructed.

Similarly, images of the human body can be reconstructed using a large number of projections from different locations (Fig. 1-1). In simplified terms, radiation passes through each cross-section in a specific way and is projected onto a detector that sends signals to a computer for processing. The computer produces clear, sharp images of the internal structure of the object.

A more complete definition of this technique has been given by Herman (1980), who stated "Image reconstruction from projections is the process of producing an image of a two-dimensional distribution (usually some physical property) from estimates of its line integrals along a finite number of lines of known locations."

Image reconstruction from projections finally found practical application in medicine in the

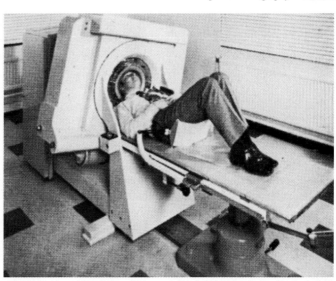

FIG. 1-2. First-generation model of a CT head scanner. (Courtesy Thorn EMI; London, England.)

1960s through the work of investigators such as Oldendorf, Kuhl, and Edwards, who studied problems in nuclear medicine. In 1963, Cormack also applied reconstruction techniques to nuclear medicine. In 1967, Hounsfield finally applied reconstruction techniques to produce the world's first clinically useful CT scanner for imaging the brain (Fig. 1-2).

These studies resulted in two types of CT systems: emission CT, in which the radiation source is inside the patient (e.g., nuclear medicine), and transmission CT, in which the radiation source is outside the patient (e.g., x-ray imaging). Both involve image reconstruction. Image reconstruction has also been used in diagnostic medical sonography and magnetic resonance imaging, which is the most recent of all imaging modalities (Fig. 1-3). This book discusses only the fundamental principles and technology of x-ray transmission CT.

Evolution of Terms

Hounsfield's work produced a technique that revolutionized medicine and diagnostic radiology. He called the technique *computerized transverse axial scanning* (tomography) in his description of the system, which was first published in the *British Journal of Radiology* in 1973. Since then a number of other terms have appeared in the literature. Terms such as "computerized transverse axial tomography," "computer-assisted tomography or computerized axial tomography," "computerized transaxial transmission reconstructive tomogra-

phy," "computerized tomography," and "reconstructive tomography" were not uncommon. The term *computed tomography* was established by the Radiological Society of North America in their major journal *Radiology*. In addition, the *American Journal of Roentgenology* accepted this term, which has now gained widespread acceptance within the radiologic community. Throughout the remainder of this book the term *computed tomography* is used.

PROCESS

The formation of CT images by a CT scanner involves three steps: data acquisition; image reconstruction; and image display, manipulation, storage, recording, and communication (Fig. 1-4).

Data Acquisition

The term *data acquisition* refers to the collection of x-ray transmission measurements from the patient. Once x-rays have passed through the patient, they fall onto special detectors that measure the transmission values, or attenuation values. Enough transmission measurements or data must be recorded to meet the requirements of the reconstruction process. In the first data collection scheme the x-ray tube and detector move in a straight line, or translate, across the patient's head, collecting a number of transmission measurements as they move from left to right (Fig. 1-5). Then the x-ray tube and detector rotated 1 degree

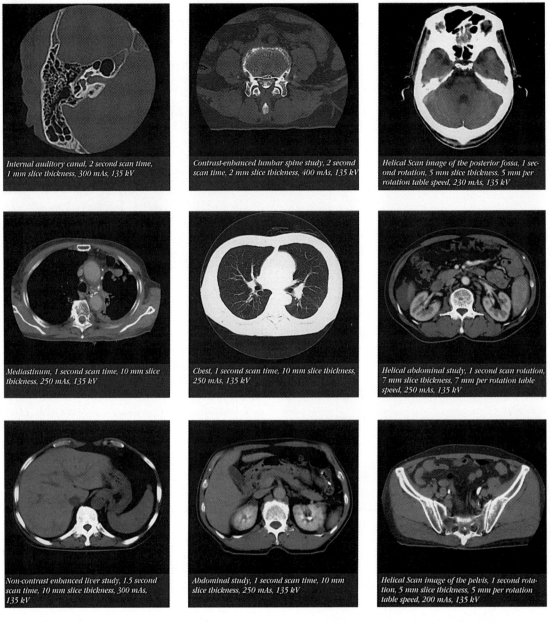

Internal auditory canal, 2 second scan time, 1 mm slice thickness, 300 mAs, 135 kV

Contrast-enhanced lumbar spine study, 2 second scan time, 2 mm slice thickness, 400 mAs, 135 kV

Helical Scan image of the posterior fossa, 1 second rotation, 5 mm slice thickness, 5 mm per rotation table speed, 230 mAs, 135 kV

Mediastinum, 1 second scan time, 10 mm slice thickness, 250 mAs, 135 kV

Chest, 1 second scan time, 10 mm slice thickness, 250 mAs, 135 kV

Helical abdominal study, 1 second scan rotation, 7 mm slice thickness, 7 mm per rotation table speed, 250 mAs, 135 kV

Non-contrast enhanced liver study, 1.5 second scan time, 10 mm slice thickness, 300 mAs, 135 kV

Abdominal study, 1 second scan time, 10 mm slice thickness, 250 mAs, 135 kV

Helical Scan image of the pelvis, 1 second rotation, 5 mm slice thickness, 5 mm per rotation table speed, 200 mAs, 135 kV

FIG. 1-3.   Examples of sectional CT images of internal anatomy after image reconstruction by the computer. (Courtesy Toshiba America Medical Systems; Tustin, Calif.)

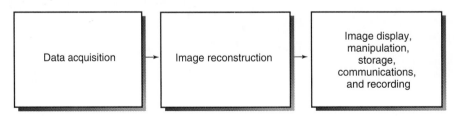

Data acquisition → Image reconstruction → Image display, manipulation, storage, communications, and recording

FIG. 1-4.   Steps in the production of a CT image.

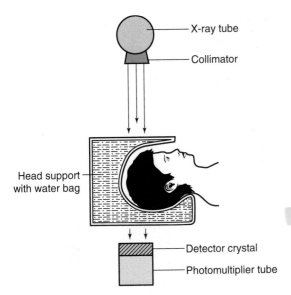

FIG. 1-5. Data collection scheme in the first CT brain scanner.

and started again to move across the patient's head, this time from right to left. This process of translate-rotate-stop-rotate, referred to as *scanning*, is repeated 180 times.

The fundamental problem with this method of data collection was the length of time required to obtain enough data for image reconstruction. Later, more efficient schemes for scanning the patient were introduced (see Chapter 5). In addition, the signals from the detectors must be converted into data that the computer can use to process the image.

Image Reconstruction

After enough transmission measurements have been collected by the detectors, they are sent to the computer for processing. The computer uses special mathematical techniques to reconstruct the CT image in a finite number of steps called *reconstruction algorithms* (see Chapter 6). For example, the reconstruction algorithm used by Hounsfield to develop the first CT scanner was called the *algebraic reconstruction technique*.

A computer is central to the CT process. In general, this involves a minicomputer and associated microprocessors for performing a number of specific functions. In some CT scanners, array processors perform high-speed calculations and specific microprocessors carry out image processing operations.

Image Display, Manipulation, Storage, Recording, and Communications

After the computer has performed the image reconstruction process, the reconstructed image can be displayed and recorded for subsequent viewing and stored for later reanalysis. The image is usually displayed on a cathode ray tube, although other display technologies are now available; for example, touch screen technology is used for scan setup and control in some scanners. However, the cathode ray tube remains the best device for the display of gray-scale imagery. Display monitors are mounted onto control consoles that allow the technologist (operator's console) and radiologist (physician's console) to manipulate, store, and record images.

Image manipulation has become popular in CT, and many computer software packages are now available. Images can be modified through image manipulation to make them more useful to the observer. For example, transverse axial images can be reformatted into coronal, sagittal, and paraxial sections. In addition, images can also be subjected to other image processing operations such as image smoothing, edge enhancement, gray-scale manipulation, and three-dimensional processing.

Images can be recorded and subsequently stored in some form of archive. Images are usually recorded on x-ray film because of its wider gray scale compared with that of instant film. Such recording is accomplished by multiformat video cameras, although laser cameras have been developed and are now common in radiology departments.

CT images can be stored on magnetic tapes and magnetic disks. More recently, optical storage technology has added a new dimension to the storage of information from CT scanners. In optical storage the stored data are read by optical means such as a laser beam. In this case, storage is referred to as *laser storage*. Optical storage media include at least three formats: disk, tape, and card (see Chapter 7).

In CT, *communications* refers to the electronic transmission of text data and images from the CT scanner to other devices such as laser printers; diagnostic workstations; display monitors in the radiology department, intensive care unit, operating and trauma rooms in the hospital; and computers outside the hospital. Electronic communications in CT require a standard protocol that facilitates connectivity (networking) among multimodalities (CT, magnetic resource imaging, digital radiography, and fluoroscopy) and multivendor equipment. The standard used for this purpose is the

Digital Imaging and Communication in Medicine (DICOM) standard established by the American College of Radiology and the National Electrical Manufacturers Association. CT departments now operate in a picture archiving and communications systems environment that allows the flow of CT data and images among devices in the radiology department. Additionally, this system can be connected to a radiology information system, which in turn is connected to the hospital information systems. (Networking is described in Chapter 2.)

HOW CT SCANNERS WORK

To enhance understanding of the early experiments and present technology, the technologist must be familiar with the way a CT scanner works (Fig. 1-6). The technologist first turns on the scanner's power and performs a quick test to ensure the scanner is in good working order. The patient is in place in the scanner opening, with appropriate positioning for the particular examination. The technologist sets up the technical factors at the control console. Scanning can now begin.

When x-rays pass through the patient, they are attenuated and subsequently measured by the detectors. The x-ray tube and detectors are inside the gantry of the scanner and rotate around the patient during scanning. The detectors convert the x-ray photons into electrical signals, or analog signals, which in turn must be converted into digital (numeric) data for input into the computer. The computer then performs the image reconstruction process. The reconstructed image is in numeric form and must be converted into electrical signals for the technologist to view on a television monitor (Fig. 1-7). Finally, the image can be stored on magnetic tapes or optical disks and recorded permanently on x-ray film.

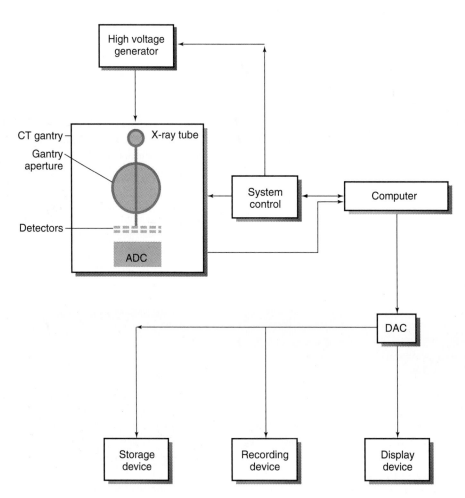

FIG. 1-6. A CT scanner showing the main components. The data communications component is not shown.

HISTORICAL PERSPECTIVES
Early Experiments

The invention of the CT scanner has revolutionized the practice of radiology. CT is so remarkable that in many cases it generates a dramatic increase in diagnostic information compared with that obtained by conventional x-ray techniques. This extraordinary invention was made possible through the work of several individuals, most notably Godfrey Newbold Hounsfield and Allan MacLeod Cormack.

Godfrey Newbold Hounsfield

Godfrey Newbold Hounsfield (Fig. 1-8) was born in 1919 in Nottinghamshire, England. He studied electronics and electrical and mechanical engineering. In 1951, Hounsfield joined the staff at EMI Limited (Electric and Musical Industries, now Thorn EMI) in Middlesex, where he began work on radar systems and later on computer technology. His research on computers led to the development of the EMIDEC 1100, the first solid-state business computer in Great Britain.

In 1967, Hounsfield was investigating pattern recognition and reconstruction techniques using the computer. (In image processing, pattern recognition involves techniques for the observer to identify, describe, and classify various features represented in an image or a signal.) From this work, he deduced that if an x-ray beam were passed through an object from all directions and measurements were made of all the x-ray transmission, information about the internal structures of that body could be obtained. This information would be presented to the radiologist in the form of pictures that would show three-dimensional representations.

With encouragement from the British Department of Health, an experimental apparatus was constructed to investigate the clinical feasibility of the technique (Fig. 1-9). The radiation used was from an americium gamma source coupled with a crystal detector. Because of the low radiation output, the apparatus took about 9 days to scan the object. The computer needed 2.5 hours to process the 28,000 measurements collected by the detector. Because this procedure was too long, various modifications were made and the gamma radiation source was replaced by a powerful x-ray tube. The results of these experiments were more accurate, but it took 1 day to produce a picture.

To evaluate the usefulness of this machine, Dr. James Ambrose, a consultant radiologist at Atkinson-Morley's Hospital, joined the study. Together, Hounsfield and Ambrose obtained readings from a specimen of human brain. The findings were encouraging in that tumor tissue was clearly differentiated from gray and white matter and controlled experiments using fresh brains from bullocks showed details such as the ventricles and pineal gland. Experiments were also done using kidney sections from pigs.

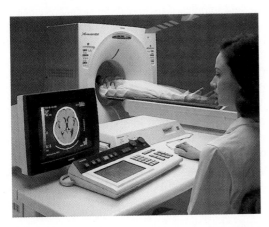

FIG. 1-7. A modern CT scanner and its control console. The reconstructed image is displayed on a television monitor for viewing by an observer. (Courtesy Toshiba America Medical Systems, Tustin, Calif.)

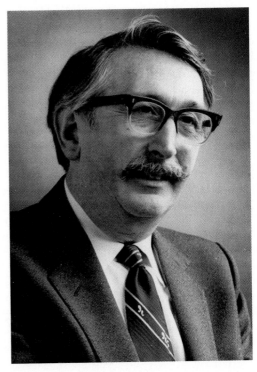

FIG. 1-8. The inventor of clinical computed tomography, Dr. Godfrey Hounsfield. (Courtesy Thorn EMI; London, England.)

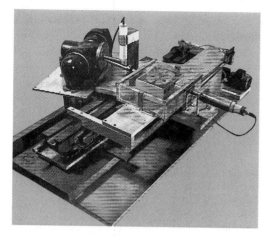

FIG. 1-9. The original lathe bed scanner used in early CT experiments by Hounsfield. (Courtesy Thorn EMI; London, England.)

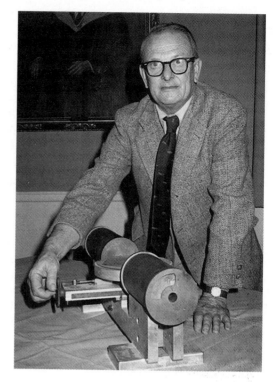

FIG. 1-10. Allan MacLeod Cormack shared the Nobel Prize with Godfrey Hounsfield for his mathematical contributions to the problem in CT. (Courtesy Tufts University; Medford, Mass.)

In 1971 the first clinical prototype CT brain scanner was installed at Atkinson-Morley's Hospital and clinical studies were conducted under the direction of Dr. Ambrose. The processing time for the picture was reduced to about 20 minutes. Later, with the introduction of minicomputers, the processing time was reduced further to 4.5 minutes.

In 1972 the first patient was scanned by this machine. This patient was a woman with a suspected brain lesion, and the picture showed clearly in detail a dark circular cyst in the brain. From this moment on and as more patients were scanned, the machine's ability to distinguish the difference between normal and diseased tissue was evident (Hounsfield, 1980).

Dr. Hounsfield's research resulted in the development of a clinically useful CT scanner for imaging the brain. For this work, Hounsfield received the McRobert Award (akin to a Nobel Prize in engineering) in 1972. In 1979, Hounsfield shared the Nobel Prize in medicine and physiology with Allan MacLeod Cormack, a physics professor at Tufts University in Medford, Massachusetts, for their contributions to the development of CT. By developing the first practical CT scanner, Hounsfield opened up a new domain for technologists, radiologists, medical physicists, engineers, and other related scientists.

Allan MacLeod Cormack

Allan MacLeod Cormack (Fig. 1-10) was born in Johannesburg, South Africa, in 1924. He attended the University of Cape Town and then studied nuclear physics at Cambridge University before returning to the University of Cape Town as a physics lecturer. He later moved to the United States and was on sabbatical at Harvard University before joining the physics department at Tufts

University. Professor Cormack developed solutions to the mathematical problems in CT.

Growth

The First 10 Years

Between 1973 and 1983 the number of CT units installed worldwide increased dramatically. Perhaps the first significant technical development came in 1974 when Dr. Robert Ledley, a professor of radiology, physiology, and biophysics at Georgetown University, developed the first whole-body CT scanner (Fig. 1-11). (Hounsfield's EMI scanner scanned only the head.)

Dr. Ledley graduated with a doctorate in dental surgery from New York University in 1948, and in 1949, he earned a master's degree in theoretical physics from Columbia University. He holds more than 60 patents on medical instrumentation and has written several books on the use of computers in biology and medicine.* In 1990 he was inducted

---

* One notable text by Dr. Ledley (co-authored by Dr. H. K. Huang) is *Cross-Sectional Anatomy: An Atlas for Computerized Tomography*, which provides radiologists and technologists with a tool to visualize sectional images. For a detailed coverage of the pioneers of CT, the reader should refer to *Naked to the Bone* by Kelves (1999).

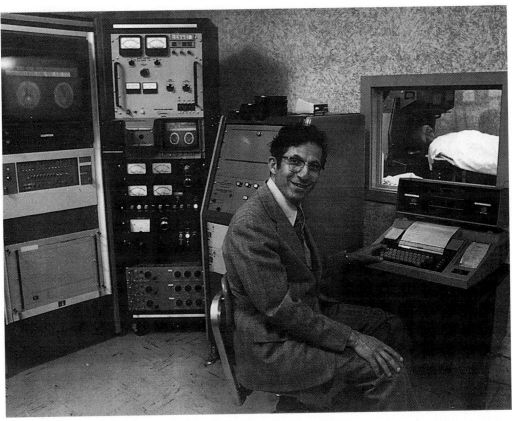

FIG. 1-11. Dr. Robert Ledley developed the first whole body CT scanner, the automatic computed transverse axial CT scanner. (Courtesy Robert Ledley; Washington, DC.)

into the National Inventors' Hall of Fame for the invention of the automatic computed transverse axial CT scanner. In 1997, Dr. Ledley won the National Medal of Technology, an honor awarded by the President of the United States for outstanding contributions to science and technology (Ledley, 1999). Currently, he is the president of the National Biomedical Research Foundation at Georgetown University Medical Center.

These pioneering works were followed by the introduction of three *generations* (a term used to refer to the method of scanning) of CT scanners. In 1974 a fourth-generation CT system was developed (Fig. 1-12).

A computer capable of performing multiple functions is central to the CT system. The CT computer has experienced several changes over time (see Chapter 7).

Image quality is another significant development as a result of technologic changes. Although earlier images appeared "blocky," images acquired later were remarkably improved (Fig. 1-13). Improvements in image quality included improved spatial resolution, decreased scan time, increased density resolution, and changes to the x-ray tube

to facilitate the increased loadability required of whole-body scanners. For example, the matrix size in 1972 was 80×80; in 1993, it was 1024×1024. In addition, the spatial resolution and scan time in 1972 were reported to be 3 line pairs/cm (lp/cm) and 5 minutes, respectively, compared with 15 lp/cm and 1 second, respectively, in 1993 (Kalender, 1993). Increased loadability resulted in scanners capable of dynamic CT examinations that took a series of scans in rapid succession. Later-model CT scanners could operate in several modes such as the prescan localization mode, which produced a survey scan of the region of interest. Rapid reformatting of the axial scans into coronal, sagittal, and oblique sections also became possible.

High-Speed CT Scanners

In 1975 the dynamic spatial reconstructor (DSR) was installed in the biodynamics unit at the Mayo Clinic. The goal of the DSR was to carry out dynamic volume scanning to accommodate imaging of the dynamics of organ systems and the functional aspects of the cardiovascular and pulmonary systems with high temporal resolution, as well as imaging anatomic details (Robb and Morin, 1991;

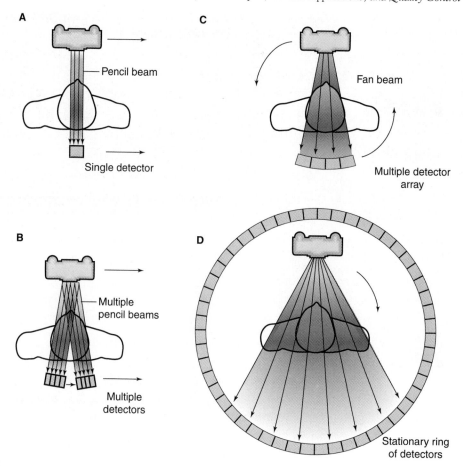

FIG. 1-12. Four basic scanning methods or systems: **A,** first generation; **B,** second generation; **C,** third generation; **D,** fourth generation.

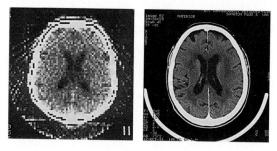

FIG. 1-13. The appearance of early CT images *(left)* compared with those produced by a more recent CT scanner *(right)*. The difference in image quality is apparent. (From Schwierz G, Kirchgeorg M: The continuous evolution of medical x-ray imaging. I. The technically driven stage of development, *Electromedica* 63:2-7, 1995.)

Ritman et al, 1991). Research on this unit has since been discontinued.

In the mid-1980s, another high-speed CT scanner was introduced using electron beam technology, a result of work by Dr. Douglas Boyd and colleagues during the late 1970s at the University of California at San Francisco. The scanner was invented to image the cardiovascular system without artifacts caused by motion. At that time the scanner was called the *cardiovascular CT scanner.* Today, this scanner is marketed by Siemens Medical Systems under the name *Evolution* and is referred to as the *electron beam CT (EBCT) scanner.* The most conspicuous difference between the EBCT scanner and conventional CT is the absence of moving parts. The EBCT scanner is capable of acquiring multislice images in as little as 50 ms and 100 ms.

Because nearly 20 manufacturers made CT scanners between 1973 and 1983, a number of developments unique to particular manufacturers were also introduced (see Appendix D). The evolution of CT continued after 1983 with nearly 10 manufacturers competing for the CT market. (The accompanying box lists milestones in CT developed by one major manufacturer.)

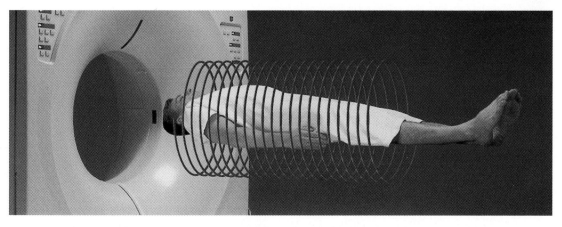

FIG. 1-14. With volume CT scanners, the x-ray tube and detectors rotate continuously as the patient moves continuously through the gantry. As a result, the x-ray beam traces a path (beam geometry) around the patient. This method of scanning the patient is referred to as *helical* or *spiral CT*. (Courtesy Toshiba America Medical Systems; Tustin, Calif.)

MILESTONES IN CT DEVELOPMENT

Data from Siemens Medical Systems, Iselin, N.J.

1974—Convolution and back-projection. Opti CT high-performance x-ray tube with compound anode technology

1976—Somatom scanner operating on fan beam principle, 5-s scan with instant image reconstruction

1978—Topogram

1981—512^2 matrix with instant image

1983—High-frequency generator technology

1984—Opti 155 CT tube with 1.75 MHU, 70-cm gantry opening, ± 25-degree gantry tilt

1986—Osteo CT (bone mineral density), xenon CT (regional cerebral blood flow)

1987—Continuous rotation flying focal spot CT tube, Dura 352 with 3.5 million heat units

1990—Spiral CT

1991—Intuitive mouse-driven Windows interface

1992—Integrated CT angiography

1994—Routine subsecond spiral CT

1996—Spiral "4" everything: neuro and high-resolution spiral

Spiral/Helical CT Scanners: Volume Scanning. In conventional CT the patient is scanned one slice at a time. The x-ray tube and detectors rotate for 360 degrees or less to scan one slice while the table and patient remain stationary. This slice-by-slice scanning is time consuming, and therefore efforts were made to increase the scanning of larger volumes in less time. This notion led to the development of a technique in which a volume of tissue is scanned by moving the patient continuously through the gantry of the scanner while the x-ray tube and detectors rotate continuously for several rotations. As a result, the x-ray beam traces a path around the patient (Fig. 1-14). Although some manufacturers call this beam geometry *spiral CT* (the beam tracing a spiral path around the patient), others refer to it as *helical CT* (the beam tracing a helical path around the patient). This book uses both terms synonymously.

The idea of this approach to scanning can be traced to three sources (Kalender, 1995). In 1989 the first report of a practical spiral CT scanner was presented at the RSNA meeting in Chicago by Dr. Willi Kalender (Fig. 1-15). Dr. Kalender has made significant contributions to the technical development and practical implementation of this approach to CT scanning. His main research interests are in the areas of diagnostic imaging, particularly the development and introduction of volumetric spiral CT.

The spiral/helical CT scanners developed after 1989 were referred to as *single-slice spiral/helical* or *volume CT scanners*. In 1992 a dual-slice spiral/helical CT scanner (volume CT scanner) was introduced to scan two slices per 360-degree rotation, thus increasing the volume coverage speed compared with single-slice volume CT scanners.

In 1998 a new generation of CT scanners was introduced at the RSNA meeting in Chicago. These scanners are called *multislice CT scanners* because they are based on the use of multidetector technology to scan more than two slices per gantry rotation, thus increasing the volume coverage speed of single-slice and dual-slice volume CT scanners.

Volume CT scanning has resulted in a wide range of applications such as CT fluoroscopy, CT angiography, three-dimensional imaging, and virtual reality imaging.

Mobile CT

A unique event in the evolution of CT technology was the development of a mobile CT scanner to image patients who are too ill or physically traumatized to be transported to a fixed CT scanner. Philips Medical Systems introduced one such scanner specifically for use in the operating room, intensive care unit, and emergency trauma unit. The portable CT scanner is compact and mounted on wheels to facilitate transportation of the unit to remote locations in the hospital for technologists (Fig. 1-16).

Clinical Efficacy Studies

The term *efficacy* is synonymous with effectiveness, efficiency, and performance. A number of investigators designed efficacy studies to test the clinical usefulness of this new diagnostic technique. Studies reported the results of scanning the brain, spinal cord, neck, thorax, abdomen, retroperitoneum, pelvis, and extremities.

CT became well established in the diagnosis of diseases of the central nervous system, and in some cases, it eliminated the need for examinations such as pneumoencephalography and reduced the frequency of cerebral angiography. Disorders such as gliomas, metastases, intracranial lesions, aneurysms, infarctions, hemorrhage, and atrophy have been successfully detected by CT. Later, whole-body clinical applications (see Chapter 21) became effective. In addition, CT proved useful in radiation treatment planning to provide accurate isodose curves and in other areas, such as determination of the mineral salt content in bones, or quantitative CT. The introduction of multislice CT scanners now requires studies to demonstrate their clinical usefulness compared with their single-slice counterparts.

Radiation Dose Studies

A fundamental goal of any new imaging technique is to provide maximum information content with the minimum radiation dose to the patient. Perry and Bridges (1973) measured both the cranial radiation dose and the gonadal radiation dose for a series of scans. Their results provided a foundation for future studies. Initially, the radiation dose to the patient was thought to be negligible because the beam

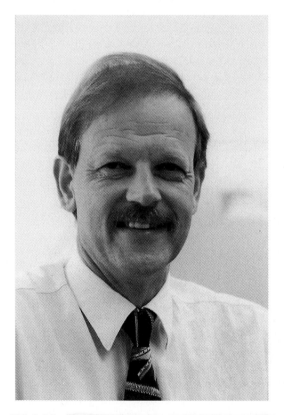

FIG. 1-16.   Dr. Willi Kalender has made significant contributions to the introduction and development of volume spiral CT scanning. (Courtesy Willi Kalender; Nürnberg, Germany.)

in CT was tightly collimated, but the patient exposure for a series of CT scans usually exceeds that of film radiography of the same area (Seeram, 1982).

Radiation dose is an integral topic in CT technology because the CT beam geometry and method of acquiring images differ from conventional radiography. Several imaging parameters in CT affect dose including slice thickness, noise, resolution detector efficiency, reconstruction algorithm, collimation, and filtration. Various dose studies have explored the ways in which these factors influence the dose.

These studies have also led to the development of special ways to measure and describe the dose (Seeram, 1999). Ionization chambers or thermoluminescent dosimeters are used to measure the dose. Dose descriptors include the single-scan dose profile, multiple-scan dose profile, CT dose index, multiple-scan average dose, and isodose curves.

Additionally, manufacturers have developed various schemes to reduce the dose in CT. One scheme uses three elements to keep the patient dose to a minimum during data acquisition: (1) combined applications to reduce exposure, a prepatient filtering technique that reduces the dose by about 15% compared with conventional CT; (2) new ultrafast ceramic detectors that reduce the dose by another 25%; and (3) online dose modulation or dose adaption, whereby the milliamperage (mA) is optimized to the patient characteristics (diameter and absorption) to reduce the dose up to about another 40% (Fig. 1-17).

Quality Control

As with any medical imaging system, CT is subject to quality control procedures and tests. Testing system performance is vital to maintain optimal image quality and minimize the production of image artifacts. Because the CT system consists of several mechanical and electronic components, many quality control tests are currently available. These range from simple tests, which the technologist can perform using phantoms provided by the manufacturers, to more complex tests that may require the expertise of the radiologic physicist or biomedical engineer.

Other Uses

CT is useful in areas other than medicine. For example, CT can be used to study internal log defects. Funt and Bryan (1987) investigated the use of CT technology in a sawmill. They developed and tested algorithms that automatically interpreted CT images of logs and stated "The computer program uses the high density and elliptical shape of knots to distinguish them from good wood, and the low density and rough texture of rotten areas to separate rotten wood from sound wood." Habermehl and Ridder (1997) detailed the use of a portable CT scanner to take images of trees to determine wood rots; locate knots, hollows, and other defects; and determine water distribution inside the tree trunk (Fig. 1-18). These portable tree CT scanners use a cesium-137 gamma radiation source with a fan beam falling on an array of about 30 sodium iodide detectors.

CT has also been used in paleoanthropology. Zonneveld and colleagues (1989) found that CT

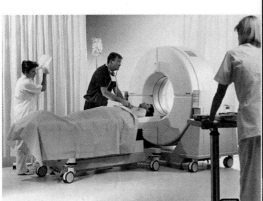
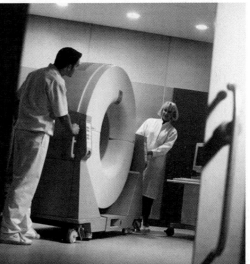

A   B

FIG. 1-16.   A, The mobile CT scanner takes images of patients who are too ill or physically traumatized to be transported to the fixed CT scanner in the main radiology department. **B,** The scanner is compact and mounted on wheels to facilitate easy transportation of the unit by technologists. (Courtesy Philips Medical Systems; Shelton, Conn.)

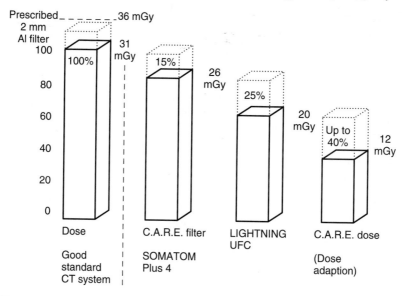

FIG. 1-17.   The Combined Application to Reduce Exposure (CARE) program is one method used to reduce the radiation dose in CT. (Courtesy Siemens Medical Systems; Iselin, NJ.)

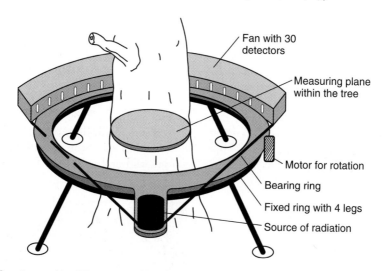

FIG. 1-18.   A portable CT scanner for imaging trees. (From Habermehl A, Ridder HW: γ-Ray tomography in forest and tree sciences. In Bonse U, ed: *Developments in x-ray tomography, proceedings of the SPIE* 3149:234-243, 1997.)

can visualize internal anatomy of completely preserved Egyptian mummies (Fig. 1-19) (Yasuda et al, 1992). Several cases report the use of CT in baggage inspection at airports and in paleoornithology, oil exploration, fat stock breeding, and other animal investigations (Fig. 1-20). In fat stock breeding, pigs are scanned to determine the meat quality defined as the best combination of water, protein, and fat, thus eliminating the need to kill the pigs for this determination (Fig. 1-21).

Sirr and Waddle (1999) used CT to evaluate bowed stringed instruments such as violins. The scans demonstrated varying degrees of internal damage (e.g., wormholes, air gaps, and plastic de-

formities of wood) or those resulting from repair (e.g., glue lines, filler substances, and wooden cleats and patches) not seen when the instruments are examined visually. The researchers also concluded that CT facilitated verification of authenticity and proof of ownership.

DIGITAL IMAGE PROCESSING

CT is an excellent example of digital image processing (Fig. 1-22). The x-ray beam passes through the patient and falls onto special detectors. These detectors convert the x-ray photons into electrical signals (analog signals) that must be converted

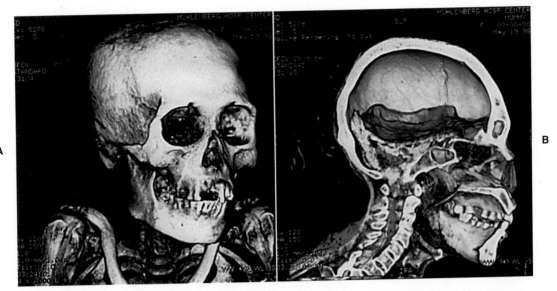

FIG. 1-19.   CT can be used to image mummies without destroying the bandages or plaster in which they are wrapped. **A,** These images are 3D CT images of a 1000-year-old Peruvian mummy using volume rendering with a bone and detail filter. **B,** A lateral view of the same mummy shows residual brain in the posterior fossa. (Courtesy John Posh; Bethlehem, Penn.)

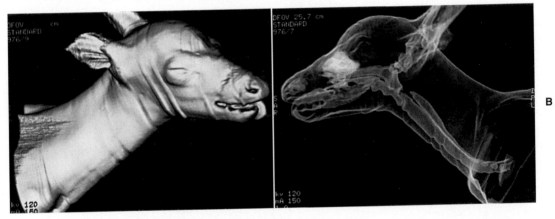

FIG. 1-20.   **A,** 3D surface rendering of a 2-month-old whitetail fawn mauled by a mountain lion. **B,** The same fawn examined by CT using 3D transparency program to demonstrate the airways and other air-filled cavities. (Courtesy John Posh; Bethlehem, Penn.)

into numeric data (digital data) for input into a digital computer.

Digital image processing involves the use of a digital computer to process and manipulate digital images. The computer receives an input of a digital image and performs specific operations on the data to produce an output image that is different from and more useful than the input image. The procedure had its origins at the National Aeronautics and Space Administration Jet Propulsion Laboratory at the California Institute of Technology, where it was used to enhance and restore images from space. Today, the space program generates and uses the largest amount of digital data.

The digital image processing of medical images dates back to the 1970s, about the time CT was introduced to the medical community. Today, digital radiography, digital fluoroscopy, digital subtraction angiography, and magnetic resonance imaging use digital image processing techniques. Currently the field of radiology generates and uses the second largest amount of digital information.

APPLICATIONS OF VOLUME SCANNING

Volume scanning from either single-slice spiral/helical or multislice spiral/helical CT generates vast amounts of data compared with slice-by-slice conventional CT scanning. Several new applications provide radiologists and other physicians with additional tools for taking images of patients using CT and enhancing their own diagnostic effectiveness. These new applications include continuous imaging or CT fluoroscopy, three-dimensional imaging and visualization, CT angiography, and virtual reality imaging.

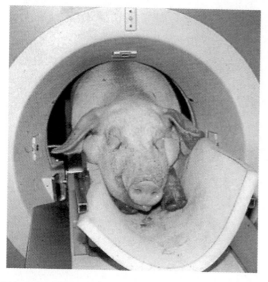

FIG. 1-21. CT scanning of pigs in fat stock breeding to determine meat quality. (Courtesy Siemens Medical Systems; Iselin, NJ.)

CT Fluoroscopy

CT fluoroscopy, or continuous imaging, depends on spiral/helical data acquisition methods, high-speed processing, and a fast image-processing algorithm for image reconstruction. In conventional CT, the time lag between data acquisition and image reconstruction makes real-time display of images impossible. CT fluoroscopy allows for the reconstruction and display of images in real-time with variable frame rates. In 1996 the United States Food and Drug Administration approved real-time CT fluoroscopy as a clinical tool for use in radiology (Katada et al, 1996).

CT fluoroscopy is based on three advances in CT technology: (1) fast, continuous scanning made possible by spiral/helical scanning principles; (2) fast image reconstruction made possible by special hardware performing quick calculations and a new image reconstruction algorithm; and (3) continuous image display using cine mode at frame rates of two to eight images per second (Daly and Templeton, 1999).

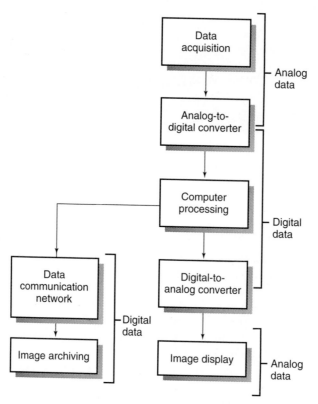

FIG. 1-22. Major components of the digital imaging system on which CT is based.

Other support tools were developed to facilitate interventional procedures in CT fluoroscopy. One such tool, the Fluoro Assisted Computed Tomography System, uses a unique flat-panel amorphous silicon digital detector coupled with an x-ray tube via a C-arm, which is a part of the CT gantry (Fig. 1-24).

Three-Dimensional Imaging and Visualization

Three-dimensional (3D) imaging is a popular technique in CT because of the availability of large amounts of digital data. 3D is now possible on CT scanners and the results have been promising. 3D CT is already used in radiation treatment planning, craniofacial imaging, surgical planning, and orthopedics.

3D images can be obtained using a hardware-based or software-based approach. The hardware-based approach uses specialized equipment such as electronic computer display units to execute algorithms for 3D imaging, and the software-based approach uses computer programs, or software-coded algorithms. These algorithms, or rendering techniques, transform the transaxial CT data into simulated 3D images. In general, two classes of techniques are available for the transformation: surface and volume-based techniques. Each technique consists of three steps: volume formation, classification, and image projection. Whereas *volume formation* involves stacking images to form a volume with some preprocessing, *classification* refers to determining the tissue types in the slices. According to Fishman

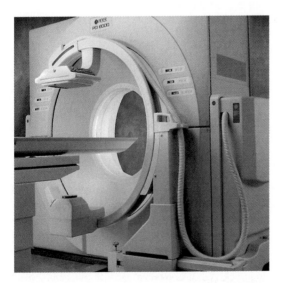

FIG. 1-23. A digital C-arm fluoro unit to assist in interventional procedures in CT fluoroscopy. (Courtesy Picker International; Cleveland, Ohio.)

(1991), image projection consists of "projecting the classified volume data in such a manner that a two-dimensional (2D) representation or simulation of the 3D volume is formed."

Computer graphics has played a role in the evolution and refinement of 3D imaging (Rhodes, 1991). Computer graphics involves the creation, manipulation, and display of pictures or images using the computer. It allows the user to express ideas and information in a visual format and includes various ways to represent data to create and display images using graphics programming languages and image processing techniques.

3D CT has created a new area of interest for technologists who have the opportunity to participate in its development. A recent article on 3D imaging by Seeram (1998) outlines the fundamental concepts and role of the technologist in this exciting new domain of CT imaging.

Visualization is a term used in the discussion of the display of images in CT. It involves the use of computer programs, or visualization tools, that provide the observer-diagnostician with additional information from the image to facilitate diagnosis. These tools can be simple (e.g., image contrast and brightness [windowing] tools) or advanced (e.g., 3D imaging, interactive, and cine visualization tools).

CT Angiography

CT angiography is defined as CT imaging of blood vessels opacified by contrast media (Kalender, 1995). During contrast injection, the entire area of interest is scanned using spiral/helical CT and images are recorded when vessels are fully opacified to show arterial or venous phase of enhancement.

CT angiography uses 3D-imaging principles to display images of the vasculature through intravenous injection of contrast media compared with those of intraarterial angiograms. Four essential elements are patient preparation; selection of acquisition parameters (total spiral/helical scan time, slice thickness, table speed) to optimize the imaging process; contrast media injection; and postprocessing techniques and visualization tools such as algorithms to display 3D images in multiplanar reconstruction, maximum intensity projection, shaded surface display, volume rendering, and interactive cine modes (Fig. 1-24).

CT Endoscopy

Virtual reality is a branch of computer science that immerses users in a computer-generated environment

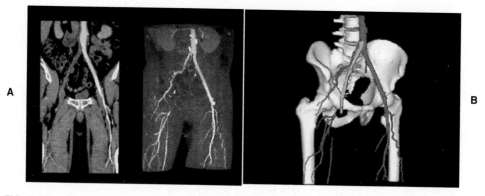

FIG. 1-24.   A, Multiplanar reconstruction (*left*) and maximum intensity projection (*right*) images. **B,** A 3D multitissue reconstruction image of an aortobifemoral bypass graft exhibiting a thrombosed right graft. (Courtesy Marconi Medical Systems; Canada.)

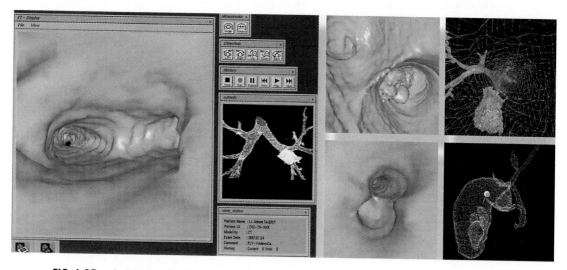

FIG. 1-25.   A virtual reality CT image. The fly-through software allows the operator to produce endoluminal images of hollow structures such as the trachea, bronchi, and blood vessels similar to those obtained by an endoscope. (Courtesy Toshiba America Medical Systems; Tustin, Calif.)

and allows them to interact with 3D scenes. The application of virtual reality concepts to the creation of inner views of tubular structures is called *virtual endoscopy* (Vining, 1999). Volume CT scanners produce large data sets (2D axial images) compared with their conventional slice-by-slice counterparts. Subsequently, volume CT scanners have allowed for improved 3D imaging, CT fluoroscopy, CT angiography, and CT virtual endoscopy (Fig. 1-25).

REFERENCES

Cormack AM: Early two-dimensional reconstruction and recent topics stemming from it, Nobel Award address, *Med Phys* 7:277–282, 1980.

Daly B, Templeton PA: Real-time CT fluoroscopy: evaluation of an interventional tool, *Radiology* 211:309–315, 1999.

Fishman EK et al: Three-dimensional imaging, *Radiology* 181:321–337, 1991.

Fu TY, Hayworth M: The digital image: its structure, storage, and transmission. In Hunter TB, ed: *The computer in radiology*, Rockville, Md, 1986, Aspen.

Funt F, Bryant EC: Detection of internal log defects by automatic interpretation of computer tomography images, *Forest Prod J* 37:56–62, 1987.

Habermehl A, Ridder H-W: γ-Ray tomography in forest and tree sciences. In Bonse U, ed: *Developments in x-ray tomography: proceedings of the SPIE*, 3149:234–243, 1997.

Herman GT: *Image reconstruction from projections: the fundamentals of computerized tomography*, New York, 1980, Academic Press.

Hounsfield GN: Computed medical imaging, Nobel Award address, *Med Phys* 7:283–290, 1980.

Kalender W: Quo vadis CT? CT in the year 2000, *Electromedica* 61:30–39, 1993.

Kalender W: *Personal communication*, 1999.

Kalender W: Spiral CT angiography. In Goldman LW, Fowlkes JB, eds: *Medical CT and ultrasound: current technology and applications*, New London, Conn, 1995, AAPM.

Katada K et al: Guidance with real-time CT fluoroscopy: early clinical experience, *Radiology* 200:851–856, 1996.

Kelves BH: *Naked to the bone*, New Brunswick, NJ, 1997, Rutgers University Press.

Ledley R: Personal communication, 1999.

Perry BJ, Bridges C: Computerized transverse axial scanning (tomography), part 3, *Br J Radiol* 46:1048–1051, 1973.

Posh J: *Personal communication*, 1999.

Rhodes ML: Computer graphics in medicine: the past decade, *IEEE Comput Graph Appl* 4:52–54, 1991.

Ritman et al: Synchronous volumetric imaging of non-invasive vivisection of cardiovascular and respiratory dynamics. Evolution of current perspectives. In Giuliani ER, ed: *Cardiology: fundamentals and practice*, St Louis, 1991, Mosby.

Robb RA, Morin RL: Principles and instrumentation for dynamic x-ray computed tomography. In Marcus ML et al, eds: *Cardiac imaging: a comparison to Braunwald's heart disease*, Philadelphia, 1991, WB Saunders.

Seeram E: 3D Imaging: basic concepts for radiologic technologists, *Radiol Technol* 69:127–148, 1998.

Seeram E: Radiation dose in CT, *Radiol Technol* 70:534–556, 1999.

Sirr SA, Waddle JR: Use of CT in detection of internal damage and repair and determination of authenticity in high-quality bowed stringed instruments, *Radiographics* 19:639–646, 1999.

Vining DJ: Virtual colonoscopy, *Semin Ultrasound CT MRI* 20:56–60, 1999.

Yasuda T et al: 3D Visualization of an ancient Egyptian mummy, *IEEE Comput Graph Appl* 2:13–17, 1992.

Zonneveld FW et al: The use of the CT in the study of the internal morphology of hominid fossils, *Medicamundi* 34:117–127, 1989.

BIBLIOGRAPHY

Dümmling K: 10 years' computed tomography: a retrospective view, *Electromedica* 52:13–28, 1984.

Hounsfield GN: Computed medical imaging, Nobel Award address, *Med Phys* 7:283–290, 1980.

Klingenbeck-Regn K, Oppelt A: Dose in CT scanning—physical relationships and potentials for dose saving, *Electromedica* 66:26–30, 1998.

Schwierz G, Kirchgeorg M: The continuous evolution of medical x-ray imaging. I. The technically driven stage of development, *Electromedica* 63:2–7, 1995.

Seeram E: *Computed tomography technology*, Philadelphia, 1982, WB Saunders.

Introduction to Computers

COMPUTER SYSTEMS

Computers are now common in every facet of human activity. In radiology, computers transmit, process, display, and archive images and information.

One reason for the increasing use of computers in radiology involves the shortcomings of film-screen technology, such as those related to imaging, storage, and cost. The computer offers several advantages because it can process, store, retrieve, and communicate information quickly and accurately—characteristics that are essential to diagnostic imaging.

Definition

A *computer* is a machine for solving problems. Specifically, the modern computer is a high-speed electronic computational machine that accepts information in the form of data and instructions through some input device and processes this information with arithmetic and logic operations from a program stored in its memory. The results of the processing can be displayed, stored, or recorded using suitable output devices or transmitted to another location.

Essentially, these same tasks can be performed by people; the word *computer* historically referred to a person. A *computer system*, on the other hand, consists of at least three elements: hardware, software, and computer users (Fig. 2-1). Whereas *hardware* refers to the physical components of the machine, *software* refers to the instructions that make the hardware work to solve problems. People are essential to computer systems because they design, develop, and operate hardware and software.

Hardware Organization

A computer processes the data or information it receives from people or other computers and outputs the results in a form suitable to the needs of the user. This is a three-step process (Fig. 2-2).

The organization of a computer includes at least five hardware components: an input device, a central processing unit (CPU), internal memory, an output device, and external memory or storage (Fig. 2-3).

Input hardware refers to input devices such as a keyboard from which information can be sent to the processor. Processing hardware includes the CPU and internal memory. The CPU is the brain of the computer; it consists of a control unit that directs the activities of the machine and an arithmetic-logic unit (ALU) to perform mathematical calculations and data comparisons. In addition, the CPU includes an internal memory, or main memory, for the permanent storage of software instructions and data.

After data are processed, results are sent to an output device in the form of hard or soft copy. One popular hard copy output device is a printer. If the results are displayed on a monitor for direct viewing, then the term *soft copy* is used. Finally, processing results can be stored on external storage devices. These include magnetic storage devices, such as disks and tapes, and optical storage devices.

Software Concepts

The hardware receives its instructions from the software. The instructions are written in steps that specify ways to solve problems. These sets of instructions are called *programs*.

The three categories of software are (1) systems software, (2) applications software, and (3) software development tools. *Systems software* refers to programs that start up the computer and coordinate the activities of all hardware components and applications software. *Applications software* refers to programs developed by computer systems users to solve specific problems. Software development tools include computer or programming languages such as BASIC, FORTRAN, COBOL, Pascal, DELPHI, C, and C++. Other tools are now available to simplify and expedite the software development process.

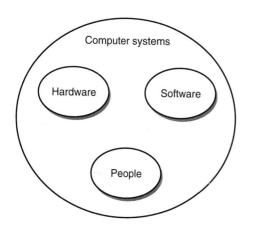

FIG. 2-1. The three essential elements of a computer system.

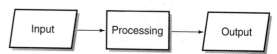

FIG. 2-2. Computer processing involves input, processing, and output.

Historical Perspectives

The history of the computer dates 2000 years to the abacus, a counting machine based on sliding beads on wires. In 1642, Blaise Pascal developed the arithmetic machine, and in 1694, Leibnitz developed a calculating machine to solve multiplication and division problems. In 1822, Charles Babbage invented the difference engine to calculate mathematical tables. He subsequently used punch card coding to develop the analytical engine, a machine that could solve mathematical problems automatically. During the United States census of 1890, Herman Hollerith introduced the first electronic tabulator based on punch card operation.

The development of computers progressed rapidly with Howard Aiken's MARK1, a large electromechanical calculator. This was followed by Eckert and Mauchly's electronic numerical integrator and calculator and electronic variable automatic computer. In 1951 the universal automatic computer became the first commercially available computer.

Today, computers are in their fifth generation. The term *generation* indicates a period of significant technical developments in hardware and software. These developments have been characterized by the following events:

- First-generation computers (1951-1958): The principal features were vacuum tubes used for memory. Punch cards and magnetic tape represented input-output media. These machines were large and slow and required an air-conditioned environment because of the amount of heat produced.

- Second-generation computers (1959-1963): These computers were characterized by solid-state devices such as transistors and magnetic cores used for internal memory. These machines were smaller and more reliable and generated less heat than first-generation computers. In addition, they required less power for operation.

- Third-generation computers (1963-1970): This period was marked by the introduction of the integrated circuit etched onto silicon chips. Magnetic disks were used for storage. These machines were smaller than second-generation computers and performed with greater speed and reliability. Major features included multiprocessing and the rapid evolution of systems and applications software.

- Fourth-generation computers (1971-1987): These computers were based on large-scale integration in which thousands of integrated circuits were set on a chip. The microprocessor was introduced in 1971.

- Fifth-generation computers (1987-present): These computers may have gallium arsenide–based circuitry instead of silicon-based circuitry. They are based on parallel processing, which uses many processors to operate on

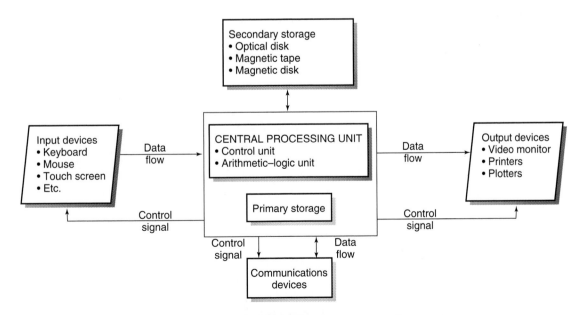

FIG. 2-3. Organization of the hardware components of a computer.

data at the same time. The processing speed of fifth-generation computers can reach 10,000 millions of floating point operations per second (MFLOPS). *Floating* refers to a scientific notation for extremely large numbers in which the decimal point is allowed to move around or "float" (Stallings et al, 1992). For example, the most powerful computer known today, the CRAY 2, operates with a speed of 200 MFLOPS.

Classification

Computers are classified according to their processing capabilities, storage capacity, size, and cost. At present, computers are grouped in four main classes: supercomputers, mainframe computers, minicomputers, and microcomputers.

Supercomputers such as the CRAY-2 are large, high-capacity computers that can process data at extremely high speeds. They are used in oil exploration studies, weather forecasts, research (especially in weapons), and scientific modeling.

Mainframe computers such as the IBM 3090/600 E are large, high-level computers capable of rigorous computations at high speeds. They have large primary memories and can support many pieces of peripheral equipment such as terminals, which enable multiple users to access the primary memory. Organizations such as banks, universities and colleges, large businesses, and governments use mainframe computers.

The *minicomputer* has been defined as "a mid-level computer built to perform complex computations while dealing efficiently with a high level of input and output from users connected via terminals. Minicomputers also frequently connect to other minicomputers on a network and distribute processing among all attached machines" (Microsoft Press, 1999). Minicomputers are used in computed tomography and magnetic resonance imaging.

Microcomputers, or personal computers, are small digital computers available in a variety of sizes such as laptops or palmtops (notebooks). According to Microsoft Press, "Technology is progressing so quickly that state-of-the-art microcomputers are as powerful as mainframes of only a few years ago at a fraction of the cost" (Microsoft Press, 1999).

Microcomputers can be built with all circuitry on a single chip or on multiple circuit boards. A central feature is a microprocessor (Fig. 2-4). The microprocessor is a digital integrated circuit that processes data and controls the general workings of the microcomputer (Capron, 2000). Its processing capability is related to the number of bits, which are binary digits (0 and 1) used to represent data. A microprocessor can be either an 8-bit processor that represents 256 (2^8) numbers or a 16-bit processor that represents 65,536 (2^{16}) numbers. The 16-bit microprocessor therefore can process more data faster than an 8-bit microprocessor. Today, 32-bit microprocessors are available for specialized and dedicated applications.

COMPUTER ARCHITECTURES AND PROCESSING CAPABILITIES

Computer architecture refers to the general structure of a computer and includes both the elements of hardware and software. Specifically, it refers to computer systems, computer chips, circuitry, and systems software.

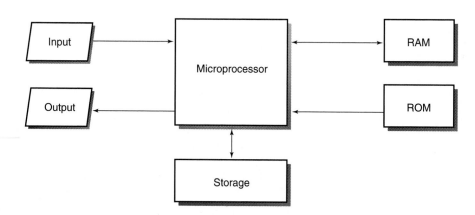

FIG. 2-4.   A microprocessor is central to a microcomputer system.

Types

Essentially, the two types of CPU architectures are complex instruction set computing (CISC) architecture and reduced instruction set computing (RISC) architecture. The CISC microprocessor design has more built-in operations compared with the RISC microprocessor design. Computers with CISC architecture include the IBM 3090 mainframe computer and nearly all microcomputers. Computers with RISC architecture are the IBM 6000, Sun Microsystems SPARC, and Motorola 88000. According to Covington (1991), "RISC is faster if memory is relatively fast so that no time is wasted fetching instructions. CISC is faster if memory is relatively slow because the same work can be done without fetching as many instruction codes."

These architectures are capable of processing operations such as serial or sequential processing, distributed processing, multiprocessing, multitasking, parallel processing, and pipelining. CT technologists should understand the meaning of these terms because they are used in the CT literature and manufacturers' brochures.

Terminology

Serial or sequential processing: Information (data and instructions) is processed in the order in which items are entered and stored in the computer. It is a simple form of processing data, one instruction at a time.

Distributed processing: The information is processed by several computers connected by a network. True distributed processing "has separate computers that perform different tasks in such a way that their combined work can contribute to a larger goal.... It requires a highly structured environment that allows hardware and software to communicate, share resources, and exchange information freely" (Microsoft Press, 1999).

Multitasking: The computer works on more than one task at a time.

Multiprocessing: Multiprocessing uses two or more connected processing units. "In multiprocessing, each processing unit works on a different set of instructions (or on different parts of the same process). The objective is increased speed or computing power, the same as in parallel processing, and the use of special units called *co-processors*" (Microsoft Press, 1999).

Parallel processing: This is a "method of processing that can run only on a type of computer containing two or more processors running simultaneously. Parallel processing differs from multiprocessing in the way a task is distributed over the available processors; in multiprocessing, a process might be divided up into sequential blocks, with one processor managing access to a database, another analyzing the data, and a third handling graphical output to the screen" (Microsoft Press, 1999). A number of processes can be carried out at the same time.

Pipelining: A "method of fetching and decoding instructions in which, at any given time, several program instructions are in various stages of being fetched or decoded. Ideally, pipelining speeds execution time by ensuring that the microprocessor does not have to wait for instructions; when it completes execution of one instruction, the next is ready and waiting.... In parallel processing, *pipelining* can also refer to a method in which instructions are passed from one processing unit to another, as on an assembly line, and each unit is specialized for performing a particular type of operation" (Microsoft Press, 1999).

DIGITAL FUNDAMENTALS

The two main types of computers are digital and analog. Digital computers operate on digital data (discrete units), and analog computers operate on continuous physical quantities that are not digital but may have any value on a continuously variable scale (analog signals). Analog signals involve physical quantities such as electrical signals (voltage), speed, pressure, temperature, and displacement. An example of an analog computer is the slide rule, which compares the length on the rule and the logarithm of a number.

Digital computers are the most common type of computers; they operate on digital data through arithmetic and logic operations. Because the digital computer is used in all radiologic applications, an understanding of the digital system is important.

The Binary Number System

An understanding of the decimal number system is necessary to then understand the binary number system. The decimal number system has a base 10, in which 10 values are represented as 0 through 9. Any decimal number can be written as a sum of these digits multiplied by a power of 10. For example, the number 321 can be written as follows:

$$(1 \times 10^0) + (2 \times 10^1) + (3 \times 10^2) = 321 =$$
$$(1 \times 1) + (2 \times 10) + (3 \times 100) = 321 =$$
$$1 + 20 + 300 = 321$$

The number 321 is thus formed from units (1), tens (20), and hundreds (300).

In the decimal system, any number can be expressed as units, tens, hundreds, thousands, tens of thousands, hundreds of thousands, millions, tens of millions, hundreds of millions, and so on. These are referred to as *powers of 10* and can be written as follows:

$$1 \times 10^0 = 1$$
$$1 \times 10^1 = 10$$
$$1 \times 10^2 = 100$$
$$1 \times 10^3 = 1000$$
$$1 \times 10^4 = 10,000$$
$$1 \times 10^5 = 100,000$$
$$1 \times 10^6 = 1,000,000$$

The binary number system, on the other hand, has a base 2, in which only two values, 0 and 1, are represented. A binary number can be 0, 1, a string of 0s, a string of 1s, or a string of 0s and 1s.

To understand the conversion of the decimal system to the binary system, consider Table 2-1. The decimal system in the first column of the table shows position values, each of which is increased 10 times (e.g., 1, 10, 100, 1000), but the position values of the binary system in the second column are only increased by a factor of 2 (e.g., 1, 2, 4, 8, 16, 32).

The decimal number 1 is represented by 0001 in the binary number system. The decimal number 7 is represented by 0111, and 10 is represented by 1010.

Decimal-to-Binary Conversion

Perform the following steps to convert decimal to binary:

1. Note the binary value closest to the decimal number to be converted.
2. Complete the sequence of binary position values from the number obtained in step 1.
3. Place a 1 under the binary position value obtained in step 1.
4. Subtract the position value of step 1 from the decimal number to be converted.
5. Place a 1 under the position value closest to the number (decimal) obtained in step 4.

TABLE 2-1

*Relationship Between Decimal and Binary Numbers**

DECIMAL NUMBERS				BINARY NUMBERS				
POSITION VALUES								
....1000	100	10	1	16	8	4	2	1
			1	0	0	0	0	1
			2	0	0	0	1	0
			3	0	0	0	1	1
			4	0	0	1	0	0
			5	0	0	1	0	1
			6	0	0	1	1	0
			7	0	0	1	1	1
			8	0	1	0	0	0
			9	0	1	0	0	1
		1	0	0	1	0	1	0
		1	1	0	1	0	1	1
		1	2	0	1	1	0	0
		1	3	0	1	1	0	1
		1	4	0	1	1	1	0
		1	5	0	1	1	1	1
		1	6	1	0	0	0	0

*See text for conversion steps.

6. Subtract this position value from step 5 from the answer obtained in step 4.
7. Repeat steps 5 and 6 until the decimal number has been converted.
8. Place 0s under all remaining binary position values.

For example, perform the following steps to convert the decimal 133 to binary:

1. The binary position value closest to 133 is 128.
2. The binary position values (sequence) from 128 are

| 128 | 64 | 32 | 16 | 8 | 4 | 2 | 1 |

3. 1 is placed under the binary position value 128:

128	64	32	16	8	4	2	1
1							

4. $133 - 128 = 5$. The binary position value closest to 5 is 4.
5. 1 is placed under the binary position value 4:

128	64	32	16	8	4	2	1
1					1		

6. $5 - 4 = 1$. The binary position value closest to 1 is 1.
7. 1 is placed under the binary position value 1:

128	64	32	16	8	4	2	1
1					1		1

8. 0s are placed under all remaining position values—that is,

128	64	32	16	8	4	2	1
1	0	0	0	0	1	0	1

The answer is 10000101, which is the binary representation of the decimal number 133.

Binary-to-Decimal Conversion

Perform the following steps to convert binary to decimal:

1. Count the digits in the binary number.
2. Set up this number of position values in the binary number system, starting from 1.
3. Perform the conversion by placing each binary digit under the appropriate position value, beginning from the right-hand side (1) and moving to the left-hand side of the position values.
4. Add the position values for every position where 1 appears.

For example, perform the following steps to convert the binary number 01010110 to decimal:

1. The number of digits in the binary number 01010110 is 8.
2. The binary position values are

| 128 | 64 | 32 | 16 | 8 | 4 | 2 | 1 |

3. Place the binary number under each of the binary position values in step 2, beginning from the right-hand side (i.e., 1) and moving toward the left (i.e., 128):

128	64	32	16	8	4	2	1
0	1	0	1	0	1	1	0

4. The sum of the binary position values under which 1 appears is

$$64 + 16 + 4 + 2 = 86$$

The answer is the binary number 01010110, which represents the decimal number 86.

Other Number Systems

Binary numbers can become very long. For example, the binary number for 1025 is 1000000001. Because this can be time-consuming with long numbers, other number systems have been developed, such as the octal and hexadecimal systems. In the octal system, groups of three binary digits are represented by one octal digit. The base of the octal system is 8, in which eight digits are represented by 0, 1, 2, 3, 4, 5, 6, and 7. The following example can help to understand the binary-to-octal conversion process.

Perform the following steps to obtain the octal number for the binary 010110100:

1. Arrange the binary number into groups of three, starting from the right-hand side of the number: 010, 110, 100
2. Refer to the steps in binary-to-decimal conversion, and represent each group by an octal digit; that is,

100 = 4
110 = 6
010 = 2

3. The octal number is thus 264.

The hexadecimal system uses four binary digits (bits) to represent one hexadecimal digit, and the base is 16 in which the 16 digits are represented by 0, 1, 2, 3, 4, 5, 6, 7, 8, 9, 10, 11, 12, 13, 14, and 15.

In this case the first 10 digits are represented by 0, 1, 2, 3, 4, 5, 6, 7, 8, and 9; and 10, 11, 12, 13, 14, and 15 are represented by the first six letters of the alphabet, A, B, C, D, E, and F, respectively.

For example, perform the following steps to obtain the hexadecimal number for the binary 11011001:

1. Arrange the binary number 11011001 into groups of four, starting from the right-hand side:

   1101, 1001

2. Convert each group of binary numbers to decimal and represent each group by the hexadecimal equivalent. That is,

   $$1001 = 8 + 1 + 1 = 9$$
   $$1101 = 8 + 4 + 1 = 13$$

3. Because the first 10 digits in the hexadecimal are represented by 0 through 9, the hexadecimal number for the decimal equivalent 13 is D.
4. The answer is D9.

One hexadecimal number represents a four-digit binary number. This number system is an efficient system for some computers.

Terminology

A binary digit, or a bit, is a single binary number. In computing, the grouping of bits is as follows:

   4 binary bits (0.5 byte) = nibble
   8 binary bits (1 byte) = byte
   16 binary bits (2 bytes) = word
   32 binary bits (4 bytes) = double word

Because binary numbers can be long, they are combined into groups of eight bits called *bytes*. A byte represents one addressable location in memory. Memory capacity is therefore measured in bytes, where

   1 thousand bytes = 1 kilobyte (K or KB)
   1 million bytes = 1 megabyte (MB)
   1 billion bytes = 1 gigabyte (GB)
   1 trillion bytes = 1 terabyte (TB)

Binary Coding Schemes

People enter information into a computer for processing in the form of characters (e.g., A, B, C), numbers (e.g., 1, 2, 3), or special characters (e.g., $, *,:, ;). These characters must be represented in binary code. Two popular binary coding schemes are extended binary coded decimal interchange code (EBCDIC) and American standard code for

information interchange (ASCII) (Table 2-2). Whereas EBCDIC, developed by IBM, is the industry standard for minicomputers and mainframe computers, ASCII is widely used by microcomputers. When a character is entered into the computer, it is automatically converted into the ASCII or EBCDIC binary code, depending on the computer system.

Elements of a Digital Signal Processor

Information is entered into a computer in analog form. If the computer is an analog computer, then the results of processing are also analog. In this case, both the input and output are in analog form. However, if the computer is a digital computer and the input is analog, an analog-to-digital converter (ADC) is needed to convert the analog input into digital data for processing. The results of digital processing are digital data that can be displayed as such but in most instances would have no meaning to an observer. Therefore an interface such as the digital-to-analog converter (DAC) is needed between the digital processor and the output display device. The ADC and DAC, coupled with a digital processor, constitute a *digital signal processor* (Fig. 2-5).

Analog-to-Digital Conversion

The ADC converts the analog signal into "a sequence of numbers having finite precision" (Proakis, 1992). This procedure is referred to as

TABLE 2-2

ASCII and EBCDIC Binary Coding Schemes for 12 Characters

CHARACTER	CODING SCHEME	
	ASCII	EBCDIC
A	0100 0001	1100 0001
B	0100 0010	1100 0010
C	0100 0011	1100 0011
D	0100 0100	1100 0100
E	0100 0101	1100 0101
F	0100 0110	1100 0110
1	0011 0000	1111 0000
2	0011 0001	1111 0001
3	0011 0010	1111 0010
4	0011 0011	1111 0100
5	0011 0100	1111 0101
6	0011 0101	1111 0110

analog-to-digital conversion (ADC). The essential parts of an ADC include a sampler, quantizer, and coder (Fig. 2-6). These components perform the following three operations: sampling, quantization, and coding.

- *Sampling* is "the conversion of a continuous-time signal into a discrete signal obtained by taking 'samples' of the continuous-time signal at discrete time instants" (Proakis, 1992).
- *Quantization* is "the conversion of a discrete-time, discrete-valued (digital) signal. The value of each signal sample is represented by a value selected from a finite set of possible values" (Proakis, 1992).
- *Coding* is the assignment of a binary bit sequence to each discrete output from the quantizer.

Digital-to-Analog Conversion

The digital signal processor outputs digital data that are subsequently converted into the analog signals needed to operate analog display devices such as television monitors. This conversion requires a DAC, which is made of solid-state electronics that generate an output voltage proportional to the input digital number.

One important characteristic of the DAC is its resolution; that is, how finely an analog voltage may be represented, which is determined by the number of digital bits. For example, an 8-bit DAC outputs 256 (2^8) analog voltage as opposed to a 12-bit DAC, which outputs 4096 (2^{12}) analog voltages and indicates significantly better resolution.

COMPUTER HARDWARE
Input Hardware

In computing, *input* refers to information entered into the computer for processing. The information can be processed immediately or stored (usually on a magnetic medium such as a magnetic tape or disk) for later processing.

Input hardware can be placed in two categories: keyboard and nonkeyboard devices.

Keyboard Devices

A keyboard is a part of a terminal, which is an input-output device with a display screen. A keyboard is a special electromechanical device that resembles a typewriter keyboard with some additional features. Keyboards are available in different sizes and shapes, but all have at least four common features: (1) regular typewriter keys with alphabet characters, (2) numeric keys (numbers), (3) special function keys called *programmable keys*, and (4) cursor movement keys (Fig. 2-7). When characters are entered from the keyboard, they are converted into binary codes and are then sent to the CPU for processing.

There are three types of terminals, as follows:

1. *Dumb terminals* cannot process information and can only display the input received from the input hardware.
2. *Smart terminals* can process and store information but cannot perform any programming operations.
3. *Intelligent terminals* are microcomputers that can process data and store it internally and externally, and therefore they can carry

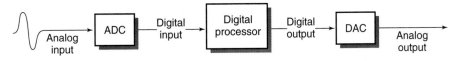

FIG. 2-5. Elements of a digital signal processor.

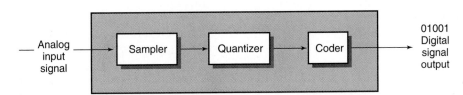

FIG. 2-6. Essential parts of an analog-to-digital converter.

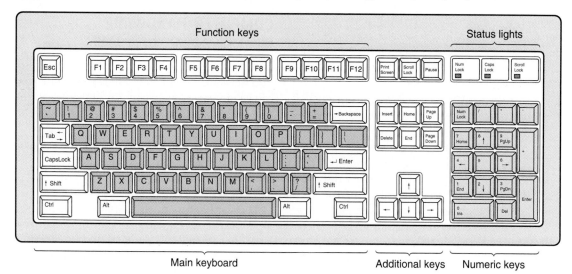

FIG. 2-7. The main features of a computer keyboard. These include function keys, main keyboard, numeric keys, and additional keys.

out programming. Communication is also possible through a communications link (a modem).

Nonkeyboard Devices

Nonkeyboard input devices include pointing devices, scanning devices, and voice input devices. Pointing devices are commonly used because pointing appears to be a basic part of human behavior. These devices include light pens, digitizers, touch screens, and the mouse. Scanning devices include image scanners, fax machines, bar code readers (common in supermarkets), and character and mark recognition devices. Voice input devices change human speech into electrical signals, which can then be digitized for processing. These systems are also referred to as *voice recognition systems* and are an integral part of the digital radiology department (Fig. 2-8).

Input devices play an important role in computer systems, as noted by Stallings et al (1992): "The conversion of data into a computer-usable form is a vital part of a computer-based information system. Input control procedures are needed to safeguard the data's integrity and to ensure the production of complete and accurate information—in other words, to ensure no 'garbage in' to avoid getting 'garbage out.'"

Processing Hardware

Speed and power are two important characteristics of computers. *Speed* refers to how fast the computer processes data. *Power* includes speed and other characteristics such as storage capacity and memory size. Several factors affect the speed of a computer, including microprocessor speed, the bus line size, cache memory, flash memory, RISC architecture, and parallel processing of data.

Microprocessor speeds can range from 1 millisecond (ms = 10^{-3} sec) to 1 microsecond (μs = 10^{-6} sec) for early computers to 1 nanosecond (10^{-9} sec) for modern computers. Research processing speeds continue to approach the picosecond (10^{-12} sec) range. These speeds are expressed in cycles per second, megahertz (MHz), or gigahertz (GHz = 10^9 cycles per second). Additionally, computer speeds can be expressed in million instructions per second (MIPS) or megaflops (MFLOPs).

The processing hardware or CPU includes the control unit, arithmetic-logic unit (ALU), registers, and memory (see Fig. 2-3).

The control unit directs the activities of the computer through programs stored in memory. For example, it indicates when information is to be moved from memory to the ALU and which operations the ALU should carry out. In addition, the control unit directs the flow of data from the CPU to the input-output hardware.

The ALU executes arithmetic and logic operations including addition, subtraction, multiplication, division, and comparisons such as "is equal to" (=), "is less than" (<), or "is greater than" (>).

Registers are temporary storage electronic devices. They hold the data for a short period and

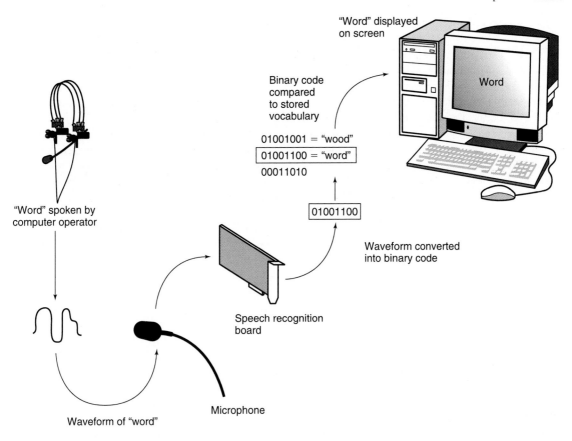

"Word" displayed
on screen

Binary code
compared
to stored
vocabulary

01001001 = "wood"
01001100 = "word"
00011010

Word

"Word" spoken by
computer operator

01001100

Waveform converted
into binary code

Speech recognition
board

Microphone

Waveform of "word"

FIG. 2-8. A voice input device works by translating the soundwaves of spoken language into binary numbers that can be interpreted by the computer. If the binary code generated by the speech recognition board finds a match in the computer's stored vocabulary, that vocabulary word is displayed on the screen.

then send it to internal memory, where it is stored temporarily.

The movement of data among these components is accomplished by the bus or bus line, which provides a path for the flow of electrical signals between units. The amount of data transported at a single moment is called the *bus width*. As noted by Capron (2000), a computer with a larger bus size will be faster because it can transfer more data at one time, will have a larger memory, and can accommodate an increase in the number and variety of instructions.

A computer may have three types of buses: a data bus (data signals), an address bus that sends data from internal memory, and a control bus that sends signals from the control unit.

A major component of processing hardware is primary storage or internal memory, or simply *memory*. Its purpose is to store (1) the information entered into the computer for processing, (2) the

program that provides the instructions for processing the input information, and (3) the results of the processing.

Internal memory is available in the form of chips, semiconductor chips, or integrated circuits. This type of memory is volatile, meaning that data are lost when the computer loses its electrical power. One semiconductor design, the complimentary metal oxide semiconductor, requires very little power to operate.

There are two basic types of internal memory chips: read-only memory (ROM) and random-access memory (RAM). Whereas ROM chips contain data and programs to make the computer hardware work and cannot be changed, erased, or lost when the computer is turned off, RAM chips provide for temporary storage of data and programs that would be lost if the computer loses power. In addition, RAM can be static (SRAM) or dynamic (DRAM). Although SRAM is faster than DRAM, it does not require refreshing of its contents by the CPU, as does DRAM.

Three additional classes of ROM chips are available: programmable read-only memory (PROM), erasable programmable read-only memory (EPROM), and electrically erasable programmable read-only memory (EEPROM). PROM chips allow users to write their own data and programs but not to change or erase these instructions. With EPROM chips, data can be erased using an ultraviolet light after the EPROM chip is removed from the computer. Finally, EEPROM chips use special software that permit data and programs to be changed electronically without removal.

The storage capacity of RAM chips is expressed in megabytes (MB). Computer programs specify the RAM capacity needed for operation.

Two other types of memory are cache memory and flash memory. Cache memory is very fast memory for the storage of information and data that are used most of the time. It can be internal or external and available on separate chips. Flash memory is nonvolatile. Flash memory chips are being developed for computers and already are used in cellular telephones and flight recorders in airplanes.

Output Hardware

After the input data and instructions have been processed by the CPU, the results can be stored permanently or made available as soft copy or hard copy output. *Hard copy* refers to printed output on permanent media, such as paper and film, and *soft copy* refers to output "information that has been produced in a seemingly intangible form" (Stallings et al, 1992).

Hard copy output devices include printers, plotters, camera output microforms such as microfiche and microfilm, and voice output devices. Printers fall into two categories: impact and nonimpact. Impact printers make contact with the paper and include letter-quality, dot matrix, and high-speed printers. Nonimpact printers include inkjet, thermal, and laser printers. Plotters produce graphics such as 3D drawings, bar charts (graphs), and maps and are categorized as drum, flat-bed, and electrostatic. Whereas drum and flat-bed plotters use pens for drawings, electrostatic plotters use electrostatic charges on a special paper to produce drawings. Voice output devices are based on prerecorded vocalized sounds, and the computer can output synthesized words in response to certain codes.

Soft copy output hardware is based on video display technology. Two common types of video display devices are the cathode ray tube (CRT) and flat-panel or flat-screen devices.

The CRT consists of an electron gun that directs a stream of electrons to strike a phosphor-coated screen located at the opposite end of the gun. Positioned in front of the screen is a shadow mask, which consists of numerous tiny holes that direct a small part of the beam to strike the screen. Each tiny spot that glows on the screen is called a *picture element,* or pixel. The displayed image on the screen is thus composed of pixels in both the horizontal and the vertical directions. The number of pixels determines the resolution, or sharpness, of the CRT image. In general, the greater the number of pixels (vertical and horizontal), the better the resolution.

Flat-screen output devices are based on flat-screen technologies and were developed primarily for portable computers. Flat-screen display technologies include the liquid crystal display (LCD), electroluminescent (EL) display, and gas plasma display. "LCDs use a clear liquid chemical trapped in tiny pockets between two pieces of glass. Each pocket of liquid is covered both front and back by very thin wires. When a small amount of current is applied to both wires, a chemical reaction turns the chemical a dark color—thereby blocking light. The point of blocked light is the pixel" (Stallings et al, 1992). An EL display panel consists of a phosphor layer that emits light when activated by a current. Two sets of electrodes are arranged with the phosphor layer to form columns and rows. A pixel glows when current flows to the electrodes that address that particular location. The gas plasma display screen is the best of the flat-screen displays. Usually a mixture of argon and neon gases is sandwiched between two glass plates with wire grids. A pixel is displayed when its address location has been charged.

Storage Hardware

Storage hardware devices include magnetic tapes and disks and optical disks. These devices constitute secondary storage (auxiliary storage), which is nonvolatile, as opposed to primary storage, which is volatile.

DATA STORAGE TECHNOLOGIES
Approaches to Secondary Storage

There are generally two approaches to secondary storage of information: the sequential access approach and the direct access method. The sequential or serial access method is analogous to finding a favorite song on an audiotape. In this method, information is stored in a specific sequence, such as alphabetically, and the information is therefore retrieved alphabetically. Tape storage is characteristic of this type of storage.

In the direct or random access method, the desired information is accessed directly and therefore this method is much faster than sequential access. Disk storage is characteristic of this type of storage.

Magnetic Tape Storage

Magnetic tape storage requires a magnetic tape unit with a magnetic tape drive. Magnetic tape is made of Mylar, a plastic-like material coated with particles that magnetize the tape to record information. The tape is threaded from a supply reel to pass by the read-write head and then moves onto a take-up reel.

The read-write head is a wire wrapped around an iron core with one or more small gaps. When information is recorded onto the tape, the electrical signal passing through the wire produces a varying magnetic field that magnetizes the particles on the tape. The direction of the magnetization on the tape represents binary code. When the tape is played back, the magnetization on the tape results in electrical signals that are sent to a display device or audio speakers. Magnetic tape used in conjunction with minicomputers and mainframes is about ½-inch wide and ½-mile long and can store about 1600 to 6400 characters (O'Leary et al, 1992).

Magnetic tape streamers, also referred to as *back-up tape cartridge units*, are also available for use with microcomputers. Popular tape cartridges use 0.25-inch wide tape and are available in 1000-foot reels. The data recording method is based on the streaming tape method. According to Stallings et al (1992), "In this method, the data [are] written onto the tape in one continuous stream. There is no starting or stopping, no gaps between blocks (or records) of data being recorded." The amount of data that can be stored on the tape is its *density*, or the number of characters per inch (cpi) or bytes per inch (bpi). Today, digital audio tape drives are available to facilitate back-up storage. These tapes are high-capacity tapes and provide very fast access to the data stored on them.

Magnetic Disk Storage

Magnetic disks include floppy disks and hard disks. Floppy disks are made of flexible Mylar plastic, whereas hard disks are metal platters. Both are coated with magnetizable particles that allow data

to be recorded and stored as binary code. Each disk consists of concentric tracks and preshaped sectors. A typical disk includes about 17 sectors per track and 512 bytes (4096 bits) of information per sector. Magnetic disks are random access devices, which means that any sector of the disk can be accessed quickly. The tracks on the disk contain dots, each of which represents a bit. The packing density of a track is about 4000 bits per inch.

Floppy disks or diskettes are available in two sizes: the 3½-inch microfloppy disk and the 5¼-inch minifloppy disk (Fig. 2-9). Both disks are made of Mylar plastic encased in plastic jacket covers. Data are stored and retrieved from these disks by means of the head window, where the read-write head of the disk drive makes contact with the disk. Microfloppy disks are commonly used in computing and can store much more data than minifloppy disks. Currently, 2-inch microfloppy disks are available in some electronic cameras and personal computers. Iomega created the Zip drive, which can hold nearly 100-megabyte disks, a capacity about 70 times that of the 3½-inch diskettes.

When data files are too large to fit on these diskettes, compression programs are available to remove certain data without loss. Compression is also important when large data files are transmitted to remote locations.

Hard disks are high-capacity storage disks capable of storing more data than floppy disks and are available as internal hard disks, hard disk car-

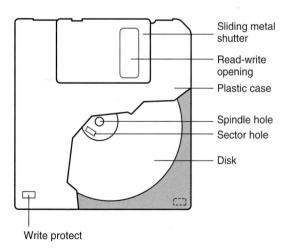

Write protect

FIG. 2-9. The external features of a 3½-inch microfloppy disk.

tridges, or hard disk packs. Internal hard disks consist of one or more metal platters positioned in a sealed container that also houses the read-write head. These common disk units are known as *Winchester disks*. Whereas internal hard disks have a fixed storage capacity, hard disk cartridges are self-contained and can be easily removed from their drives. In addition, they facilitate the storage of an unlimited amount of data. Hard disk packs have several stacked platters with read-write heads positioned so that as one head reads the underside of the disk above it, the other reads the surface of the disk below it. Hard disks are hermetically sealed to prevent smoke, dust, or other particles from entering the container. These particles may cause a head crash, in which case data are lost.

Redundant Array of Independent Disks

Safety is one problem of data and information storage on single disk systems. The redundant array of

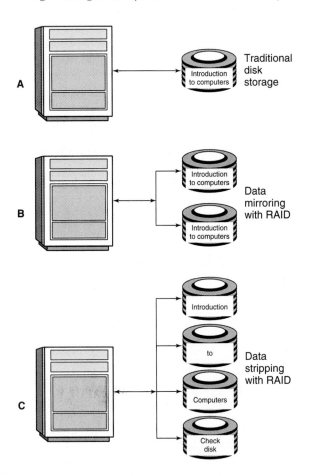

FIG. 2-10.   The concept of RAID storage compared with traditional storage. (From Capron HL: *Computers: tools for an information age,* Upper Saddle River, NJ, 2000, Prentice Hall.)

independent disks (RAID) system overcomes this problem through the use of hard disk technology.

There are several levels of RAID organization (Fig. 2-10). The first level uses disk mirroring in which data are copied onto another set of disks (Fig. 2-10, *B*). Should one disk fail in this situation, the data are not lost because they are stored on the other disk system. Another level uses data stripping (Fig. 2-10, *C*). The data are now distributed across several disks "with one disk used solely as a check disk, to keep track of what data is where. If a disk fails, the check disk can reconstitute the data" (Capron, 2000). RAID is now common in the digital imaging department, where vast amounts of data from several imaging modalities are stored in a safe and secure environment.

Optical Disk Storage

The most recent storage technology is optical storage, which is based on the use of optical rather than magnetic technology. It is a technology in which stored data are read by optical means (Bradley, 1989).

Optical disk storage involves the use of a laser beam (e.g., from a helium-neon laser) to write the data on the surface of a metallic disk. The laser beam is tightly focused to form a spot of light, or the optical stylus, which burns tiny pits onto the concentric tracks (rings) on the disk to write data. The laser beam scans the pits, which reflect light from the disk to a photodetector to read data. The output electrical signal from the detector depends on the geometry and distribution of the pits.

Optical disks are available in diameters of 3½, 4¾, 5¼, 8, 12, and 14 inches. Three types of optical disks are available: compact disc, read-only memory (CD-ROM); write once, read many (WORM); and erasable optical disks. Information can only be read from a CD-ROM by optical means and cannot be recorded or erased. WORM optical disks can write data once to be read multiple times but not erased, which makes this disk suitable for information archives.

Erasable optical disks are made of magnetooptic materials (e.g., gadolinium, terbium, or iron). To write data on the disk, a focused laser beam heats a small region of magnetized ferromagnetic film and causes it to lose its magnetization. The region becomes magnetized in the opposite direction during cooling and in the presence of a magnetic field. In addition, the power of the laser used to write the data is much greater than that used to read the data, which ensures that stored data are not destroyed.

Storage Capacity

The storage capacity of the different storage devices is determined by the number of bytes that the device can hold. Storage capacities are expressed in kilobytes (K), megabytes (MB), gigabytes (GB), and terabytes (TB). For example, secondary storage capacities for desktop microcomputers are now in the GB range.

COMPUTER SOFTWARE
Programming

The programmer follows a six-step developmental procedure for programming: (1) define the problem, (2) make or buy the decision, (3) design the program, (4) code the program, (5) debug the program, and (6) document (Fig. 2-11). Step 3 deserves a brief description. Programming techniques such as top-down program design, pseudocode, flow charting, and logic structures are used to arrive at a solution. Whereas the first two techniques concern major processing steps and a story or narrative of the program logic, respectively, flow charting involves the use of graphic symbols to indicate the sequence of operations needed to solve the problem. The program flow chart includes at least three logic structures: sequence (a program statement), decision, and a loop (the repetition of a process when the condition is true).

The program is coded or written in a programming language available to the computer system. Five generations of programming languages are now available, as follows (see box below, top):

Machine language, or machine code, is the only language that a computer can understand. It is a low-level language based on sequences of 0s and 1s, which can be represented by on (1) and off (0) switches.

Assembly language is another low-level language that uses abbreviations to develop the program. These must subsequently be converted into machine code using a special program called an *assembler*.

Procedural languages are considered high-level languages because they are similar to human languages (see box below, bottom).

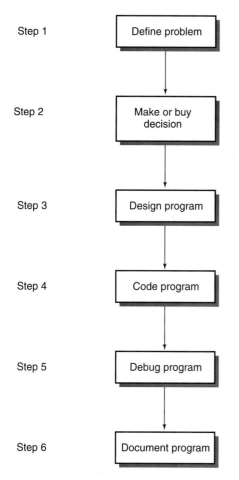

FIG. 2-11. The programming procedure involves at least six steps.

Step 1 — Define problem

Step 2 — Make or buy decision

Step 3 — Design program

Step 4 — Code program

Step 5 — Debug program

Step 6 — Document program

PROGRAMMING LANGUAGES

Machine—first generation (least advanced)
Assembly—second generation
Procedural—third generation
Problem oriented—fourth generation
Natural—fifth generation (most advanced)

PROCEDURAL LANGUAGES

BASIC (Beginners' all-purpose symbolic instruction code)—Developed in the mid-1960s at Dartmouth College; common in microcomputing

COBOL (Common business-oriented language)—A language common to business applications

FORTRAN (Formula translation)—Developed 1954-1958; a compiled structured language; used specifically for scientific and engineering applications

Pascal—A popular language for use in microcomputing, developed by Niklaus Wirth (1967-1971); a compiled structured language

C—Popular for microcomputers; a compiled language developed by Dennis Ritchie at Bell Laboratories in 1972

According to O'Leary (1992), procedural languages are so named because "they are designed to express the logic—the procedures—that can solve general problems." Procedural languages include BASIC, COBOL, and FORTRAN, which must be converted into machine code that the computer can process. This conversion is accomplished by either a compiler or an interpreter. A compiler converts the programmer's procedural language program, or source code, into a machine language code called the *object code*. This object code can then be saved and run later.

Problem-oriented languages were developed to simplify the programming process and are intended for use in specific applications. Examples are dBASE and Lotus 1-2-3.

Natural languages are the highest level of programmable languages. These are fifth-generation languages such as Clout and Intellect. The goal of these languages is to resemble human speech. Natural language is now applied to expert systems and artificial intelligence applications.

Applications Software

Applications software refers to programs developed to perform specific types of work such as the creation of text and images, manipulation of words and numbers, or communication of information. Five general-purpose applications programs are common. These are intended for word processing, spreadsheets, graphics, database management, and communications. If all these applications programs are available in one package, the package is referred to as *integrated software*. Examples include Microsoft Works, First Choice, Framework, and Symphony.

MAJOR OPERATING SYSTEMS

- Apple DOS—Apple Disk Operating System
- CP/M—Control Program/Microcomputers
- MS-DOS—Microsoft Disk Operating System
- Mac OS—Operating system (for Macintosh computers only)
- OS/2—Operating system for microcomputers and networking
- UNIX—A portable operating system that can be shared by several users simultaneously

Systems Software

An operating system (OS) is a program that controls "the allocation and usage of computer hardware resources such as memory, central processing unit (CPU) time, disk space, and peripheral devices" (see box below) (Microsoft Press, 1999). *Systems software* are programs and data that comprise and relate to the OS. Systems software include at least four types of programs: (1) a bootstrap loader, (2) diagnostic routines, (3) input-output system programs, and (4) the OS.

The *bootstrap loader* is a program stored in ROM that starts up the computer and loads the OS into primary memory. Diagnostic routines ensure the CPU, primary memory, and other internal hardware are in proper working order. In addition, input-output system programs interpret and input characters and send these characters to output devices. The OS performs system initialization, memory and file management, and input-output control. It also facilitates multitasking and multiprocessing, depending on its capabilities.

Software Interfacing

As defined in the *Microsoft Press Computer Dictionary* (1999), an *interface* is the point at which a connection is made between two elements so they can work together.

Software provides the connection between computer users. Essentially, there are three types of software interfaces: command-driven, menu-driven, and graphic interfaces. A command-driven interface is characteristic of command-driven programs, which require the user to type in commands from the computer console to initiate the operation of the system. The user must therefore learn and remember a set of commands for various programs. For example, the command *DIR*, or *dir*, enables the user of an IBM or IBM-compatible microcomputer to look at the system's directory.

Menu-driven programs use menu-driven interfaces that allow the user to select commands from a displayed list, menu list, displayed bar, or menu bar. This makes it easier for people to use the system because they do not have to remember numerous commands. In this respect, menu-driven programs are considered user friendly and easier to learn than command-driven programs.

A graphic user interface enables the user to choose commands, start programs, and see lists of files and other options by pointing to pictorial representations (icons) and lists of menu items on the screen (Microsoft Press, 1999). The concept of a graphic interface was developed at Xerox (Palo Alto Research Center) and originally used by Apple to develop the Macintosh operating system (Arnold, 1991). It is also available for IBM microcomputers as Microsoft Windows, or Windows.

Windows can be found on most personal computers. Two important characteristics of Windows are its (1) plug-and-play technology and (2) object-linking and embedding technology. Plug-and-play enables the computer to automatically configure itself when anything new is added; object linking and embedding allows the user to link or embed documents.

Windows NT is noted for its stability and is best suited to networked environments, making it a candidate for use in the digital radiology department. Windows NT is already used in several workstations for medical imaging.

DATA COMMUNICATIONS
Data Transmission Media

Data communications involves the transmission of data from one location to another through the use of pathways. These pathways are referred to as *transmission media* or *channels* and include telephone lines, coaxial cable, microwaves, satellites and radio waves, and optical fibers.

The choice of communication channel depends on several factors, of which data transmission speed is relatively important. Data transmission speed is influenced by the baud rate and the bandwidth of the communications channel (Arnold, 1991). The *baud rate* refers to the number of discrete signal elements (bauds) transmitted per second. The *bandwidth* refers to the frequency capacity of the channel and is expressed in bits per second (bps) (Arnold, 1991). There are essentially three types of bandwidths: voice band (e.g., a telephone line), which can transmit about 110 to 9600 bps; medium band, which can transmit 9600 to 256,000 bps; and broad band (e.g., coaxial, fiberoptics, and microwave), which can transmit 256,000 to 1,000,000 bps.

Data Communications Hardware

A typical data communications scheme sends data from computer A to computer B through the telephone line (Fig. 2-12). The modem modulates, or converts digital data to analog signals, and demodulates, or converts analog signals to digital data; both signals are to be transmitted and received.

Other hardware components include multiplexers, concentrators, controllers, and front-end processors. A multiplexer allows several computers to share a single communications line. A concentrator allows many devices to share a single communications line and is more "intelligent" than a multiplexer because it can store and forward transmissions (Capron, 2000). A controller supports a group of devices such as terminals and printers connected to a computer (Capron, 2000). A front-end processor is a small computer that performs several data management and communications functions, thus relieving the host or main computer of these processing tasks. Telephone companies are now replacing analog phone networks with integrated services digital networks (ISDN), which can handle data communications and also

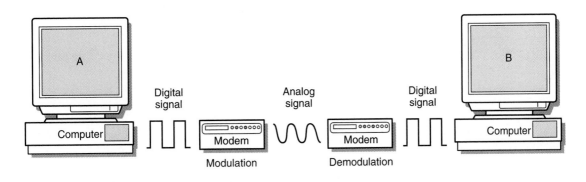

FIG. 2-12. Typical scheme for data communication using computers.

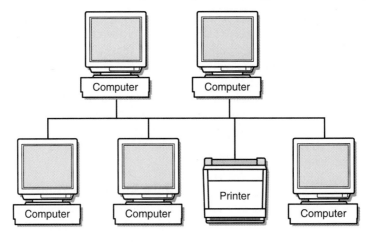

FIG. 2-13.   Bus network.

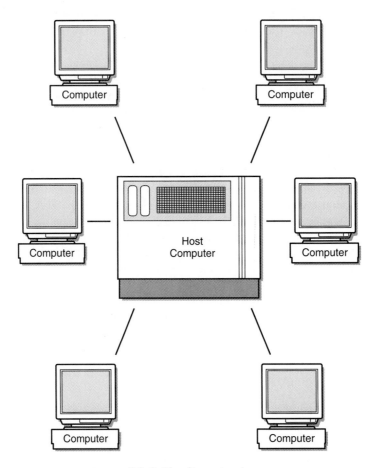

FIG. 2-14.   Star network.

allow audio and video signals to be transmitted simultaneously over cable.

Network Topologies

There are four network topologies or configurations: bus, star, ring, and hierarchical. In a bus network (Fig. 2-13), devices such as computers and printers are connected so that each is responsible for its own communications control. The bus cable connects the devices, and there is no host computer or file server. The star network (Fig. 2-14) is characterized by a host computer or file server to which several computers are connected. In a ring network topology, the devices (mostly mainframes) are connected to form a ring without a

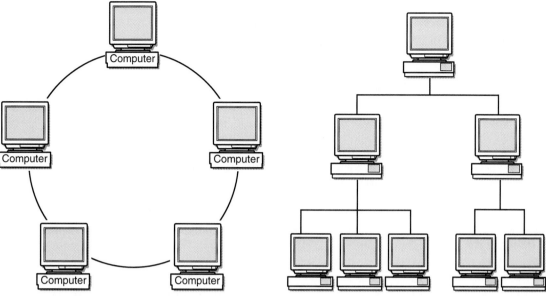

FIG. 2-15. Ring network.

FIG. 2-16. Hierarchical network.

host computer or file server (Fig. 2-15). The hierarchical network (Fig. 2-16) consists of a central host computer to which other computers are connected. These computers then serve as hosts to several smaller machines. In a typical system, a host computer represents a mainframe that plays host to two minicomputers, which in turn play host to several microcomputers (Capron, 2000).

When computers and other hardware located in the same building are linked through a topology, they create a local area network (LAN) (Fig. 2-17). Fig. 2-17 also includes a network gateway that allows the LAN to be connected to other LANs. If the LANs are connected across a region or city, a metropolitan area network (MAN) is created. Similarly, a wide area network (WAN) is created when computers are connected across the country.

LANs, MANs, and WANs require a technology that allows fast communication of the signals. One such technology common to LANs is Ethernet. Ethernet is based on a bus topology in which computers share the same cable to send data. Other technologies include Bitnet and Internet, which are characteristic of WANs.

THE INTERNET
History

The Internet is the largest computer network system in existence because it connects users all over the world. Concern that a single bomb could destroy the computing facilities of the United States Department of Defense led to the creation and devel-

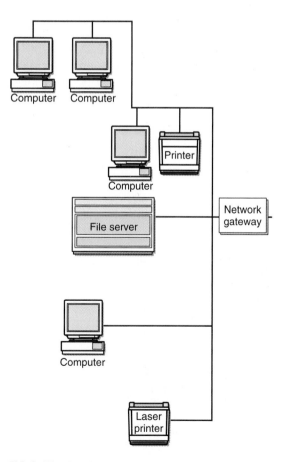

FIG. 2-17. Local area network using a bus topology. The network gateway allows the network to connect to other networks.

opment of the Internet in 1959. Efforts were made to rely on one computer system at a single location and a large number of computers at remote locations. Communications between these computers breaks down messages into packets, each of which has a specific destination address and is subsequently reassembled when it arrives at its destination address. Software was then developed to facilitate the communication process. This software is referred to as *transmission control protocol/Internet protocol* (TCP/IP). TCP manages the packets and their reassembly, and the IP component ensures the packets arrive at their appropriate remote computers.

In 1990, Dr. Berners-Lee developed the worldwide web (www) to facilitate communications with remote computers through a set of links. (The name *web* refers to his vision of these links as a spider's web.) Dr. Berners-Lee's goal was to communicate more easily with his colleagues by linking with their computers.

Major Components

The Internet user must first access a server computer called the *Internet service provider* (ISP) using a phone line or direct cable connection. The server computer relays the user's message to the Internet. Finally, the Internet returns electronic mail (e-mail) or requested information to the user through the ISP server (Fig. 2-18).

A web browser allows the user to use a mouse to point and click on text, drawings, and pictures to facilitate an Internet search. Two popular browsers are Netscape and Internet Explorer. Websites can be located with a uniform resource locator (URL) that must conform to a specific format to ensure successful communications. The URL is the address of the site or file on the Internet. An example of a URL is as follows:

http://www.med.harvard.edu/AANLIB/home.html

The parts of the URL that enable users to access a web page or file include the protocol for communicating links (http:// [hypertext transfer protocol]); the ISP address or domain name (www.med.harvard.edu); and the final portion of the domain name, or top-level domain, which demonstrates the type and purpose of the organization. In the above URL, *edu* indicates an educational institution. The URL ends with path, directory, and file name (AANLIB/home.html). This site features "The Whole Brain Atlas."

The Internet also features search engines to help users find information in a systematic and organized manner. Examples of search engines include Alta Vista, Lycos, Yahoo!, Excite, Infoseek, HotBot, Northern Light, and WebCrawler.

OTHER TOPICS

Many other topics in computer science are gaining attention in medical imaging. For example, computer graphics is the basis for 3D rendering techniques such as shaded surface displays and

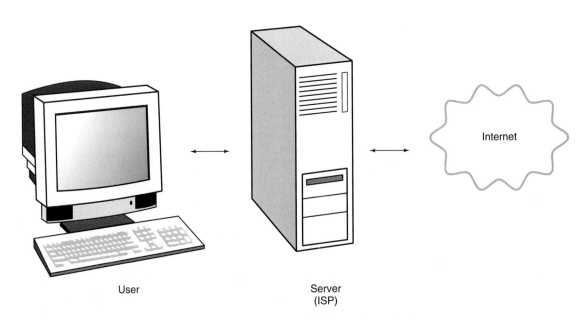

User

Server
(ISP)

Internet

FIG. 2-18. The major components of connecting to the Internet.

volume rendering, which have become common in 3D CT.

 GLOSSARY OF *Topics*

Artificial intelligence The branch of computer science that deals with enabling computers to emulate such aspects of intelligence as speech recognition, deduction, inference, creative response, the ability to learn from past experience, and the ability to make reasonable inferences from incomplete information. Artificial intelligence is a complex arena that includes work in two related areas—one involved with understanding how living things think and the other with finding ways to impart similar capabilities to computer programs. Some tasks that used to be considered very difficult for a computer to perform, such as playing chess, have turned out to be relatively easy to program; and some tasks that were once thought easy to program, such as speech recognition and language translation, have turned out to be extremely difficult. Practical applications in this area include computer-based chess games and diagnostic aids, called *expert systems,* that are used by physicians and other professionals (Microsoft Press, 1999).

Computer graphics Broadly, the display of "pictures" as opposed to only alphabetic and numeric characters on a computer screen. The term *computer graphics* encompasses different methods of generating, displaying, and storing information (Microsoft Press, 1999).

Expert system A type of application program that makes decisions or solves problems in a particular field, such as finance or medicine, by using knowledge and analytical rules defined by experts in the field. Human experts solve problems by using a combination of factual knowledge and reasoning ability. In an expert system, these two essentials are contained in two separate but related components, a knowledge base and inference engine. The knowledge base provides specific facts and rules about the subject, and the inference engine provides the reasoning ability that enables the expert system to form conclusions (Microsoft Press, 1999).

Virus (computer) A set of illicit instructions that passes itself onto other programs with which it comes into contact (Capron, 2000).

Virtual reality A system in which the user is immersed in a computer-created environment so that the user physically interacts with the computer-produced 3D scene (Capron, 2000).

COMPUTERS IN RADIOLOGY

In 1955, computers were used to calculate radiation dose distributions in cancer patients. Today, computer applications in radiology include two categories: imaging and nonimaging applications (Seeram, 1989).

Imaging Applications

Imaging applications are those modalities in which the information acquired from the patient is subject to computer processing. Such processing involves digital image processing techniques to produce computer-generated or digital images. These digital images can be stored on a magnetic tape or optical disk, displayed on a monitor for observation, or printed on film for interpretation.

Several methods exist for creating digital images: computed radiography, digital fluoroscopy, radiographic film digitization, computed tomography, and magnetic resonance imaging.

Nonimaging Applications

Information Systems

Nonimaging applications refer to radiology information systems (RIS) such as patient admissions, scheduling, accounting, billing, film library functions, word processing, statistics, database management, and data communications. RIS can connect to a hospital information system (HIS), which addresses the needs of all departments in the hospital including laboratory, pharmacy, finance, admissions, and hospital administration.

Picture Archiving and Communications Systems

An electronic system for archiving, transmitting, viewing, and manipulating images is now essential to the digital radiology department (Huda and Szeverenyi, 1999). Such a system is referred to as a *picture archiving and communications system* (PACS) (Fig. 2-19). The accompanying box shows the major components of a PACS.

Communication Protocol Standards

Connectivity refers to a measure of the effectiveness and efficiency of computers and computer-based devices to communicate and share information and messages without human intervention (Laudon, 1994).

The use of communication protocol standards is integral to achieving connectivity. Whereas a

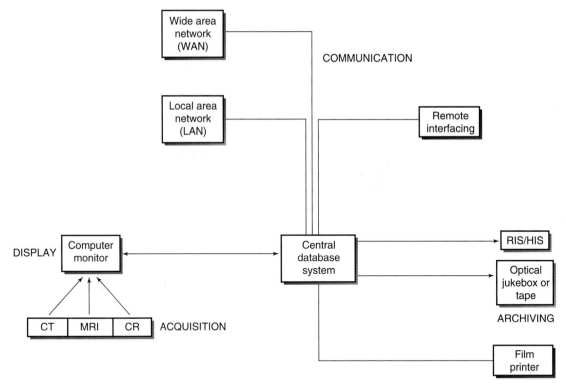

FIG. 2-19. Picture archiving and communications system showing major components.

MAJOR COMPONENTS OF A PICTURE ARCHIVING AND COMMUNICATIONS SYSTEM

- *Image acquisition:* This includes imaging modalities that acquire data from the patient's internal structures, such as CT, MRI, digital radiography and fluoroscopy, digital angiography, ultrasound, and nuclear medicine. For example, data acquired from a patient's tissues that have been injected with contrast media during CT, are reconstructed by the computer to produce images of internal anatomy.
- *Storage and retrieval:* Images from an optical jukebox or tape storage system require a central database system that also allows electronic interaction with the hospital information system and radiology information system.

- *Display and output:* Images can be displayed on diagnostic workstations, viewing workstations, and personal workstations.
- *Communications and networking:* Communications is through local area or wide area networks.
- *PACS/RIS interfacing:* Integration with a radiology information system or hospital information system is essential to merge patient demographics, health records. and also images from various imaging modalities so that information can be shared.

protocol deals with the specifics of how a certain task will be done, a *standard* is an "approved reference model and protocol determined by standard-setting groups for building or developing products and services" (Laudon, 1994).

In health care, HIS, RIS, and PACS, integration is based on different communication protocol standards. Two such popular standards are health level 7 (HL-7) and digital imaging and communi-

cations in medicine (DICOM). HL-7 is the standard application protocol for use in most HIS and RIS; DICOM is the imaging communication protocol for PACS (Creighton, 1999). DICOM was developed by the American College of Radiology and the National Electrical Manufacturers Association. Today, manufacturers of digital imaging equipment, including CT scanners, list their products as DICOM compliant.

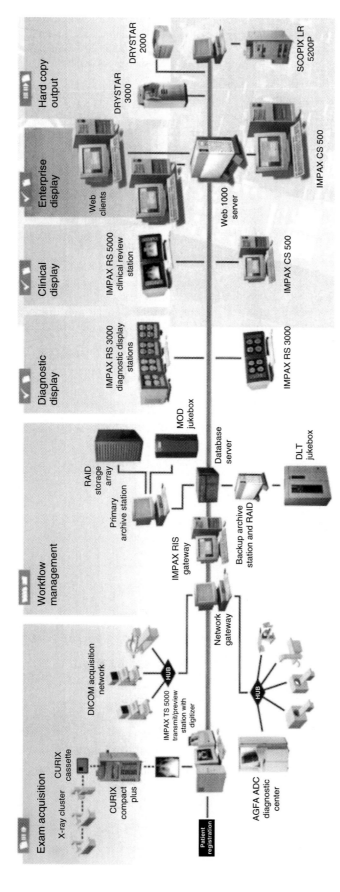

FIG. 2-20.   The IMPAX image management system consists of several functional units working together to provide total solutions to information systems integration. It is DICOM compliant and compatible with HIS and RIS. (Courtesy Technical Imaging Systems, Agfa Division, Bayer Corporation; Ridgefield Park, NJ.)

Essential features of an image management and archiving system that is compliant with DICOM, and compatible with HIS, and RIS include examination acquisition (acquisition of patient demographics) and image acquisition; workflow management; diagnostic, clinical, and enterprise display; and hard copy output (Fig. 2-20). The enterprise display component allows users to view, retrieve, and distribute image data and radiology reports online using the DICOM webserver. The nature of possible network systems in radiology is complex.

REFERENCES

Arnold DO: *Computers and society: impact*, New York, 1991, Mitchell McGraw-Hill.

Bradley AC: *Optical storage for computers*, West Sussex, England, 1989, Ellis Horwood Ltd.

Capron HL: *Computers: tools for an information age*, Upper Saddle River, NJ, 2000, Prentice Hall.

Covington MA: *Computer science—outline notes*, New York, 1991, Barron's.

Creighton C: A literature review on communications between picture archiving and communications systems and radiology information systems and/or hospital information systems, *J Dig Imaging* 12:138-143, 1999.

Dwyer S: Network wise, *Appl Radiol* 2:13-15, 1999.

Huda W, Szeverenyi NM: The filmless radiology department: a primer, *Appl Radiol* 2:30-34, 1999.

Laudon KC: *Management information systems: organization and technology*, Englewood Cliffs, NJ, 1994, MacMillan.

Lodwick G, Edwards M: Computers in radiology, *Appl Radiol* 2:27-30, 1983.

Microsoft Press: *Computer dictionary*, Redmond, Calif., 1999, Microsoft Press.

O'Leary TJ, Williams BK, O'Leary LI: *McGraw-Hill computing essentials, 1992-1993*, New York, 1992, Mitchell McGraw-Hill.

Proakis JG: *Digital signal processing: principles, algorithms, and applications*, New York, 1992, Macmillan.

Seeram E, ed: *Computers in diagnostic radiology—a book of selected readings*, Springfield, Ill, 1989, Charles C. Thomas.

Stallings WD et al: *Computers: the user perspective*, ed 3, St Louis, 1992, Mosby.

Digital Image
Processing

CT is classified as a digital imaging system because it uses computers to process images. X-rays pass through the patient and land on suitable detectors that convert the x-ray photons into electrical signals, or analog signals. These signals are then sampled and digitized (converted into numeric form) for subsequent processing by the computer. The method of digitization of patient data and the types of processing operations carried out by the computer belong to the domain of digital image processing.

Digital image processing is therefore relevant to CT from two perspectives:

1. During analysis of patient data, the steps that apply to digitizing an image are similar to those applied to CT. If the fundamental steps in digitizing an image are understood, the principles of CT are better understood.

2. In CT, a number of digital image processing operations are used, of which *windowing* is perhaps the most important. An understanding of the rudiments of these operations helps the appreciation of image manipulation in CT.

This chapter explores these two topics through a brief history of digital image processing, image representation, the digitizing process, image processing operations, and image processing hardware considerations.

HISTORICAL PERSPECTIVES

The history of digital image processing dates to the early 1960s, when the National Aeronautics and Space Administration (NASA) was developing its lunar and planetary exploration program. The Ranger spacecraft returned images of the lunar surface to Earth. These analog images taken by a television camera were converted into digital images and subsequently processed by the digital computer to obtain more information about the moon's surface.

The development of digital image processing techniques can be attributed to work at NASA's Jet Propulsion Laboratory at the California Institute of Technology. The technology of digital processing continues to expand rapidly and its applications extend into fields such as astronomy, geology, forestry, agriculture, cartography, military science, and medicine. (An overview of the history of digital image processing technology is shown in Fig. 3-1.) The technology has found widespread applications in medicine and particularly in diagnostic imaging, where it has been suc-

cessfully applied to ultrasound, digital radiography, nuclear medicine, CT, and magnetic resonance imaging (Huang, 1999). Digital image processing is a multidisciplinary subject that includes physics, mathematics, engineering, and computer science.

IMAGE FORMATION AND REPRESENTATION

An understanding of images is necessary to define digital image processing. Castleman (1996) has classified images based on their form or method of generation. He used set theory to explain image types. According to this theory, images are a subset of all objects. Within the set of images, there are other subsets such as visible images (e.g., paintings, drawings, or photographs), optical images (e.g., holograms), nonvisible physical images (e.g., temperature, pressure, or elevation maps), and mathematical images (e.g., continuous functions and discrete functions). The sine wave is an example of a continuous function (analog signal), whereas a discrete function represents a digital image. Castleman (1996) has noted that "only the digital images can be processed by computer."

Analog Images

Analog images are continuous images. For example, a black-and-white photograph of a chest x-ray is an analog image because it represents a continuous distribution of light intensity as a function of position on the radiograph.

In photography, images are formed when light is focused on film. In radiography, x-rays pass through the patient and are projected onto x-ray film. In both cases, films are processed in chemical solutions to render them visible and the images are formed by a photochemical process. Images can also be formed by photoelectronic means, in which the images may be represented as electrical signals (analog signals) that emerge from the photoelectronic device.

Digital Images

Digital images are numeric representations or images of objects. The formation of digital images requires a digital computer. Any information that enters the computer for processing must first be converted into digital form, or numbers (Fig. 3-2). An important component is the analog-to-digital converter (ADC), which converts continuous sig-

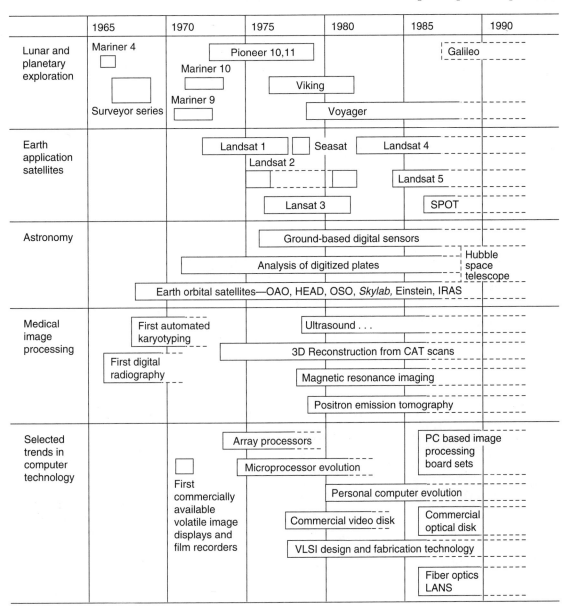

FIG. 3-1. Overview of the first 20 years of important developments in digital image processing. (From Green WB: *Digital image processing: a systems approach,* ed 2, New York, 1989, Van Nostrand Reinhold.)

nals to discrete signals, or digital data (Luiten, 1995).

The computer receives the digital data and performs the necessary processing. The results of this processing are always digital and can be displayed as a digital image (Fig. 3-3) (Seeram, 1985).

DEFINITIONS

In image processing, it is necessary to convert an input image into an output image. If both the input image and output image are analog, this is re-

ferred to as *analog processing.* If both the input image and output image are discrete, this is referred to as *digital processing.* In cases where an analog image must be converted into digital data for input to the computer, a digitization system is required. CT is based on a reconstruction process, whereby a digital image is changed into a visible physical image (Fig. 3-4).

Castleman (1996) defined a *process* as "a series of actions or operations leading to a desired result; thus, a series of actions or operations are performed upon an object to alter its form in a desired

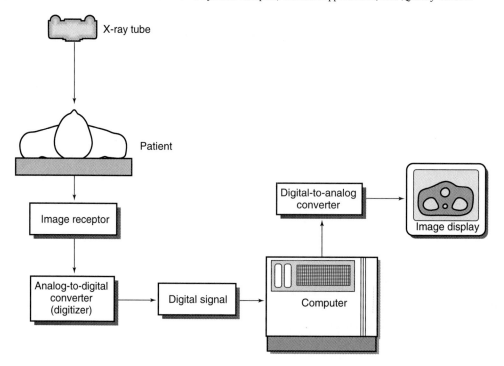

FIG. 3-2. The conversion of analog data into digital data for input to a digital computer.

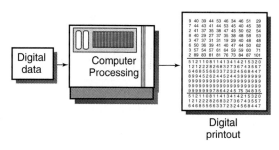

FIG. 3-3. Input digital data can be displayed in digital form after computer processing.

IMAGE PROCESSING OPERATIONS

Image generation
Image modification
    Image enhancement
    Image combination
    Image restoration
Image analysis
    Pattern recognition
    Image interpretation
    Feature extraction

manner." Castleman also defined *digital image processing* as "subjecting numerical representations of objects to a series of operations in order to obtain a desired result."

Given the variety of possible operations (Baxes, 1994), image processing has emerged as a discipline in itself (see box above).

IMAGE DIGITIZATION

The primary objective during image digitization is to convert an analog image into numeric data for processing by the computer (Seibert, 1995). Digitization consists of three distinct steps: scanning, sampling, and quantization.

Scanning

Consider an image or transparency of a beautiful scene (Fig. 3-5). The first step in digitization is the division of the picture into small regions, or scanning. Each small region of the picture is a picture element, or pixel. Scanning results in a grid characterized by rows and columns. The size of the grid usually depends on the number of pixels on each side of the grid. In Fig. 3-5, the grid size is 9 × 9, which results in 81 pixels. The rows and columns identify a particular pixel by providing an address for that pixel. The rows and columns comprise a matrix; in this case, the matrix is 9 × 9. As the number of pixels in the image matrix increases, the image becomes more recognizable and facilitates better perception of image details (Fig. 3-6).

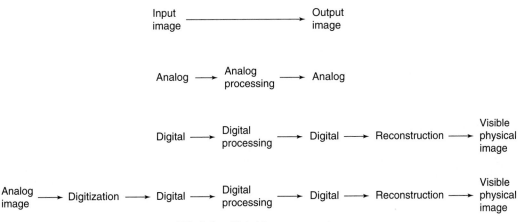

FIG. 3-4. Digital image processing.

Sampling

The second step in image digitization is sampling, which measures the brightness of each pixel in the entire image (Fig. 3-7). A small spot of light is projected onto the transparency and the transmitted light is detected by a photomultiplier tube positioned behind the picture. The output of the photomultiplier tube is an electrical (analog) signal.

Quantization

Quantization is the final step, in which the brightness value of each sampled pixel is assigned an integer (0, or a positive or negative number) called a *gray level*. The result is a range of numbers or gray levels, each of which has a precise location on the rectangular grid of pixels. The total number of gray levels is called the *gray scale*, such as a four-level gray scale (Fig. 3-8). The gray scale is based on the value of the gray levels; 0 represents black and 4 represents white. The other numbers, 1, 2, and 3, represent shades of gray. In the case of two gray levels, the picture would show only black and white. An image can therefore be composed of any number of gray levels.

In quantization, the electrical signal obtained from sampling is assigned an integer based on the strength of the signal. In general, the value of the integer is proportional to the signal strength (Seibert, 1995).

The result of the quantization process is a digital image, an array of numbers representing the analog image that was scanned, sampled, and quantized. This array of numbers is sent to the computer for further processing.

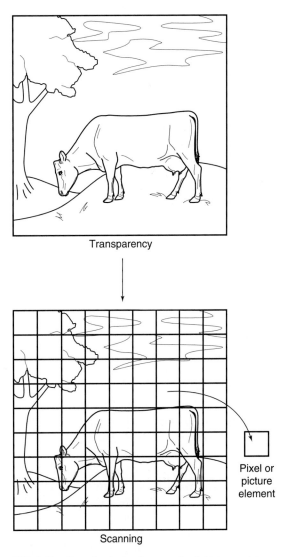

Transparency

Scanning

Pixel or picture element

FIG. 3-5. Scanning is the first step in digitizing a picture.

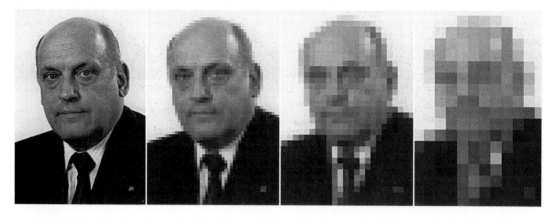

FIG. 3-6. An increased number of pixels in the image matrix improves the picture quality and enhances the perception of details in the image. (From Luiten AL: Digital: discrete perfection, *Medicamundi* 40:95-100, 1995.)

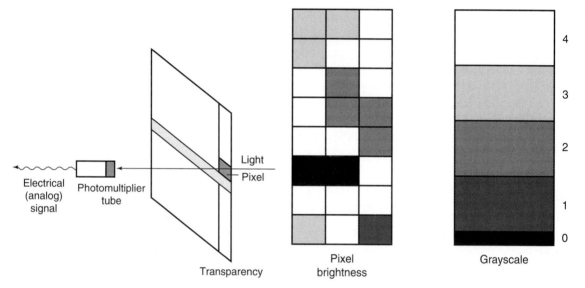

FIG. 3-7. Sampling is the second step in digitizing a picture.

FIG. 3-8. Quantization is the final step in digitizing a picture.

Analog-to-Digital Conversion

The conversion of analog signals to digital information is accomplished by the analog-to-digital converter (ADC). The ADC samples the analog signal at various times to measure its strength at different points. The more points sampled, the better the representation of the signal. This sampling process is followed by quantization.

Two important characteristics of the ADC are speed and accuracy. *Accuracy* refers to the sampling of the signal. The more samples taken, the more accurate the representation of the digital image (Fig. 3-9). If not enough samples are taken, the representation of the original signal will be inaccurate after computer processing (Fig. 3-10). This

sampling error is referred to as *aliasing,* and it appears as an artifact on the image. Aliasing artifacts appear as moiré patterns on the image (Baxes, 1994).

The sampling results in the division of the signal. The more parts to the signal, the greater the accuracy of the ADC. The measurement unit for these parts is the bit. Recall that a bit can be either 0 or 1. In a 1-bit ADC, the signal is divided in two parts ($2^1 = 2$). A 2-bit ADC generates four equal parts ($2^2 = 4$). An 8-bit ADC generates 256 equal parts ($2^8 = 256$). The higher the number of bits, the more accurate the ADC.

The ADC also determines the number of levels or shades of gray represented in the image. A

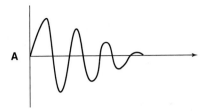

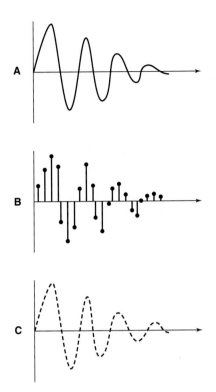

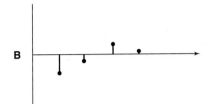

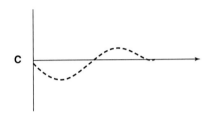

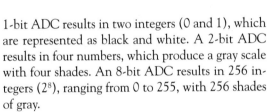

FIG. 3-9. Good sampling (**B**) of original analog signal (**A**) produces an accurate representation of the original signal (**C**) after computer processing.

FIG. 3-10. Poor sampling (**B**) misrepresents the shape of the original (**A**) after computer processing (**C**).

1-bit ADC results in two integers (0 and 1), which are represented as black and white. A 2-bit ADC results in four numbers, which produce a gray scale with four shades. An 8-bit ADC results in 256 integers (2^8), ranging from 0 to 255, with 256 shades of gray.

The other characteristic of the ADC is *speed*, or the time taken to digitize the analog signal. In the ADC, speed and accuracy are inversely related—that is, the greater the accuracy, the longer it takes to digitize the signal.

Why Digitize Images?

The major goal of digitization is that digital images can be processed by a computer, resulting in numerous advantages, as follows:

- Image enhancement: The image can be made to look more pleasing to the observer. Certain characteristics such as contours and shapes can be enhanced to improve the overall quality of the image.
- Image restoration: Poor images can be filtered to remove unwanted "noise." Filtering can also help remove unnecessary fine detail in the image, a technique known as *smoothing*.
- Image analysis: Also referred to as *scene analysis*, this process "seeks to extract the information contained in the various objects in a scene without placing any interpretation on them" (Marion, 1991).
- Image detection: Detection allows the observer to look for specific shapes, contours, or textures while disregarding the other features in the image.
- Pattern recognition: The computer can "see" structures and identify patterns.
- Geometric transformation: Images can be rotated or scaled by changing the position of the pixels.
- Data compression: The compression of digital images reduces the amount of data that comprise the image, which is important in data storage and transmission.

IMAGE PROCESSING TECHNIQUES

In general, image processing techniques are based on three types of operations: point operations (point processes), local operations (area processes), and global operations (frame processes). The image processing algorithms on which these operations are based alter the pixel intensity values. The exception is the geometric processing algorithm, which changes the position (spatial position or arrangement) of the pixel.

Point Operations

Point operations are perhaps the least complicated and most frequently used image processing technique. The value of the input image pixel is mapped on the corresponding output image pixel (Fig. 3-11). The algorithms for point operations enable the input image matrix to be scanned, pixel by pixel, until the entire image is transformed.

The most commonly used point processing technique is called *gray-level mapping*. This is also referred to as "contrast enhancement," "contrast stretching," "histogram modification," "histogram stretching," or "windowing." Gray-level mapping uses a look-up table (LUT), which plots the output and input gray levels against each other (Fig. 3-12).

LUTs can be implemented with hardware or software for gray-level transformation. Fig. 3-13 illustrates the transformation process. Gray-level mapping changes the brightness of the image and results in the enhancement of the display image.

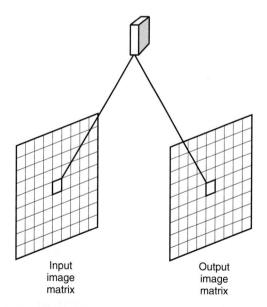

FIG. 3-11. In a point operation, the value of the input image pixel is mapped onto the corresponding output image pixel.

Gray-level mapping results in a modification of the histogram of the pixel values. A histogram is a graph of the pixels in all or part of the image, plotted as a function of the gray level. A histogram can be created as follows:

1. Observe the image matrix (Fig. 3-14) and create a table of the number of pixels with a specific intensity value, as shown.
2. Plot a graph (Fig. 3-15) of the number of pixels versus the gray levels (intensity or density values).

Histograms indicate the overall brightness and contrast of an image. If the histogram is modified or changed, the brightness and contrast of the image can be altered, a technique referred to as *histogram modification*, or histogram stretching. This is also an example of a point operation in digital image processing. If the histogram is wide, the resulting image has high contrast. If the histogram is narrow, the resulting image has low contrast. On the other hand, if the histogram values are closer to the lower end of the range of values, the image appears dark, as opposed to a bright image, in which the values are weighted toward the higher end of the range of values.

Local Operations

A *local operation* is an image processing operation in which the output image pixel value is determined from a small area of pixels around the corresponding input pixel (Fig. 3-16). These operations are also referred to as *area processes* or *group processes* because a group of pixels is used in the transformation calculation.

Spatial frequency filtering is an example of a local operation that concerns brightness information in an image. If the brightness of an image changes rapidly with distance in the horizontal or vertical direction, the image is said to have *high spatial frequency*. (An image with smaller pixels has higher frequency information than an image with larger pixels.) When the brightness changes slowly or at a constant rate, the image is said to have *low spatial frequency*. Spatial frequency filtering can alter images in several ways such as image sharpening, image smoothing, image blurring, noise reduction, and feature extraction (edge enhancement and detection).

There are two places to perform spatial frequency filtering: (1) in the frequency domain, which considers the Fourier transform, or (2) in the spatial domain, which uses the pixel values (gray levels) themselves. Convolution, a general purpose algorithm, is a technique of filtering in the space domain (Fig. 3-17) (Greenfield and Hubbard, 1984; Lindley, 1991).

The value of the output pixel depends on a group of pixels in the input image that surround the input pixel of interest: in this case, pixel P5. The new value for P5 in the output image is calculated by obtaining its weighted average and that of its surrounding pixels. The average is computed using a group of pixels called a *convolution kernel,* in which each pixel in the kernel is a weighting factor, or convolution coefficient. In general, the size of the kernel is a 3 × 3 matrix. Depending on the type of processing, different types of convolution kernels can be used, in which case the weighting factors are different.

During convolution, the convolution kernel moves across the image, pixel by pixel. Each pixel in the input image, its surrounding neighbors, and the kernels are used to compute the value of the corresponding output pixel—that is, each pixel is multiplied by its respective weighting factor and then summed. The resulting number is the value of the center output pixel. This process is applied to all pixels in the input image; each calculation requires nine multiplications and nine additions. This can be time consuming, but special hardware can speed up this process.

Global Operations

In global operations, the entire input image is used to compute the value of the pixel in the output image (Fig. 3-18). A common global operation is Fourier domain processing, or the Fourier transform, which uses filtering in the frequency domain rather than the space domain (Baxes, 1994). Fourier domain image processing techniques can provide edge enhancement, image sharpening, and image restoration.

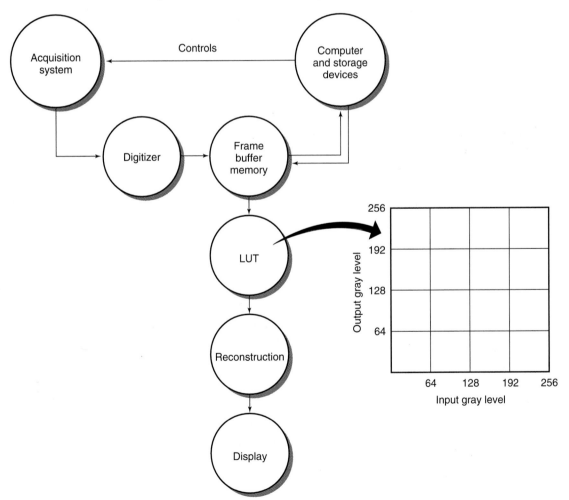

FIG. 3-12. Gray level mapping. The look-up (LUT) table plots the input gray level against the output gray level.

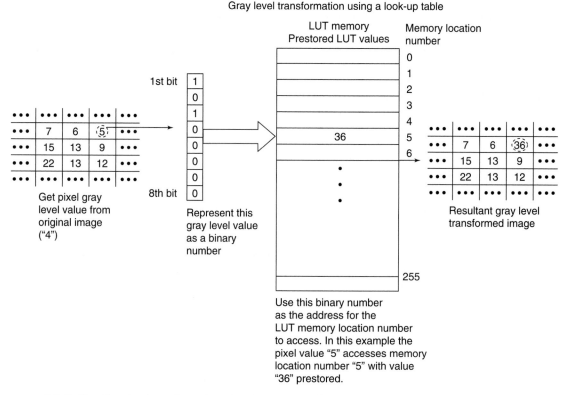

FIG. 3-13. Gray level transformation of an input image pixel. The algorithm uses the look-up table to change the value of the input pixel (5) to 36, the new value of the output pixel. (From Huang HK: *Elements of digital radiology*, Englewood Cliffs, NJ, 1987, Prentice-Hall.)

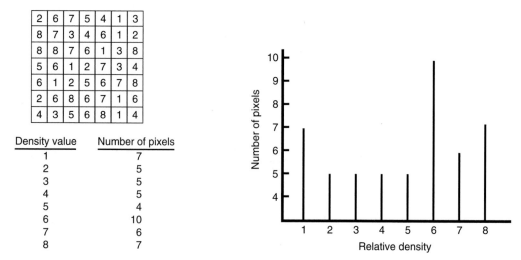

FIG. 3-14. To create a histogram, total the number of pixels in the image (intensity value) that have the same pixel value (density value).

FIG. 3-15. Plot of the histogram using the table values in Fig. 3-14.

Geometric Operations

Geometric operations are intended to modify the spatial position or orientation of the pixels in an image. These algorithms change the position rather than the intensity of the pixels, which is also a characteristic of point, local, and global operations. Geometric operations can result in the scaling and sizing of images and image rotation and translation (Castleman, 1996).

IMAGE PROCESSING HARDWARE

A basic image processing system consists of several interconnected components (Fig. 3-19). The major components are the analog-to-digital converter, image storage, image display, image processor, host computer, and digital-to-analog converter.

- Digitizer: As can be seen in Fig. 3-19, the analog signal is converted into digital form by the digitizer, or analog-to-digital converter (ADC).
- Image memory: The digitized image is held in storage for further processing. Several components are connected to the image store and provide input and output. The size of this memory depends on the image. For example, a $512 \times 512 \times 8$ bit image requires a memory of 2,097,152 bits.
- Digital-to-analog converter (DAC): The digital image held in the memory can be displayed on a television monitor. However, because monitors work with analog signals, it is necessary to convert the digital data to analog signals with a DAC.
- Internal image processor: This processor is responsible for high-speed processing of the input digital data.

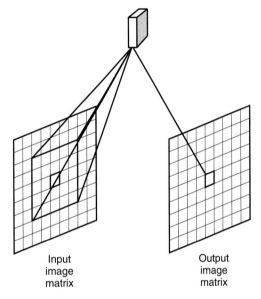

FIG. 3-16. In the local operation, the value is determined from a small area of pixels surrounding the corresponding input pixel.

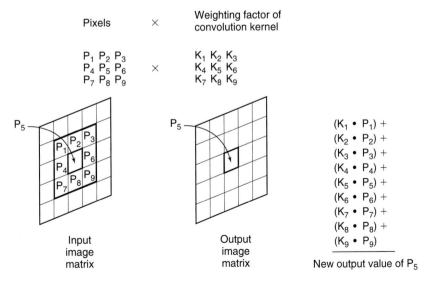

FIG. 3-17. In convolution, the value of the output pixel is calculated by multiplying each input pixel by its corresponding weighting factor of the convolution kernel (usually a 3×3 matrix). These products are then summed.

- Host computer: In digital image processing, the host computer is a primary component capable of performing several functions. For example, the host computer can read and write the data in the image store and provide for archival storage on tape and disk storage systems. The host computer plays a significant role in applications that involve the transmission of images to another location, such as medical imaging.

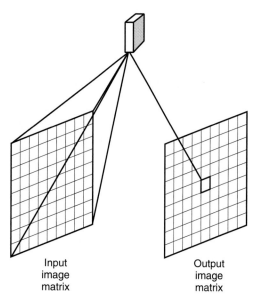

FIG. 3-18. In a global operation, the entire input image is used to compute the value of the pixel in the output image.

CT AS A DIGITAL IMAGE PROCESSING SYSTEM

A number of imaging modalities in radiology use image processing techniques, including digital radiography and fluoroscopy, nuclear medicine, magnetic resonance imaging, ultrasound, and computed tomography. The future of digital imaging is promising in that a wide variety of applications have received increasing attention, such as 3D imaging (Huang, 1999). The major image-processing operations in medical imaging that are now common in the radiology department are presented in Table 3-1.

The basic components of a digital imaging system were illustrated in Fig. 1-22. As a digital image processing system, CT fits into this scheme. Similar steps in image digitization can be applied to the CT process, as follows:

1. First, divide the picture into pixels. In CT, the slice of the patient is divided into small regions called *voxels* (volume element) because the dimension of depth (slice thickness) is added to the pixel. The patient is scanned as the x-ray tube moves around the patient.
2. Next, sample the pixels. In CT, the voxels are sampled when x-rays pass through them. This measurement is performed by detectors. The signal from the detector is in analog form and must be converted into digital form before it can be sent to the computer for processing.
3. The final step is quantization. In CT, the analog signal is also quantized and changed into a digital array for input into the computer.

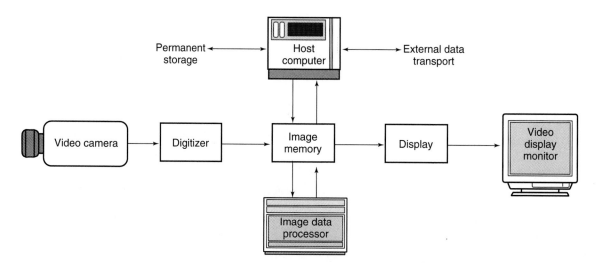

FIG. 3-19. The essential hardware components of a generalized digital image processing system.

TABLE 3-1

Essential Image-Processing Operations Used in Digital Imaging Technologies

IMAGING MODALITY	PRINCIPAL IMAGE-PROCESSING OPERATIONS	OBJECTIVES
Radionuclide imaging	Processing of image sequences, slice reconstruction, filtration, quantitative processing	Display quality, tomography, extraction of physiologic data
Digital radiography	Modification of display parameters using contrast reproduction curve, spatial filtration, histogram transformation; selection of particular information out of a sequence of basic images (e.g., dual energy)	Display optimization harmonization of image, extraction of quantitative or semiquantitative information
Digital subtraction angiography	Subtraction of images out of a sequence, analytic processing	Immediate display of subtraction images, evaluation of perfusion and/or blood flow, removal of artifacts arising from patient movement, extraction of physiologic data, contrast enhancement
Computed tomography	Level and window adjustment, image comparison, magnification, ROI (region of interest) processing, reconstruction, reconstruction of perpendicular slices	Display of very large contrast range; display, adaptation to human observer, and hard copy; extraction of quantitative and statistical information; image formation
Magnetic resonance imaging	Level and window adjustment, image comparison, magnification, image synthesis	Adaptation to display and human observer; creation of new images showing tendency on T1, T2, local density, and flow
Ultrasonic imaging	Processing of image sequences, filtration	Display quality, extraction of physiologic data

From Buchmann F et al: Digital image processing, *Medicamundi* 30:37–45, 1985.

The digital data resulting from quantization are processed by the computer through a series of operations or techniques to modify the input image. In CT, the digital data are also subject to several processing algorithms so the output image can be displayed in a form suitable for human observation.

REFERENCES

Baxes GA: *Digital image processing: principles and applications*, New York, 1994, John Wiley & Sons.

Castleman KR: *Digital image processing*, Englewood Cliffs, NJ, 1996, Prentice Hall.

Greenfield GB, Hubbard LB: *Computers in radiology*, New York, 1984, Churchill Livingstone.

Huang HK: *PACS: basic principles and applications*, New York, 1999, Wiley-Liss.

Lindley CA: *Practical image processing in C*, New York, 1991, John Wiley & Sons.

Luiten AL: Digital: discrete perfection, *Medicamundi* 40:95–100, 1995.

Marion A: *Introduction to image processing*, London, 1991, Chapman and Hall.

Seeram E: *X-ray imaging equipment. An introduction*, Springfield, Ill, 1985, Charles C Thomas.

Seibert JA: Digital image processing: basics. In Balter S, Shope TB, eds: *A categorical course in physics: physical and technical aspects of angiography and interventional radiology*, Oak Brook, Ill, 1995, RSNA.

BIBLIOGRAPHY

Buchmann F et al: Digital image processing, *Medicamundi* 30:37–45, 1985.

Bushong S: *Magnetic resonance imaging: physical and biological principles*, St Louis, 1996, Mosby.

Delp EJ, Buda AJ: Digital image processing. In Green WB, ed: *Digital image processing*, New York, 1983, Van Nostrand Reinhold.

Green WB: *Digital image processing: a systems approach*, ed 2, New York, 1989, Van Nostrand Reinhold.

4

Physical Principles of Computed Tomography

The information presented in a CT image differs from a conventional radiographic image in several respects. The most obvious is that CT shows cross-sectional (transaxial) views of patient anatomy (Fig. 4-1). Other significant differences in CT imaging will become apparent in the following chapters. In this presentation of the principles of CT, a review of conventional tomography and the limitations of radiography is helpful to understand the CT image.

LIMITATIONS OF RADIOGRAPHY AND TOMOGRAPHY

In both radiography and tomography, x-rays pass through the patient and are absorbed in different ways by the body's tissues. For example, because bone is denser, it absorbs more x-rays than the less-dense soft tissues. This differential absorption is contained in the x-ray beam that passes through the patient and is recorded on film.

Limitations of Radiography

The major shortcoming of radiography is the superimposition of all structures on the film, which makes it difficult and sometimes impossible to distinguish a particular detail (Fig. 4-2). This is especially true when structures differ only slightly in density, as is often the case with some tumors and their surrounding tissues. Although multiple views such as laterals and obliques can be taken to localize a structure, the problem of superimposition in radiography still persists.

A second limitation is that radiography is a qualitative rather than quantitative procedure (Fig. 4-3). It is difficult to distinguish between a homogeneous object of nonuniform thickness and a heterogenous object (Fig. 4-3 includes bone, soft tissue, and air) of uniform thickness (Marshall, 1976).

Limitations of CT

The problem of superimposition in radiography can be somewhat overcome by conventional tomography (Bocage, 1974; Vallebona, 1931). The most common method of conventional tomography is sometimes referred to as *geometric tomography* to distinguish it from computed tomography (Fig. 4-4). When the x-ray tube and film are moved simultaneously in opposite directions, un-

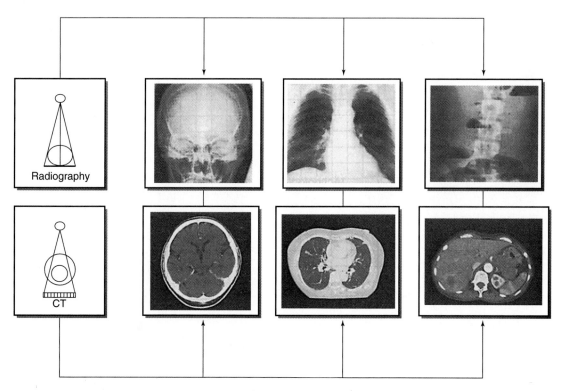

FIG. 4-1. The most conspicuous difference between conventional radiographic imaging and CT imaging is that CT shows cross-sectional or transaxial anatomy.

wanted sections can be blurred while the desired layer or section is kept in focus.

The immediate goal of tomography is to eliminate structures above and below the focused section, or the focal plane. However, this is difficult to achieve, and under no circumstances can all unwanted planes be removed. The limitations of tomography include persistent image blurring that cannot be completely removed, degradation of image contrast because of the presence of scattered radiation created by the open geometry of the x-ray beam, and other problems resulting from film-screen combinations.

In addition, both radiography and tomography fail to adequately demonstrate slight differences in subject contrast, which are characteristic of soft tissue. The differences for soft tissues such as human fat, water, human cerebrospinal fluid, human plasma, monkey pancreas, monkey white matter, monkey gray matter, monkey liver, monkey muscle, and human red cells are 0.194, 0.222, 0.227, 0.227, 0.230, 0.230, 0.235, 0.236, 0.238, and 0.246, respectively (Ter-Pogossian et al, 1974). Ra-

diographic film is not sensitive enough to resolve these small differences because typical films can only discriminate x-ray intensity differences of 5% to 10%.

The limitations of radiography and tomography result in the inability of film to image very small differences in tissue contrast. In addition, contrast cannot be adjusted after it has been recorded on the film.

Enter CT

The goal of CT is to overcome the limitations of radiography and tomography by achieving the following (Hounsfield, 1973):

1. Minimal superimposition
2. Improved image contrast
3. The recording of very small differences in tissue contrast

The basic methodologic approach to these three tasks is shown in Fig. 4-5. A few important points can be noted from this figure, as follows:

1. A beam of x-rays is transmitted through a specific cross-section of the patient. This procedure removes the problem of superimposition of structures above and below the specific cross-section or slice of tissue.
2. The beam of x-rays is highly collimated into a thin beam that only passes through the cross-section of tissue to be imaged. This procedure is intended to minimize scatter production and therefore improve the contrast of the image.
3. When the x-ray beam passes through the patient, it strikes special detectors positioned opposite the x-ray tube. These detectors are quantitative and can measure very small differences in tissue contrast. However, film is considered a qualitative detector and cannot record these small differences. In addition, the data from the detectors are processed by a digital computer that uses special algorithms to reconstruct an image of the cross-section.

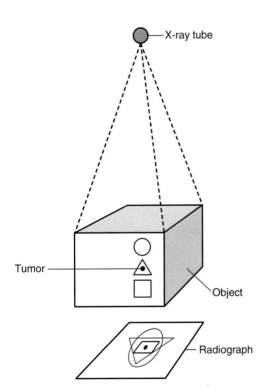

FIG. 4-2. The major shortcoming of radiography is that the superimposition of all structures on the radiograph makes it difficult to discriminate whether the tumor is in the circle, triangle, or square. (From Seeram E: *Computed tomography technology,* Philadelphia, 1982, WB Saunders.)

PHYSICAL PRINCIPLES

CT can be described in terms of physical principles and technologic considerations. The physical principles involve physics and mathematical concepts to understand the way the image is produced, and the technologic considerations involve the practical implementation of scientific and engineering principles such as computer sci-

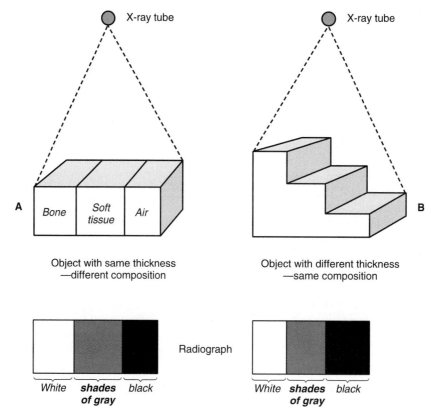

FIG. 4-3. Radiography is a qualitative rather than quantitative procedure. Two radiographs can appear the same even though the two objects, **A** and **B,** are entirely different. (From Seeram E: *Computed tomography technology,* Philadelphia, 1982, WB Saunders.)

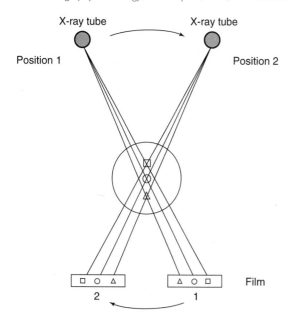

FIG. 4-4. Basic principles of conventional tomography. The x-ray tube and film move simultaneously and in opposite directions to ensure that the desired section (O) of the patient is imaged by blurring out structures above (□) and below (△) the plane of interest (O). (From Seeram E: *Computed tomography technology,* Philadelphia, 1982, WB Saunders.)

ence and technology. The physical principles and technology of CT include the three processes referred to in Chapter 1: data acquisition; data processing; and image display, storage, and documentation. This section discusses each process in basic terms; they are described in more detail in later chapters.

Data Acquisition

Data acquisition refers to the systematic collection of information from the patient to produce the CT image. The two methods of data acquisition are slice-by-slice data acquisition and volume data acquisition (Fig. 4-6).

In conventional slice-by-slice data acquisition, data are collected through different beam geometries to scan the patient. Essentially, the x-ray tube rotates around the patient and collects data from the first slice. The tube stops, and the patient moves into position to scan the next slice. This process continues until all slices have been individually scanned.

In volume data acquisition, a special beam geometry referred to as *spiral* or *helical geometry* is

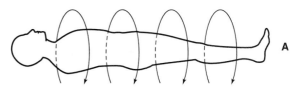

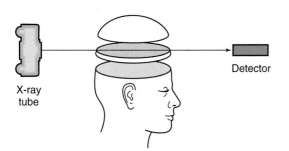

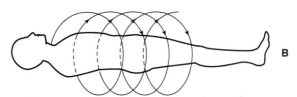

FIG. 4-5. In CT a thin beam is transmitted through a specific cross-section, striking special detectors opposite the x-ray tube.

FIG. 4-6. **A,** Conventional slice-by-slice scanning. **B,** Volume scanning.

used to scan a volume of tissue rather than one slice at a time (Fig. 4-6). In spiral/helical CT, the x-ray tube rotates around the patient and traces a spiral/helical path to scan an entire volume of tissue while the patient holds a single breath. This method generates a single slice per one revolution of the x-ray tube. More recently, multislice spiral/helical CT has become available for faster imaging of patients. Multislice CT generates multiple slices per one revolution of the x-ray tube.

The first step in data acquisition is scanning (Fig. 4-7). During scanning, the x-ray tube and detectors rotate around the patient to collect views. The detectors measure the radiation transmitted through the patient from various locations. As a result, relative transmission values (Hounsfield, 1973) or attenuation measurements (Sprawls, 1995) can be calculated as follows:

$$\text{Relative transmission} = \text{Log} \frac{\text{intensity of x-rays at the source (I}_0\text{)}}{\text{intensity of x-rays at the detector (I)}}$$

The relative transmission values are sent to the computer and stored as raw data.

A large number of penetration measurements are needed to reconstruct the CT image. In general, several hundred views are obtained. Each view is composed of a number of rays, and the total penetration measurement for each scan is given by the following relationship (Sprawls, 1995):

$$\text{Total number of transmission measurements} = \text{Number of views} \times \text{number of rays in each view}$$

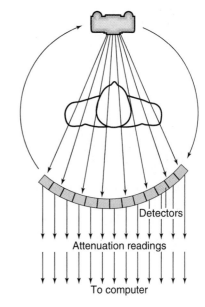

FIG. 4-7. During scanning, the x-ray tube and detectors rotate around the patient to collect views.

Attenuation

The problem in CT is to determine the attenuation in the tissues and use this information to reconstruct an image of the slice of tissue. The solution to this problem is complex and involves physics, mathematics, and computer science. This book takes a fundamental approach to the problem and its solution. The study begins with an understanding of attenuation of radiation in general and attenuation in CT in particular.

Attenuation is the reduction of the intensity of a beam of radiation as it passes through an object—some photons are absorbed, but others are scattered. Attenuation depends on the electrons per gram, atomic number, tissue density, and radiation energy used. In addition, because there are two types of radiation beams (homogeneous and heterogeneous) a study of how each of these beams is attenuated is important to understand the problem in CT. Attenuation in CT depends on the effective atomic density (atoms/vol), the atomic number (Z) of the absorber, and the photon energy.

In a homogeneous beam, all the photons have the same energy, whereas in a heterogeneous beam, the photons have different energies. A homogeneous beam is also referred to as a *monochromatic* or *monoenergetic beam,* and a heterogeneous beam is referred to as a *polychromatic beam.*

When Hounsfield invented the CT scanner, he used a homogeneous beam (Fig. 4-8) in his initial experiments because such a beam satisfies the requirements of the Lambert-Beer law, an exponential relationship that describes what happens to the photons as they travel through the tissues using the following attenuation:

$$I = I_0 e^{-\mu x} \tag{4-1}$$

where I is the transmitted intensity, I_0 is the original intensity, x is the thickness of the object, e is Euler's constant (2.718), and μ is the linear attenuation coefficient.

The goal of CT is to calculate the linear attenuation coefficient μ, which indicates the amount of attenuation that has occurred. Therefore it is a quantitative measurement with a unit of per centimeter (cm^{-1})—hence the term *linear* (Curry et al, 1990).

The equation $I = I_0 e^{-\mu x}$ can be solved to find the value of μ:

$$I = I_0 e^{-\mu x}$$
$$I/I_0 = e^{-\mu x}$$
$$\ln I/I_0 = -\mu x$$
$$\ln I_0/I = \mu x$$
$$\mu = (1/x) \cdot (\ln I_0/I) \tag{4-2}$$

where *ln* is the natural logarithm. In CT, the values of I and I_0 are known (these are measured by the detectors), and x is also known. Hence μ can be calculated.

Fig. 4-8 shows the attenuation of a homogeneous beam of radiation. Each section of the absorber attenuates the beam by equal amounts; that is, each 1-cm section removes 20% of the photons remaining in the beam. The initial beam intensity of 1000 photons is reduced to 410 photons. In other words, the quantity of photons is reduced. In a homogeneous beam the quality of the beam, or beam energy, does not change. If the starting beam energy is 88 keV (kiloelectron volt), the transmitted photons all have an energy of 88 keV.

In the early experiments conducted by Hounsfield, the radiation was from a gamma source and the attenuation was that of a homogeneous beam. One problem he encountered was that it took too long to scan and produce an image, and therefore he substituted a beam produced by a conventional x-ray tube. This beam is a heterogeneous beam of radiation that consists of a range of energies. The attenuation of a heterogeneous or polychromatic beam is somewhat different from that of a homogeneous beam, and therefore Hounsfield had to make several assumptions and adjustments to determine the linear attenuation coefficients.

During the attenuation of a heterogeneous beam (Fig. 4-9), as the beam passes through equal thicknesses of material, the attenuation is not exponential, but rather both the quantity and quality of the photons change. In Fig. 4-9, the initial quantity of photons is 1000 with a mean beam quality (energy) of 40 kV. Each block of water removes different quantities of photons, and the mean energy of the transmitted photons increases to 57 kV. The first centimeter of water attenuates more photons than subsequent 1-cm blocks of water. Also, the lower energy photons are absorbed, which allows the higher-energy photons to pass through. As a re-

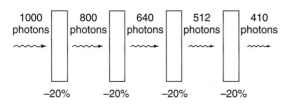

FIG. 4-8.   Attenuation of a homogeneous beam of radiation through water. The absorber is 1 cm of water.

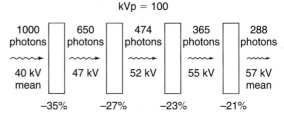

FIG. 4-9.   Attenuation of a heterogeneous beam of radiation through water.

sult, the penetrating power of the photons increases and the beam becomes harder.

The equation $I = I_0e^{-\mu x}$ applies only to a homogeneous beam. It then follows that in CT, which is based on the use of a heterogeneous beam, it is necessary to make the heterogeneous beam approximate a homogeneous beam to satisfy the equation.

It was stated earlier that attenuation is the result of absorption and scattering. X-rays can be attenuated because of the photoelectric effect, or they can be attenuated and scattered by the Compton effect. The total attenuation is then given by

$$I = I_0e^{-(\mu_p + \mu_c)x} \qquad (4-3)$$

where μ_p is the linear attenuation coefficient that results from photoelectric absorption, and μ_c is the linear attenuation coefficient that results from the Compton effect.

The photoelectric effect occurs mainly in tissues with a high atomic number, Z (such as bone, contrast medium) and occurs minimally in some soft tissues and substances with a lower Z. The Compton effect occurs in soft tissues, and differences in density result in differences in Compton interactions. In addition, the photoelectric effect depends on the beam energy (kV); however, the Compton effect is less likely to dominate as the beam energy increases and "the energy dependence is not nearly as dramatic as it is with the photoelectric effect" (Morgan, 1983).

Equation 4-2, like Equation 4-1, holds true only for a homogeneous beam of radiation. Because a heterogeneous beam is used in CT, how is the linear attenuation coefficient determined in CT? The concern is with the number of photons, N, that pass through the tissue during scanning, rather than with the intensity, I. Equation 4-1 can therefore be expressed as

$$N = N_0e^{-\mu x} \qquad (4-4)$$

where N is the number of transmitted photons, N_0 is the number of photons entering the tissue (incident photons), x is the thickness of the tissue, μ is $\mu_p + \mu_c$ (linear attenuation coefficients of the tissue), and e is the base of the natural logarithm.

Equation 4-3 applies to a homogenous block of tissue. However, a slice of tissue in the patient through which the radiation passes is not homogeneous because the tissue is composed of several different substances. In this case, the slice is divided into a number of small regions, "each characterized by its own linear attenuation coefficient" (Morgan, 1983). This can be shown as

$$N_0 \rightarrow \boxed{\mu_1}\,\boxed{\mu_2}\,\boxed{\mu_3}\,\boxed{\mu_4}\,\boxed{\mu_5} \;//\; \boxed{\mu_n} \rightarrow N$$

In this situation, the linear attenuation coefficients can be determined as follows:

$$N = N_0e^{-(\mu_1 + \mu_2 + \mu_3 + \mu_4 + \mu_5 \ldots + \mu_n)x} \qquad (4-5)$$

Data Acquisition Geometries

The way that the x-ray tube and detectors are arranged to collect transmission or penetration measurements describes the data acquisition geometry of the CT system (Fig. 4-10). In Fig. 4-10, A, the x-ray tube and detectors are coupled and rotated 360 degrees around the patient to collect transmission measurements using a fan beam of radiation. In Fig. 4-10, B, the x-ray tube rotates 360 degrees around the patient and is positioned

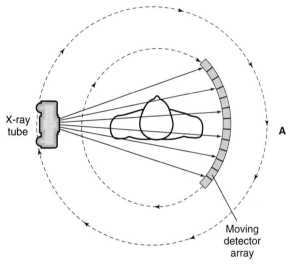

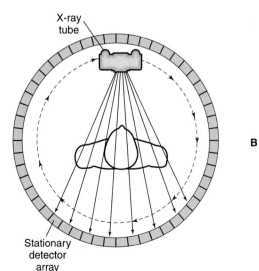

FIG. 4-10. Two data acquisition geometries. **A,** Continuous rotation. **B,** Stationary detectors.

inside a stationary ring of detectors. The radiation beam also describes a fan.

Data Processing

Data processing essentially constitutes the mathematical principles involved in CT. Data processing is a three-step process (Fig. 4-11). First, the raw data undergo some form of preprocessing, in which corrections are made and some reformatting of the data occurs. This is necessary to facilitate the next step in data processing, image reconstruction (Fig. 4-12). In this step, the scan data, which represent attenuation readings, are converted into a digital image characterized by CT numbers.

Conversion of the attenuation readings into a CT image is accomplished by mathematical procedures referred to as *reconstruction techniques* or *reconstruction algorithms*. Reconstruction techniques include simple back-projection, iterative methods, and analytic methods.

The final step in data processing is image storage of the reconstructed digital image. This image is held in a disk memory as short-term storage.

CT Numbers

As shown in Fig. 4-12, each pixel in the reconstructed image is assigned a CT number. CT numbers are related to the linear attenuation coefficients (μ) of the tissues that comprise the slice (Table 4-1) and can be calculated as follows:

$$\text{CT number} = \frac{\mu_t - \mu_w}{\mu_w} \cdot K \qquad (4\text{-}6)$$

where μ_t is the attenuation coefficient of the measured tissue, μ_w is the attenuation coefficient of water, and K is a constant or contrast factor.

The value of K determines the contrast factor, or scaling factor. In the first EMI scanner, the value of K was 500, which resulted in a contrast scale of 0.2% per CT number. The CT numbers obtained with a contrast factor of 500 were referred to as *EMI numbers*. Later, the contrast factor was doubled to give a factor of 1000, and the CT numbers obtained with this factor are referred to as the *Hounsfield (H) scale*. The H scale expresses μ more precisely because the contrast scale is now 0.1% per CT number. (Both the H and EMI scales are shown in Fig. 4-13.) CT numbers are established on a relative basis with the attenuation of water as a reference. Thus the CT number for water is always 0, whereas those for bone and air are $+1000$ and -1000, respectively, on the H scale.

The computer calculates the CT numbers, which can be printed as a numeric image (Fig. 4-14). This image must be converted into a gray-scale image (Fig. 4-15) because it is more useful to the radiologist than a numeric printout. To facilitate this conversion, brightness levels that correspond with the CT numbers must be established (Fig. 4-16). In Fig. 4-16, the upper ($+1000$) and lower (-1000) limits of the scale represent white and black, respectively. All other values represent various shades of gray.

The relationship between the CT numbers and shades of gray is variable and is referred to as *windowing*. Fig. 4-12 depicts the relationship be-

TABLE 4-1

Linear Attenuation Coefficients for Various Body Tissues*

TISSUES	LINEAR ATTENUATION COEFFICIENT (cm^{-1})
Bone	0.528
Blood	0.208
Gray matter	0.212
White matter	0.213
Cerebrospinal fluid	0.207
Water	0.206
Fat	0.185
Air	0.0004

*At 60 keV.

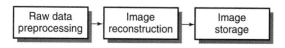

FIG. 4-11. The three data processing steps in CT.

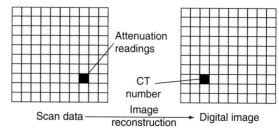

FIG. 4-12. Data acquired by scanning an object measures beam penetration. A digital image is created by converting these data into CT numbers.

tween the tissue voxel from which the linear attenuation data are collected and the image pixel for which a CT number is computed and subjected to windowing.

CT and Energy Dependence

The linear attenuation coefficient (μ) is affected by several factors including the energy of the radiation. For example, the linear attenuation coefficients for water at 60, 84, and 122 keV are 0.206, 0.180, and 0.166, respectively. It then follows that photon energy also affects CT numbers because they can be calculated based on the attenuation coefficients by the equation

$$\ln I_0/I = \int \mu(E,x)\, dx \qquad (4\text{-}7)$$

In this summation equation, E represents the photon energy and demonstrates that the attenuation coefficient changes with the beam energy.

In the original CT scanner, CT numbers were calculated on the basis of 73 keV, which is the effective energy of a 230 kVp beam after passing through 27 cm of water (Zatz, 1981). At 73 keV, the linear attenuation coefficient for water is 0.19 cm^{-1}. For example, if the linear attenuation coefficients for bone and water are 0.38 and 0.19 cm^{-1}, respectively, and the scaling factor (K) of the scanner is 1000, the CT numbers for bone and water can be calculated:

$$
\begin{aligned}
CT_{bone} &= \frac{\mu_{bone} - \mu_{water}}{\mu_{water}} \cdot K \\[6pt]
&= \frac{0.38 - 0.19}{0.19} \cdot 1000 \\[6pt]
&= \frac{0.19}{0.19} \cdot 1000 \\[6pt]
&= 1000
\end{aligned}
$$

Thus the CT number for bone is 1000.

$$
\begin{aligned}
CT_{water} &= \frac{\mu_{water} - \mu_{water}}{\mu_{water}} \cdot K \\[6pt]
&= \frac{0.19 - 0.19}{0.19} \cdot 1000 \\[6pt]
&= \frac{0}{0.19} \cdot 1000 \\[6pt]
&= 0
\end{aligned}
$$

Thus the CT number for water is 0.

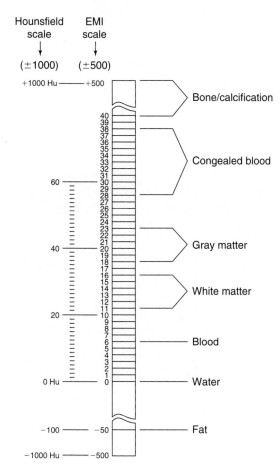

Hounsfield scale ($\pm$1000)   EMI scale ($\pm$500)

+1000 Hu —— +500 — Bone/calcification

—— Congealed blood

—— Gray matter

—— White matter

—— Blood

0 Hu —— 0 —— Water

−100 —— −50 —— Fat

−1000 Hu —— −500

FIG. 4-13. Distribution of CT numbers on the Hounsfield and EMI scales. (From Seeram E: *Computed tomography technology*, Philadelphia, 1982, WB Saunders.)

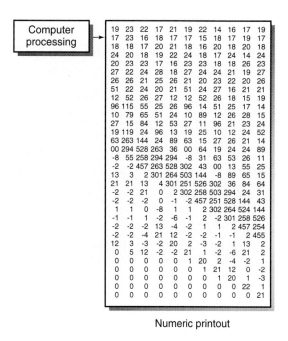

Numeric printout

FIG. 4-14. Appearance of the CT image after computer processing. This is a numeric printout of the processed image.

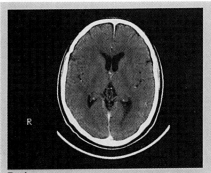

Brain
2-sec scan of 10-mm slice

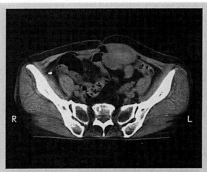

Pelvis
1-sec scan of 10-mm slice

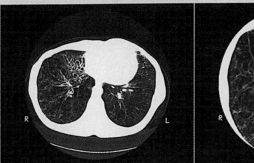

Lung
1-sec scan of 10-mm slice

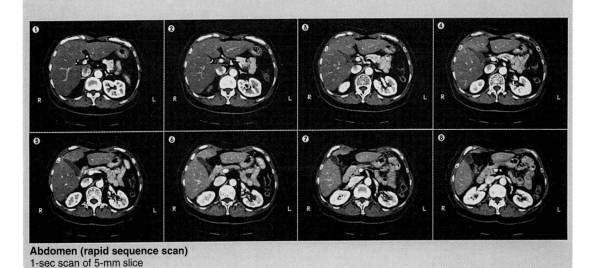

Abdomen (rapid sequence scan)
1-sec scan of 5-mm slice

FIG. 4-15. Gray-scale CT images serve a more useful purpose to the radiologist than a numeric print-out. (Courtesy Toshiba America Medical Systems; Tustin, Calif.)

In CT, a high-kV technique (about 120 kV) is generally used for the following reasons:

1. To reduce the dependency of attenuation coefficients on photon energy
2. To reduce the contrast of bone relative to soft tissues
3. To produce a high radiation flux at the detector

These reasons are important to ensure optimum detector response (e.g., to reduce artifacts caused by changes in skull thickness, which can conceal small changes in attenuation in soft tissues, and to minimize artifacts resulting from beam hardening effects).

CT numbers may vary because of their energy dependence. It is therefore essential that the CT system ensure the accuracy and reliability of these numbers because the consequences can be disastrous and might lead to a misdiagnosis. The system incorporates a number of correction schemes to maintain the precision of the CT numbers.

Image Display

The third and final step in the CT process involves image display, storage, and documentation. After the CT image has been reconstructed, it exits the computer in digital form (see Figs. 4-12 and 4-14). This must be converted to a form that is suitable for viewing and meaningful to the observer (Seeram, 1982).

In CT the digital reconstructed image is converted into a gray scale image (see Fig. 4-15) for interpretation by the radiologist. Because a diagnosis is made from this image, it is important to present this image in a way that facilitates diagnosis.

Display Device. The gray scale image is displayed on a cathode ray tube (CRT), or television monitor, which is an essential component of the control or viewing console (Fig. 4-17). Fig. 4-17 shows two monitors, one for text information and one for images.

In the display and manipulation of gray scale images for diagnosis, it is important to optimize im-

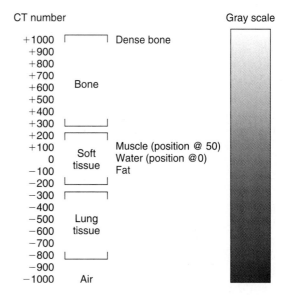

FIG. 4-16. The relationship between CT number and the brightness level.

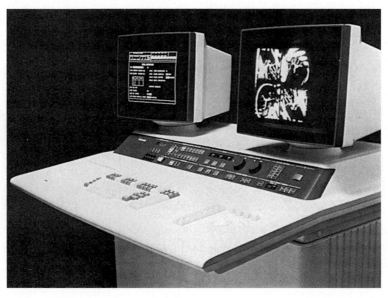

FIG. 4-17. Two gray-scale CRT display monitors positioned on the control console of a CT system. (Courtesy Toshiba America Medical Systems, Tustin, Calif.)

age fidelity (i.e., the faithfulness with which the device can display the image). This is influenced by physical characteristics such as luminance, resolution, noise, and dynamic range.

A gray scale monitor is a funnel-shaped, evacuated glass envelope with an electron gun at the narrow end of the tube. The expanded end of the tube forms a screen, the inner surface of which is coated with a phosphor that emits light when struck by electrons (Seeram, 1985).

In CT the digital image from the computer must be converted into analog signals by the digital-to-analog converter. These signals produce an electron beam that scans the phosphor screen. The gray scale monitor can then display the input digital image, pixel by pixel.

Resolution is an important physical parameter of the gray scale display monitor and is related to the size of the pixel matrix, or matrix size. The display matrix can range from 64×64 to 1024×1024, but high-performance monitors can display an image with a 2048×2048 matrix (Dwyer, et al, 1992).

Windowing. The CT image is composed of a range of CT numbers (e.g., $+1000$ to -1000, for a total of 2000 numbers) that represent varying shades of gray (see Fig. 4-16). The range of numbers is referred to as the *window width* (WW), and the center of the range is the *window level* (WL). Both the WW and WL are located on the control console; in Fig. 4-17, they are the two knobs located just below the image monitor. These controls can alter the image contrast. With a WW of 2000 and a WL of 0, the entire gray scale is displayed and the ability of the observer to perceive small differences in soft tissue attenuation will be lost because the human eye can perceive only about 40 shades of gray (Castleman, 1994).

The process of changing the CT image gray scale in this way is referred to as *windowing* (Fig. 4-18). Fig. 4-18 shows the way in which contrast can be altered to highlight a brain tumor.

Format of the CT Image. The original clinical CT scans were composed of an 80×80 matrix for a total of 6400 pixels.

The size of the matrix is chosen by the technologist before the CT examination and depends on the anatomy under study. The technologist must select the field of view (FOV) or reconstruction circle, which is a circular region from which the transmission measurements are recorded during scanning. This region is specifically referred to as the *scan FOV*.

During data collection and image reconstruction, a matrix is placed over the scan FOV to cover the slice to be imaged. In general, a technologist can select the FOV appropriate to the examination within three to four scan FOVs.

Because the slice to be scanned has the dimension of depth, the pixel is transformed into a voxel, or volume element. The radiation beam passes through each voxel and a CT number is then generated for each pixel in the displayed image. The display FOV can be equal to or less than the scan FOV.

The pixel size can be computed from the FOV and the matrix size through the following relationship:

$$\text{Pixel size, } d = \text{field of view/matrix size}$$

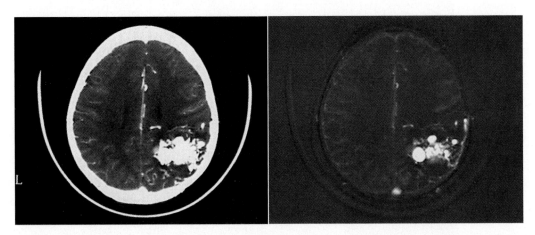

FIG. 4-18. Effect of windowing. The contrast of bone and soft tissue in the image on the left is changed to that shown on the image on the right. The tumor is highlighted on the image on the right, with a loss of image contrast for bone and soft tissue. (Courtesy Toshiba America Medical Systems; Tustin, Calif.)

For example, if the reconstruction circle (FOV) is 25 cm and the matrix size is 512^2, the pixel size can be determined as follows:

$$\text{Pixel size} = 25 \cdot 10 \text{ mm} / 512$$
$$= 250 \text{ mm} / 512$$
$$= 0.488 \text{ mm}$$
$$= 0.49 \text{ mm}$$
$$= 0.5 \text{ mm}$$

The pixel size generally ranges from 1 to 10 mm on most scanners. Thus voxel size depends not only on the thickness of the slice but also on the matrix size and the field of view (Fig. 4-19).

Finally, each pixel in the CT image can have a range of gray shades. The image can have 256 (2^8), 512 (2^9), 1024 (2^{10}), or 2048 (2^{11}) different gray scale values. Because these numbers are represented as bits, a CT image can be characterized by the number of bits per pixel. CT images can have 8, 9, 10, 11, or 12 bits per pixel. The image therefore consists of a series of bit planes referred to the *bit depth* (Fig. 4-20) (Seibert, 1995). The numeric value of the pixel represents the brightness of the image at that pixel position. A 12-bits-per-pixel CT image would represent numbers ranging from −1000 to 3095 for a total of 4096 (2^{12}) different shades of gray (Barnes and Lakshminarayanan, 1989).

TECHNOLOGIC CONSIDERATIONS

The ultimate goal of a CT scanner is to produce high-quality CT images with minimal radiation dose and physical discomfort to the patient. Whether this is achieved depends on the design of the CT system, which influences the performance of the system's components. In this section, *design* refers to the technology necessary to produce a CT image.

The technology of a CT scanner encompasses a number of subsystems (Fig. 4-21). The major subsystems are described briefly to demonstrate the flow of data through the system.

Data Flow in a CT Scanner

The subsystems shown in Fig. 4-21 include the x-ray tube, power supply, and cooling system; beam geometry, defined by collimators and characterized by tube scanning motion; detectors, detector electronics, preprocessors, host computer with fast-access memory, high-speed array processor, image processor, storage, display, and system control.

The flow of data from Fig. 4-21 is summarized in Fig. 4-22. The language that describes some of the events (e.g., *convolution* and *back-projection*) will be explained further in subsequent chapters.

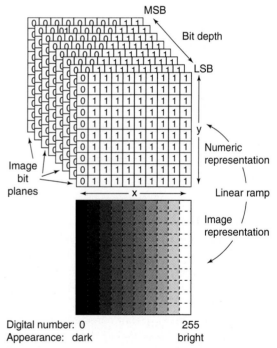

FIG. 4-20. Representation of the digital image as a stack of bit planes. Encoding of the least significant bit (LSB) to the most significant bit (MSB) as bit planes is shown. The corresponding gray-scale image indicates digital value and brightness relationships. (From Seibert JA: Digital image processing basics. In Balter S, Shope TB, eds: *RSNA categorical course in physics. Physical and technical aspects of angiography and interventional radiology,* Oak Brook, Ill, 1995, RSNA.)

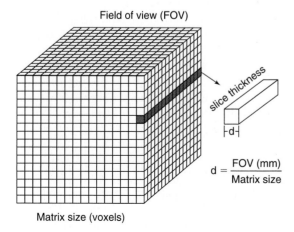

$$d = \frac{\text{FOV (mm)}}{\text{Matrix size}}$$

FIG. 4-19. Voxel size depends on slice thickness, matrix size, and field of view.

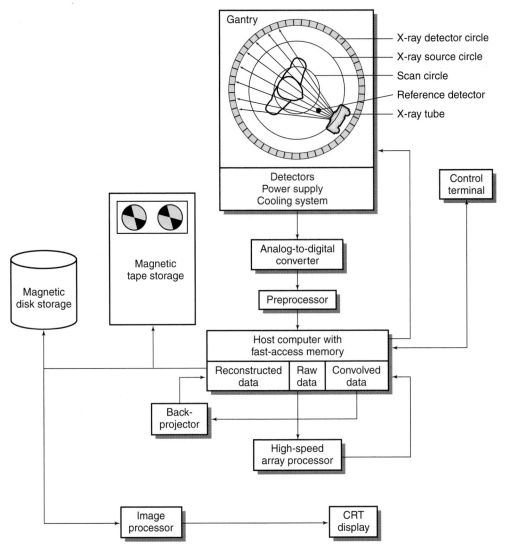

FIG. 4-21. Fourth-generation CT scanner configuration with major subsystems.

Sequence of Events

The events represented in the data flow are as follows:

1. The x-ray tube (and detectors) rotate around the patient, who is positioned in the gantry aperture for the CT examination. This step is characterized by the beam geometry and method of scanning and involves the passage of x-rays through the patient. The x-ray beam is highly collimated by prepatient collimators.

2. The radiation is attenuated as it passes through the patient. The transmitted photons are measured by two sets of detectors, a reference detector, which measures the intensity of radiation from the x-ray tube, and another set that records x-ray transmission through the patient.

3. The transmitted beam and reference beam are both converted into electrical current signals that are amplified by special circuits. This is followed by logarithmic amplification, in which the relative transmission readings (I_0/I) are changed into attenuation (μ) and thickness (x) data through the use of Equation 4-2:

$$\mu = \frac{1}{x} \ln I_0 / I$$

4. Before the data are sent to the computer, they must be converted into digital form. This is done by the analog-to-digital converters (ADCs), or *digitizers*. Steps 2, 3, and 4 constitute the second step in the data acquisition process.

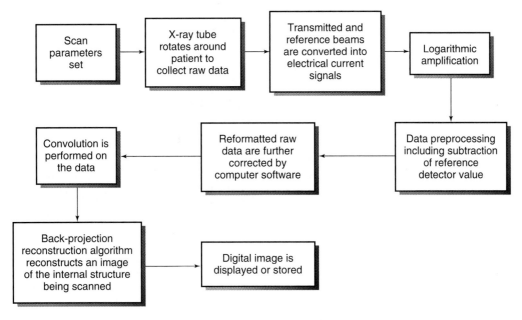

FIG. 4-22. Data flow in a CT system.

5. Data processing begins. The digital data undergo some form of preprocessing, which includes corrections and reformatting. "Some of the corrections to the data will include subtraction of the air reference detector signal to normalize the attenuation data, obtaining local averages of detectors to determine if any detectors are outside a predetermined standard deviation which help locate bad detectors, and corrections due to dead time losses (i.e., detection response time losses) by the individual detectors." (Huang, 1987). The data are now referred to as *reformatted raw data*. Additional data corrections are performed on the data using computer software.

6. As shown in Fig. 4-22, convolution is performed on the data by the array processors.

7. The back-projection reconstruction algorithm then reconstructs an image of the internal anatomic structures under examination.

8. The reconstructed image can then be displayed, recorded on film with a laser camera, or stored on magnetic or optical tape or disks.

9. The image processor shown in Fig. 4-21 allows the performance of various image processing operations on the displayed image. Fig. 4-21 does not show the digital-to-analog converter (DAC), a component positioned between the image processor and CRT display or between the host computer and control terminal, which has a CRT display unit.

10. The control terminal is usually an operator's control console, which completely controls the CT system.

ADVANTAGES AND LIMITATIONS OF CT

Advantages

The main advantages of CT stem from the fact that the technique overcomes the limitations of radiography and conventional tomography. Compared with radiography and conventional tomography, CT offers the following advantages:

1. Excellent low-contrast resolution is possible because (1) a highly collimated beam is used to take an image of a cross-sectional slice of the patient and (2) special detectors are used to measure the radiation transmitted through the slice.

2. By changing the WW and WL settings in image windowing, the contrast scale of the image can be varied to suit the needs of the observer.

3. With spiral data acquisition, CT scanning in spiral geometry has overcome several limitations of conventional start-stop acquisition. Its advantages include volume data acquisition in a single breath rather

than slice-by-slice acquisition, improvements in 3D imaging, multiplanar image reformatting, and other applications, such as continuous imaging, CT angiography, and virtual reality imaging, or CT endoscopy.

4. CT has made available a variety of techniques intended to facilitate the diagnostic process such as xenon CT (the use of inhaled, stable xenon to study blood flow), quantitative CT (determination of bone mineral content), dynamic CT (rapid-sequence CT scanning to study physiology), perfusion CT, and high spatial resolution CT scanning to optimize the spatial resolution. In addition, CT can assist in radiation treatment planning.

5. With regard to image manipulation and analysis, the digital nature of the CT image makes it a candidate for digital image processing. Through the application of certain image processing algorithms, the image can be modified to enhance its information content or analyzed to obtain information about the shape and texture of lesions.

Limitations

CT is not without its limitations. Compared with radiography and tomography, the following disadvantages can be noted:

1. The spatial resolution of CT is "notably poorer" (Hendee and Ritenour, 1992).
2. The dose in CT is generally higher for similar anatomic regions.
3. CT is limited to transverse axial slices because of the hardware of the scanner, although the gantry can be angled to take images of slices up to 30 degrees to the transverse section.
4. In CT, it is difficult to image anatomic regions in which soft tissues are surrounded by large amounts of bone, such as the posterior fossa, spinal cord, pituitary and the interpetrous space (Oldendorf and Oldendorf, 1991).
5. The presence of metallic objects on the patient produces streak artifacts on CT images. CT also creates other artifacts not common to radiography.

By no means have these limitations hindered the development of CT or restricted its use. In fact, they have opened avenues for problem solving and research. At present, CT continues to be a useful diagnostic tool in medicine, and studies are under way to improve the performance of CT scanners.

REFERENCES

Barnes GT, Lakshminarayanan AV: Computed tomography: physical principles and image quality considerations. In Lee JT et al, eds: *Computed tomography with MRI correlation*, ed 2, New York, 1989, Raven Press.

Bocage EM: Patent No. 536, 464, Paris. Quoted in Massiot J: History of tomography, *Medicamundi* 19:106-115, 1974.

Castleman KR: *Digital image processing*, ed 2, Englewood Cliffs, NJ, 1994, Prentice-Hall.

Curry TS III, Dowdey JE, Murry RC Jr: *Christensen's physics of diagnostic radiology*, ed 4, Philadelphia, 1990, Lea & Febiger.

Dwyer SJ et al: Performance characteristics and image fidelity of gray-scale monitors, *Radiographics* 12:765-772, 1992.

Hendee WR, Ritenour ER: *Medical imaging physics*, ed 3, St Louis, 1992, Mosby.

Hounsfield GH: Computerized transverse axial scanning (tomography). I. Description of the system, *Br J Radiol* 46:1016-1022, 1973.

Huang HK: *Elements of digital radiology*, Englewood Cliffs, NJ, 1987, Prentice-Hall.

Marshall CH: Principles of computed tomography, *Postgrad Med* 59:105-109, 1976.

Morgan CL: *Basic principles of computed tomography*, Baltimore, 1983, University Park Press.

Oldendorf W, Oldendorf W Jr: *MRI primer*, New York, 1991, Raven Press.

Seeram E: *Computed tomography technology*, Philadelphia, 1982, WB Saunders.

Seeram E: *X-ray equipment. An introduction*, Springfield, Ill, 1985, Charles C Thomas.

Seibert JA: Digital image processing basics. In Balter S, Shope TB, eds: *RSNA categorical course in physics. Physical and technical aspects of angiography and interventional radiology*, Oak Brook, Ill, 1995, RSNA.

Sprawls P: *Physical principles of medical imaging*, ed 2, Rockville, Md, 1995, Aspen.

Ter-Pogossian MM et al: The extraction of the yet unused wealth of information in diagnostic radiology, *Radiology* 113:515-520, 1974.

Vallebona A: Radiography with great enlargement (microradiography) and a technical method for radiographic dissociation of the shadow, *Radiology* 17:340-341, 1931.

Zatz LM: Basic principles of computed tomography scanning. In Newton TH, Potts DG, eds: *Radiology of the skull and brain*, St Louis, 1981, Mosby.

5

Data Acquisition Concepts

BASIC SCHEME FOR DATA ACQUISITION

In CT, transmission measurements, or projection data, are systematically collected from the patient. Several schemes are available for such data collection, each based on a specific "geometrical pattern of scanning" (Villafana, 1987).

Data acquisition refers to the method by which the patient is scanned to obtain enough data for image reconstruction. *Scanning* is defined by the beam geometry, which characterizes the particular CT system and also plays a central role in spatial resolution and artifact production.

Two elements in a basic scheme for data acquisition (Fig. 5-1) are the beam geometry and the components comprising the scheme. *Beam geometry* refers to the size, shape, and motion of the beam and its path, and *components* refer to those physical devices that shape and define the beam, measure its transmission through the patient, and convert this information into digital data for input into the computer.

The following points should be noted from Fig. 5-1:

1. The x-ray tube and detector are in perfect alignment.
2. The tube and detector scan the patient to collect a large number of transmission measurements.
3. The beam is shaped by a special filter as it leaves the tube.
4. The beam is collimated to pass through only the slice of interest.
5. The beam is attenuated by the patient and the transmitted photons are then measured by the detector.
6. The detector converts the x-ray photons into an electrical signal (analog data).
7. These signals are converted by the analog-to-digital converter (ADC) into digital data.
8. The digital data are sent to the computer for image reconstruction.

Terminology

Consider the first data acquisition scheme used by Hounsfield and others early in the development of CT (Fig. 5-2). The x-ray tube and detector move across the object or patient in a straight line, or translate, to collect several transmission measurements. After the first translation, the tube and detector rotate by 1 degree to collect more measure-

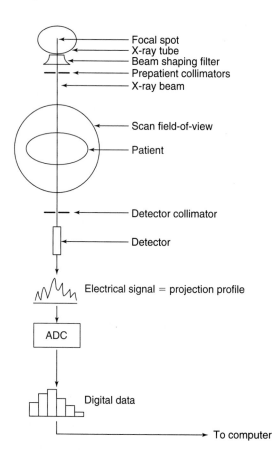

FIG. 5-1. Basic data acquisition scheme in CT.

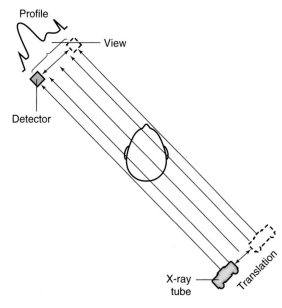

FIG. 5-2. In CT, a *ray* is the part of the x-ray beam that falls onto one detector. A *view* is a collection of these rays for one translation across the object. The view generates what is called a *profile*.

ments. This sequence is repeated until data are collected for at least 180 degrees for one slice of the anatomy. Scanning also includes the movement of the patient through the gantry to scan the next slice. This sequence is repeated until all slices have been scanned.

The x-ray beam that emanates from the tube consists of several rays. In CT, a *ray* is the part of the beam that falls on one detector. In Fig. 5-2, the line from the x-ray tube to the detector is considered a single ray, and a collection of these rays for one translation across the object constitutes a *view*.

Projection data are collected by the detector because each ray is attenuated by the patient and subsequently transmitted and projected on the detector. The detector in turn generates an electrical signal, which represents a signature of the attenuation as the ray moves across the slice. This signal represents a profile. Whereas a view generates a profile, a ray generates only a small part of the profile. In addition, each transmission measurement is referred to as a *data sample*.

The production of a CT image of one slice of the anatomy requires a large set of data samples taken at different locations to satisfy the image reconstruction process. The total number of data samples (DS_{total}) per scan is given by the following expression:

DS_{total} = number of detectors · number of data samples per detector $\qquad$ (5-1)

or

DS_{total} = number of data samples per view · number of views $\qquad$ (5-2)

DATA ACQUISITION GEOMETRIES

Three primary types of acquisition geometries are parallel beam geometry, fan beam geometry, and CT scanning in spiral geometry, which is the most recently developed geometry. As a result, a simple categorization of CT equipment has evolved based on the scanning geometry, scanning motion, and number of detectors, as follows (Fig. 5-3):

1. First-generation scanners were based on the parallel beam geometry and translate-rotate scanning motion.
2. Second-generation scanners were based on the fan beam geometry and translate-rotate motion.
3. Third-generation scanners were based on fan beam geometry and complete rotation of the tube and detectors.
4. Fourth-generation scanners were based on fan beam geometry and complete rotation

of the x-ray tube around a stationary ring of detectors.

5. Fifth-generation scanners were developed primarily for high-speed CT scanning. These scanners are based on special configurations intended to facilitate very fast scanning.

First-Generation Scanners

Parallel beam geometry was first used by Hounsfield. The first EMI brain scanner and other earlier scanners were based on this concept.

Parallel beam geometry is defined by a set of parallel rays that generates a projection profile (see Fig. 5-2). The data acquisition process is based on a translate-rotate principle in which a single, highly collimated x-ray beam and one or two detectors first translate across the patient to collect transmission readings. After one translation, the tube and detector rotate by 1 degree and translate again to collect readings from a different direction. This is repeated for 180 degrees around the patient. This method of scanning is referred to as *rectilinear pencil beam scanning*.

First-generation CT scanners took at least 4.5 to 5.5 minutes to produce a complete scan of the patient, which restricted patient throughput. The

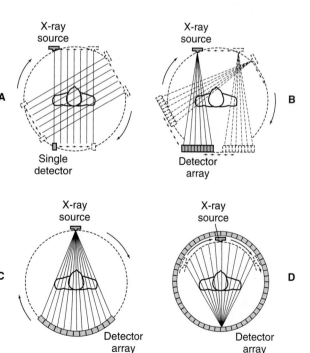

FIG. 5-3. The geometries of the first four generations of CT scanners. **A,** First generation, parallel beam, translate and rotate. **B,** Second generation, fan beam, translate, and rotate. **C,** Third generation, fan beam, rotate only. **D,** Fourth generation, fan beam, stationary circular detector.

image reconstruction algorithm for first-generation CT scanners was based on the parallel beam geometry of the image reconstruction space (a square or circle in which the slice to be reconstructed must be positioned).

Second-Generation Scanners

Second-generation scanners were based on the translate-rotate principle of first-generation scanners with a few fundamental differences such as a linear detector array (about 30 detectors) coupled to the x-ray tube and multiple pencil beams. The result is a beam geometry that describes a small fan whose apex originates at the x-ray tube. This is the fan beam geometry shown in Fig. 5-3, *B, C,* and *D.*

Also, the rays are divergent instead of parallel, resulting in a significant change in the image reconstruction algorithm, which must be capable of handling projection data from the fan beam geometry.

In second-generation scanners, the fan beam translates across the patient to collect a set of transmission readings. After one translation, the tube and detector array rotate by larger increments (compared with first-generation scanners) and translate again. This process is repeated for 180 degrees and is referred to as *rectilinear multiple pencil beam scanning.* The x-ray tube traces a semicircular path during scanning.

The larger rotational increments and increased number of detectors result in shorter scan times that range from 20 seconds to 3.5 minutes. In general, the time decrease is inversely proportional to the number of detectors. The more detectors, the shorter the total scan time.

Third-Generation Scanners

Third-generation CT scanners were based on a fan beam geometry that rotates continuously around the patient for 360 degrees (see Fig. 5-3). The x-ray tube is coupled to a curved detector array that subtends an arc of 30 to 40 degrees or greater from the apex of the fan. As the x-ray tube and detectors rotate, projection profiles are collected and a view is obtained for every fixed point of the tube and detector. This motion is referred to as *continuously rotating fan beam scanning.* The path traced by the tube describes a circle rather than the semicircle characteristic of first-generation and second-generation CT scanners. Third-generation CT scanners collect data faster than the previous units

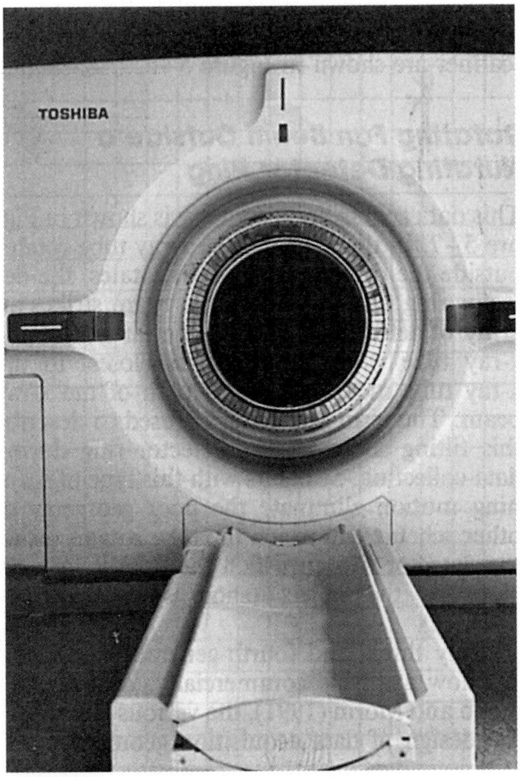

FIG. 5-4. Stationary circular detector array. (Courtesy Toshiba America Medical Systems, Tustin, Calif.)

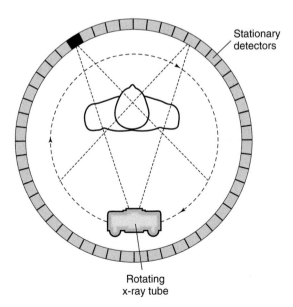

FIG. 5-5. In a fourth-generation scanner, each detector position gives rise to a fan.

(generally within a few seconds). This scan time increases patient throughput and limits the production of artifacts caused by respiratory motion.

Fourth-Generation Scanners

Essentially, fourth-generation CT scanners feature two types of beam geometries: a rotating fan beam within a stationary ring of detectors, and a nutating fan beam in which the apex of the fan (x-ray tube) is located outside a nutating ring of detectors.

Rotating Fan Beam Within a Circular Detector Array

The main data acquisition features of a fourth-generation CT scanner are as follows:

1. The x-ray tube is positioned within a stationary, circular detector array (Fig. 5-4).
2. The beam geometry describes a wide fan.
3. The apex of the fan now originates at each detector (Fig. 5-5). Fig. 5-5 shows two fans that describe two sets of views.
4. As the tube moves from point to point within the circle, single rays strike a detector. These rays are produced sequentially during the point's circular travel.

5. Scan times are very short and vary from scanner to scanner, depending on the manufacturer.
6. The x-ray tube traces a circular path.
7. The image reconstruction algorithm is for a fan beam geometry in which the apex of the fan is now at the detector, as opposed to the x-ray tube in the third-generation systems.

Rotating Fan Beam Outside a Nutating Detector Ring

In this scheme, the x-ray tube rotates outside the detector ring (Fig. 5-6). As it rotates, the detector ring tilts so that the fan beam strikes an array of detectors located at the far side of the x-ray tube while the detectors closest to the x-ray tube move out of the path of the x-ray beam. The term *nutating* describes the tilting action of the detector ring during data collection. Scanners with this type of scanning motion eliminate the poor geometry of other schemes, in which the tube rotates inside its detector ring, near the object. However, nutate-rotate systems are not currently manufactured.

CT Scanning in Spiral-Helical Geometry

Scanning in spiral-helical geometry is the most recent development in CT data acquisition. The need for faster scan times and improvements in 3D and multiplanar reconstruction have encouraged the development of continuous rotation scanners, or volume scanners, in which the data is collected in volumes rather than individual slices. CT scanning in spiral/helical geometry is based on slip-ring technology, which shortens the high-tension cables to the x-ray tube to allow continuous rotation of the gantry. The path traced by the x-ray tube, or fan beam, during the scanning process describes a spiral (Fig. 5-7) or helix. The terms *spiral geometry*

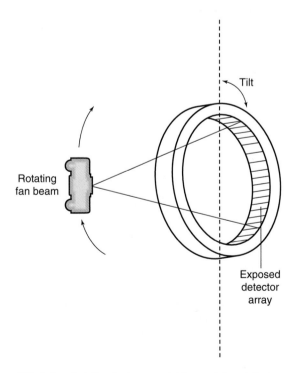

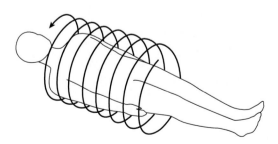

FIG. 5-6. Rotating fan beam outside a nutating detector ring. *Nutating* refers to how the detector ring tilts to expose an array of detectors to the x-ray beam. Nutate-rotate systems are no longer manufactured.

FIG. 5-7. The path traced by the x-ray tube in CT scanning describes a spiral or helix. These terms are used interchangeably.

(Siemens) and *helical geometry* (Toshiba) are commonly and synonymously used to describe the data acquisition geometry of continuous rotation scanners. This geometry is obtained during the scanning process. As the tube rotates, the patient is transported through the gantry aperture for a single breath hold. Because this results in a volume of the patient being scanned, the term *volume CT* is also used.

Fifth-Generation Scanners

Fifth-generation scanners are classified as high-speed CT scanners because they can acquire scan data in milliseconds. Two such scanners are the electron beam CT scanner (EBCT) (Fig. 5-8) and the dynamic spatial reconstructor scanner. In the electron beam CT scanner, the data acquisition geometry is a fan beam of x-rays produced by a

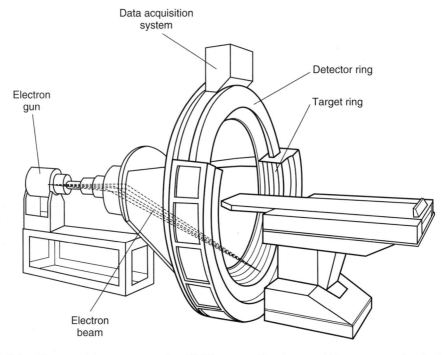

FIG. 5-8. The essential components of an EBCT scanner. The data acquisition geometry is a fan beam of x-rays produced by the electron beam striking the tungsten targets.

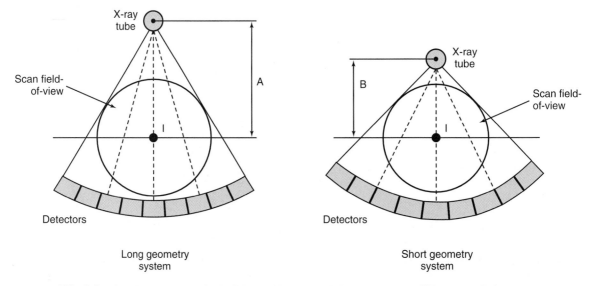

FIG. 5-9. Imaging the same field-of-view with long and short geometry CT systems. **I,** Isocenter; **A,** source-to-isocenter distance; **B,** source-to-isocenter distance; $\left(\frac{A}{B}\right)^2$, x-ray efficiency improvement.

beam of electrons that scans several stationary tungsten target rings. The fan beam passes through the patient and the x-ray transmission readings are collected for image reconstruction. The dynamic spatial reconstructor (DSR) is a highly specialized fifth-generation, high-speed scanner capable of producing dynamic three-dimensional (3D) images of volumes of the patient.

Long and Short Geometry Systems

Several factors influence the external dimensions of the CT gantry, including the source-to-isocenter distance, source-to-detector distance, scan field-of-view, and fan angle. These factors also help define long and short geometries for CT systems (Fig. 5-9). Each geometry has its advantages and disadvantages.

In the short geometry system, the distance between the x-ray tube and the patient at the isocenter is shorter than in the long geometry system. This arrangement results in improved x-ray efficiency, and more photons are available for image production. For example, the increase from a 40-degree fan angle in a long geometry system to a 50-degree fan angle for a short geometry system will result in the arrival of 25% more photons at each detector. Subsequently, image noise is reduced by about 12% per milliamperes (mA) (Arenson, 1995).

However, the concentration of photons per unit area increases for short geometry systems and therefore patient dose increases. Additionally, image blur increases for short geometry systems.

Long geometry systems are necessary to improve image blur and decrease radiation dose. As a result, the external dimensions of the gantry must be increased.

SLIP-RING TECHNOLOGY

Spiral-helical CT is made possible through the use of slip-ring technology, which allows for continuous gantry rotation. Slip rings (Fig. 5-10) are "electromechanical devices consisting of circular electrical conductive rings and brushes that transmit electrical energy across a rotating interface" (Brunnett et al, 1990). Today, most CT scanners incorporate slip-ring design and are referred to as *continuous rotation*, *volume CT*, or *slip-ring* scanners. Slip-ring technology has been applied previously in CT. For example, the Varian V-360-3 CT scanner was based on slip-ring design to achieve continuous rotation of the gantry. Such rotation

results in very fast data collection, which is mandatory for procedures such as dynamic CT scanning and CT angiography.

Design and Power Supply

Two slip-ring designs are the disk (Fig. 5-11) and cylinder. In the disk design, the conductive rings form concentric circles in the plane of rotation.

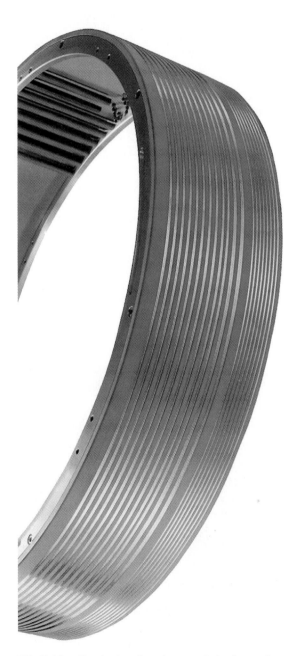

FIG. 5-10. Conductive rings (*upper strips*) of one slip-ring system. Each strip carries voltage to components such as the generator, x-ray tube, and collimators. (Courtesy Elscint; Hackensack, NJ.)

The cylindric design includes conductive rings positioned along the axis of rotation to form a cylinder (see Fig. 5-10). The brushes that transmit electrical power to the CT components glide in contact grooves on the stationary slip ring (Fig. 5-12).

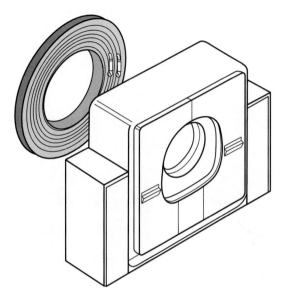

FIG. 5-11. Slip ring based on the disk design concept. The rings are positioned as concentric circles within the plane of rotation. This is a characteristic design of the Siemens Somatom Plus CT scanner.

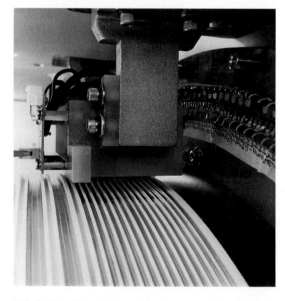

FIG. 5-12. Slip ring based on the cylindric design characteristic of the Picker PQ-2000 CT scanner. The brushes glide in contact grooves on the stationary slip ring. (Courtesy Picker International; Cleveland, Ohio.)

Two common brush designs are the wire brush and composite brush. The wire brush uses conductive wire as a sliding contact. "A brush consists of one or more wires arranged such that they function as a cantilever spring with a free end against the conductive ring. Two brushes per ring are often used to increase either communication reliability or current carrying capacity" (Brunnett et al, 1990). The composite brush uses a block of some conductive material (e.g., a silver-graphite alloy) as a sliding contact. "A variety of different spring designs are commonly used to maintain contact between the brush and ring including cantilever, compression, or constant force. Again two brushes per ring are frequently used" (Brunnett et al, 1990).

Slip-ring scanners provide continuous rotation of the gantry through the elimination of the long high-tension cables to the x-ray tube used in conventional start-stop scanners, which must be unwound after a complete rotation. In conventional scanners, these cables originate from the high-voltage generator, usually located in the x-ray room. The high-voltage generators of slip-ring scanners are located in the gantry. Scanners with either low-voltage or high-voltage slip rings are available based on the power supply to the slip ring (Fig. 5-13).

Low-Voltage Slip Ring. In a low-voltage slip-ring system, 480 AC power and x-ray control signals are transmitted to slip rings by means of low-voltage brushes that glide in contact grooves on the stationary slip ring. The slip ring then provides power to the high-voltage transformer, which subsequently transmits high voltage to the x-ray tube

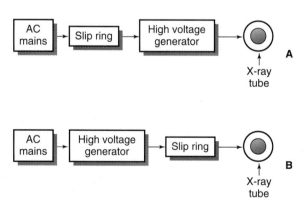

FIG. 5-13. Basic differences between low-voltage (**A**) and high-voltage (**B**) slip-ring CT scanners in terms of high-voltage power to the x-ray tube.

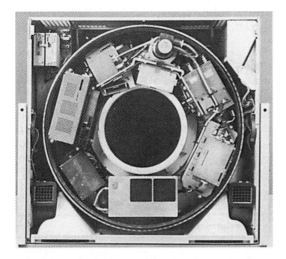

FIG. 5-14. Low-voltage slip-ring scanner showing an open gantry. In this scanner, the x-ray tube, high-voltage generator, and other controls are mounted on the orbital scan frame. The x-ray tube and generator can now rotate continuously because of the elimination of the long high-voltage cable. A short cable connects the x-ray tube and generator. (Courtesy Picker International; Cleveland, Ohio.)

(Fig. 5-13, *A*). In this case, the x-ray generator, x-ray tube, and other controls are positioned on the orbital scan frame (Fig. 5-14).

High-Voltage Slip Ring. In a high-voltage slip-ring system (Fig. 5-13, *B*), the AC delivers power to the high-voltage generator, which subsequently supplies high voltage to the slip ring. The high voltage from the slip ring is transferred to the x-ray tube. In this case, the high-voltage generator does not rotate with the x-ray tube.

Advantages

The major advantage of slip-ring technology is that it facilitates continuous rotation of the x-ray tube so that volume data can be acquired quickly from the patient. As the tube rotates continuously, the patient is translated continuously through the gantry aperture. This results in CT scanning in spiral geometry. Other advantages are as follows:

1. Faster scan times and minimal interscan delays
2. Capacity for continuous acquisition protocols in the future
3. Elimination of the start-stop process characteristic of conventional CT scanners
4. Removal of the cable wrap-around process

X-RAY SYSTEM

In his initial experiments, Hounsfield used low-energy, monochromatic gamma ray radiation. He later conducted experiments with an x-ray tube because of several limitations imposed by the monochromatic radiation source, such as the low radiation intensity rate, large source size, low source strength, and high cost. Subsequently, CT scanners were manufactured to function with x-ray tubes to provide the high radiation intensities necessary for clinical, high-contrast CT scanning. However, the heterogeneous beam was problematic because it did not obey the Lambert-Beer exponential law (see Equation 4-1).

The components of the x-ray system include the x-ray generator, x-ray tube, x-ray beam filter, and collimators (see Fig. 5-1).

X-Ray Generator

CT scanners use three-phase power for the efficient production of x-rays. In the past, generators for CT scanners were based on the 60-Hertz (Hz) voltage frequency and the high-voltage generator was a bulky piece of equipment located in a corner of the x-ray room. A long, high-tension cable ran from the generator to the x-ray tube in the gantry.

CT scanners now use high-frequency generators, which are small, compact, and more efficient than conventional generators. These generators are located inside the CT gantry. In some scanners, the high-frequency generator is mounted on the rotating frame with the x-ray tube (Fig. 5-14); in others it is located in a corner of the gantry and does not rotate with the tube.

In a high-frequency generator (Fig. 5-15), the circuit is usually referred to as a *high-frequency inverter circuit*. The low-voltage, low-frequency current (60 Hz) from the main power supply is converted to high-voltage, high-frequency current (500 to 25,000 Hz) as it passes through the components, as shown in Fig. 5-15. Each component changes the low-voltage, low-frequency alternating current (AC) waveform to supply the x-ray tube with high-voltage, high-frequency direct current (DC) of almost constant potential. After high-voltage rectification and smoothing, the voltage ripple from a high-frequency generator is less than 1%, compared with 4% from a three-phase, 12-pulse generator. This makes the high-frequency generator more efficient at x-ray production than its predecessor. The x-ray exposure technique obtained from these generators depends on the generator power output. Current CT generators have maximum power ratings of about 50 kilowatts (kW) that allow kVp settings in the range of 80 to 140kVp and tube currents in the range of 100 to 400 mA.

X-Ray Tubes

The radiation source requirement in CT depends on two factors: (1) radiation attenuation, which is a function of radiation beam energy, the atomic number and density of the absorber, and the thickness of the object; and (2) the quantity of radiation

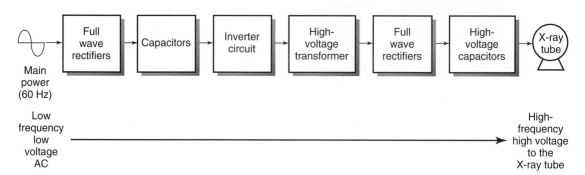

FIG. 5-15.   The basic components of a high-frequency generator used in modern CT scanners.

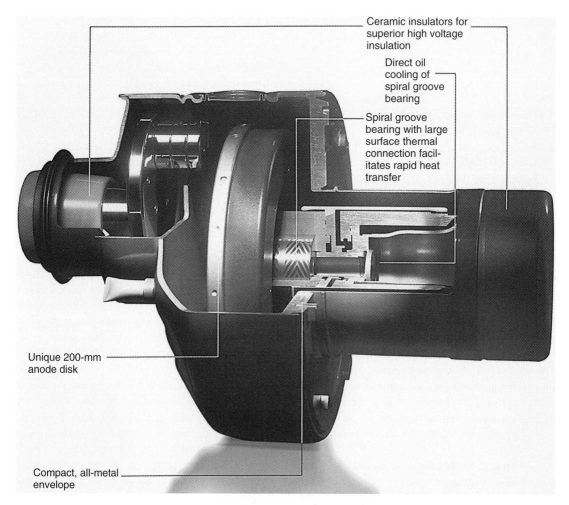

FIG. 5-16.   A modern rotating anode x-ray tube used in CT scanners. (Courtesy Philips Medical Systems; Shelton, Conn.)

required for transmission. X-ray tubes satisfy this requirement.

First-and second-generation scanners used fixed-anode, oil-cooled x-ray tubes, but rotating anode x-ray tubes have become common in CT because of the demand for increased output (Fig. 5-16). These rotating anode tubes produce a heterogeneous beam of radiation from a large-diameter anode disk with focal spot sizes to facilitate the spatial resolution requirements of the scanner. The disk is usually made of a rhenium, tungsten, and molybdenum (RTM) alloy and other materials with a small target angle (usually 12 degrees) and a rotation speed of 3600 rpm to 10,000 rpm (high-speed rotation).

The introduction of spiral-helical CT with continuous rotation scanners has placed new demands on x-ray tubes. Because the tube rotates continually for a longer period compared with conventional scanners, the tube must be able to sustain higher power levels. Several technical advances in component design have been made to achieve these power levels and deal with the problems of heat generation, heat storage, and heat dissipation. For example, the tube envelope, cathode assembly, anode assembly including anode rotation, and target design have been redesigned (Fox, 1995; Homberg and Koppel, 1997).

The glass envelope ensures a vacuum, provides structural support of anode and cathode structures, and provides high-voltage insulation between the anode and cathode. Internal getters (ion pumps) remove air molecules to ensure a vacuum. Although the borosilicate glass provides good thermal and electrical insulation, electrical arcing results from tungsten deposits on the glass caused by vaporization. Tubes with metal envelopes are now common and solve this problem. Ceramic insulators (Fig. 5-16) isolate the metal envelope from the anode and cathode voltage. Metal envelope tubes have larger anode disks; for example, the tube shown in Fig. 5-16 has a disk with a 200-mm diameter, compared with the 120 to 160 mm diameter typical of conventional tubes. This feature allows the technologist to use higher tube currents. Heat storage capacity is also increased with an improvement in heat dissipation rates.

The cathode assembly consists of one or more tungsten filaments positioned in a focussing cup. The getter is usually made of barium to ensure a vacuum by the absorption of air molecules released from the target during operation.

The anode assembly consists of the disk, rotor stud and hub, rotor, and bearing assembly. The large anode disk is thicker than conventional

disks; the three basic designs are the conventional all-metal disk (Fig. 5-17), brazed graphite disk, and chemical vapor deposition (CVD) graphite disk. In conventional tubes, the all-metal disk (Fig. 5-17, A) consists of a base body made of titanium, zirconium, and molybdenum with a focal track layer of 10% rhenium and 90% tungsten. It can transfer heat from the focal track very quickly. Unfortunately, tubes with this all-metal design cannot meet the needs of spiral/helical CT imaging because of their weight.

The brazed graphite anode disk (Fig. 5-17, B) consists of a tungsten-rhenium focal track brazed to a graphite base body. Graphite increases the heat storage capacity because of its high thermal capacity, which is about 10 times that of tungsten. As noted by Fox (1995), the material used in the

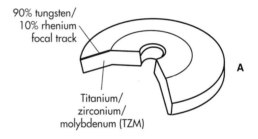

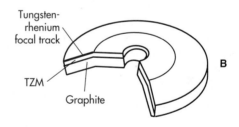

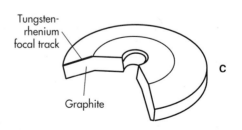

FIG. 5-17. Three types of disk designs for modern x-ray tubes used in CT scanners: **A,** conventional all-metal disk; **B,** brazed graphite anode disk; and **C,** CVD graphite anode disk.

brazing process influences the operating tempera-ture of the tube, and the higher temperatures result in higher heat storage capacities and faster cooling of the anode. Tubes for spiral/helical CT scanning are based mostly on this type of design.

The final type of anode design (Fig. 5-17, C) is also intended for use in spiral/helical CT x-ray tubes. The disk consists of a graphite base body with a tungsten-rhenium layer deposited on the focal track by a chemical vapor process. This de-sign can accommodate large, lightweight disks with large heat storage capacity and fast cooling rates (Fox, 1995).

The purpose of the bearing assembly is to pro-vide and ensure smooth rotation of the anode disk. In CT, high-speed anode rotation allows the use of higher loadability. Rotation speeds of 10,000 rpm are possible with increased frequency to the stator windings. Smooth rotation of the disk is possible because of the ball bearings lubricated with silver; however, because ball-bearing technology results in mechanical problems and limits x-ray tube per-formance, a liquid-bearing method to improve an-ode disk rotation was introduced (Fig. 5-18).

The stationary shaft of the anode assembly consists of grooves that contain gallium-based liq-uid metal alloy. During anode rotation, the liquid is forced into the grooves and results in a hy-droplaning effect between the anode sleeve and

liquid (Homberg and Koppel, 1997). The purpose of this bearing technology is to conduct heat away from the x-ray tube more efficiently than conven-tional ball bearings with improved tube cooling. Additionally, the liquid bearing technology is free of vibrations and noise.

As noted by Fox (1995), the rotor hub and ro-tor stud also prevent the transmission of heat from the disk to the bearings. The rotor is a copper cylinder "brazed to an inner steel cylinder with a ceramic coating around the outside to enhance heat radiation" (Fox, 1995).

The working life of the tubes can range from about 10,000 to 40,000 hours, compared with 1000 hours, which is typical of conventional tubes with conventional bearing technology.

Filtration

Radiation from x-ray tubes consists of long and short wavelengths. The original experiments in the development of a practical CT scanner used monochromatic radiation to satisfy the Lambert-

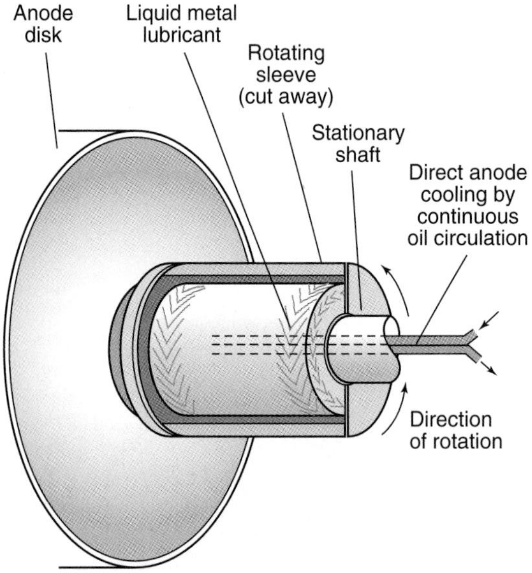

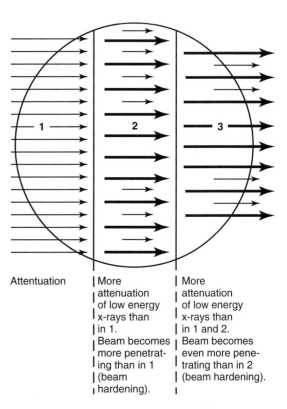

FIG. 5-18. The anode assembly of a modern x-ray tube used in CT imaging. The main parts of the assembly are the disk, rotor, and bearing assembly that contains liquid metal lubricant.

FIG. 5-19. Attenuation of radiation through a circular object. The beam becomes more penetrating (harder) in section 3 because of differences in attenuation in sections 1 and 2. The heavier arrows indicate less attenuation and more penetrating rays.

Beer exponential attenuation law. However, in clinical CT, the beam is polychromatic. Because it is essential that the polychromatic beam have the appearance of a monochromatic beam to satisfy the requirements of the reconstruction process, a special filter must be used.

In CT, filtration serves a dual purpose, as follows:

1. Filtration removes long wavelength x-rays because they do not play a role in CT image formation but instead contribute to patient dose. As a result of filtration, the mean energy of the beam increases and the beam becomes "harder," which may cause beam-hardening artifacts.
2. Filtration shapes the energy distribution across the radiation beam to produce uniform beam hardening when x-rays pass through the filter and the object (Fig. 5-19).

In Fig. 5-19, the attenuation differs in sections 1, 2, and 3 and the penetration increases in sections 2 and 3. This results from the absorption of the soft radiation in sections 1 and 2 and it is referred to as *hardening of the beam*. Because the detector system does not respond to beam-hardening effects for the circular object shown, "the problem can be solved by introducing additional filtration into the beam" (Seeram, 1982). In the original EMI scanner, this problem was solved with a water bath around the patient's head. Today, specially shaped filters conform to the shape of the object (Fig. 5-20). These filters are positioned between the x-ray tube and patient, and they shape the beam to produce more uniformity at the detectors.

Collimation

The purpose of collimation in conventional radiography and fluoroscopy is to protect the patient by restricting the beam to the anatomy of interest only. In CT, collimation is equally important because it affects patient dose and image quality (Fig. 5-21). The basic collimation scheme in CT is shown in Fig. 5-21, *A*, in which prepatient collimators and postpatient collimators, or predetector collimators, are apparent. These detectors must be perfectly aligned to optimize the imaging process.

Prepatient collimation design is influenced by the size of the focal spot of the x-ray tube because

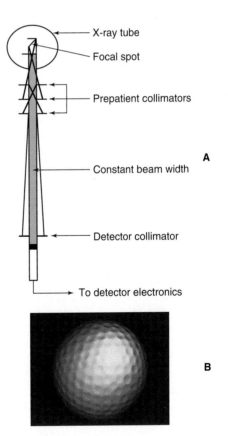

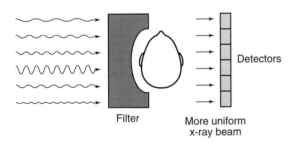

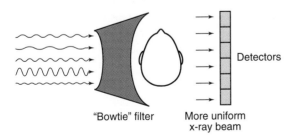

FIG. 5-20. Two types of beam-shaping filters for use in CT. These filters attenuate the beam so that a more uniform (monochromatic) beam falls onto the detectors. This uniform beam reduces the dynamic range of the electronics (analog-to-digital converters).

FIG. 5-21. **A,** Collimation scheme typical of CT scanning. **B,** The removal of scattered radiation by the two sets of collimators improves the resolution of the golf ball dimples. (Courtesy Shimadzu Medical Systems, Seattle, Wash.)

of the penumbra effect associated with focal spots. The larger the focal spot, the greater the penumbra and the more complicated the design of the collimators.

In general, a set of collimator sections is carefully arranged to shape the beam, which is proximal to the focal spot. Both proximal and distal (predetector) collimators are arranged to ensure a constant beam width at the detector. Detector collimators also shape the beam and remove scattered radiation. Such removal improves axial resolution as illustrated in Fig. 5-21, *B*, in which the golf ball dimples are apparent. The collimator section at the distal end of the collimator assembly also helps define the thickness of the slice to be imaged. Slice thickness can range from 0.5 to 10 mm, depending on the scanner.

CT DETECTOR TECHNOLOGY

The position of the CT detection system is shown in Fig. 5-22. CT detectors capture the radiation beam from the patient and convert it into electrical signals, which are subsequently converted into binary coded information.

Detector Characteristics

A detector must exhibit several characteristics essential for CT image production: efficiency, response time, dynamic range, high reproducibility, and stability.

Efficiency refers to the ability to capture, absorb, and convert x-ray photons to electrical signals. CT detectors must possess high capture efficiency, absorption efficiency, and conversion efficiency. *Capture efficiency* refers to the efficiency with which the detectors can obtain photons transmitted from the patient; the size of the detector area facing the beam and distance between two detectors determine capture efficiency. *Absorption efficiency* refers to the number of photons absorbed by the detector and depends on the atomic number, physical density, size, and thickness of the detector face (Villafana, 1987).

Stability refers to the steadiness of the detector response. If the system is not stable, frequent calibrations are required to render the signals useful.

The *response time* of the detector refers to the speed with which the detector can detect an x-ray event and recover to detect another event. Response times should be very short (i.e., microseconds) to avoid problems such as afterglow and detector "pile-up."

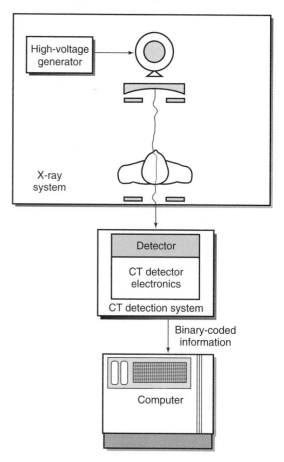

FIG. 5-22. Relationship of the CT detection system to the x-ray system and computer.

The *dynamic range* of a CT detector is the "ratio of the largest signal to be measured to the precision of the smallest signal to be discriminated (i.e., if the largest signal is 1 μA and the smallest signal is 1 nA, the dynamic range is 1 million to 1)" (Parker and Stanley, 1981). The dynamic range for most CT scanners is about 1 million to 1. The total detector efficiency, or dose efficiency, is the product of the capture efficiency, absorption efficiency, and conversion efficiency (Villafana, 1987).

Types

The conversion of x-rays to electrical energy in a detector is based on two fundamental principles (Fig. 5-23). Scintillation detectors convert x-ray energy into light, and then the light is converted into electrical energy (Fig. 5-23, *A*). Gas ionization detectors convert x-ray energy directly to electrical energy (Fig. 5-23, *B*).

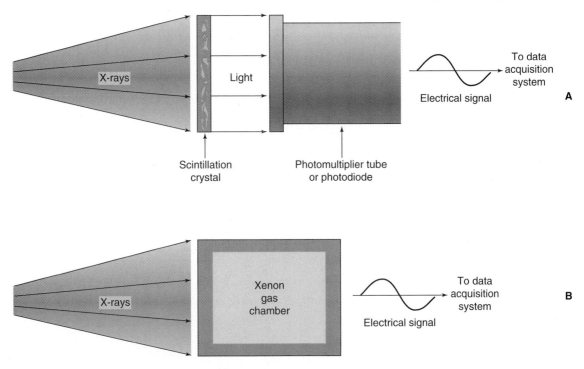

FIG. 5-23. Two methods to convert x-ray photons into electrical energy. **A,** Scintillation crystal detection and conversion scheme. **B,** Conversion of x-rays into electrical energy through gas ionization.

Scintillation Detectors

Scintillation detectors consist of a scintillation crystal coupled to a photomultiplier tube (Fig. 5-24). When x-rays fall onto the crystal, flashes of light, or scintillations, are produced. The light is then directed to the photomultiplier, or PM tube. As illustrated in Fig. 5-24, the light from the crystal strikes the photocathode of the PM tube, which then releases electrons. These electrons cascade through a series of dynodes that are carefully arranged and maintained at different potentials to result in a small output signal.

In the past, early scanners used sodium iodide crystals coupled to PM tubes. Because of afterglow problems and the limited dynamic range of sodium iodide, other crystals such as calcium fluoride and bismuth germanate were used in later scanners. Today, solid-state photodiode multiplier scintillation crystal detectors are used (Fig. 5-25). The photodiode is a semiconductor (silicon) whose *p-n* junction allows current flow when exposed to light. A lens is an essential part of the photodiode and is used to focus light from the scintillation crystal to the *p-n* junction, or semiconductor junction.

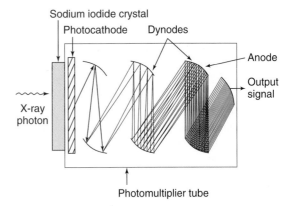

FIG. 5-24. Schematic representation of a scintillation detector based on the photomultiplier tube.

When light falls on the junction, electron hole pairs are generated and the electrons move to the *n* side of the junction while the holes move to the *p* side. The amount of current is proportional to the amount of light. Photodiodes are normally used with amplifiers because of the low output

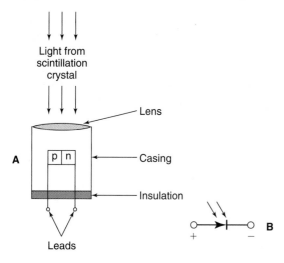

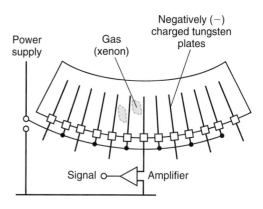

FIG. 5-25. **A,** Basic structure of a photodiode. **B,** The electronic symbol of a photodiode.

FIG. 5-26. The basic configuration of a gas ionization detector consists of a series of individual gas chambers separated by tungsten plates.

from the diode. In addition, the response time of a photodiode is extremely fast (about 0.5 to 250 nanoseconds, depending on its design).

Two scintillation materials currently used with photodiodes are cadmium tungstate and a ceramic material made of high-purity, rare earth oxides based on doped rare earth compounds such as yttria and gadolinium oxide ultrafast ceramic (Hahn et al, 1997; Hupke et al, 1997). Usually these crystals are optically bonded to the photodiodes. The advantages and disadvantages of these two scintillation materials can be discussed in terms of the detector characteristics described earlier. The conversion efficiency and photon capture efficiency of cadmium tungstate are 99% and 99%, respectively, and the dynamic range is 1 million to 1. On the other hand, the absorption efficiency of the ceramic rare earth oxide is 99%, whereas its scintillation efficiency is three times that of cadmium tungstate.

Gas Ionization Detectors

Gas ionization detectors are based on the principle of ionization and were introduced in third-generation scanners. The basic configuration of a gas ionization detector consists of a series of individual gas chambers, usually separated by tungsten plates carefully positioned to act as electron collection plates (Fig. 5-26). When x-rays fall on the individual chambers, ionization of the gas (usually xenon) results and produces positive and negative ions. The positive ions migrate to the negatively charged plate, whereas the negative ions are attracted to the positively charged plate. This migra-

tion of ions causes a small signal current that varies directly with the number of photons absorbed.

The gas chambers are enclosed by a relatively thick ceramic substrate material because the xenon gas is pressurized to about 30 atmospheres to increase the number of gas molecules available for ionization. Xenon detectors have excellent stability and fast response times and exhibit no afterglow problems. However, their quantum detection efficiency (QDE) is less than that of solid-state detectors. Whereas the QDE is 95% to 100% for crystal solid-state scintillation detectors and 94% to 98% for ceramic solid-state detectors, it is only 50% to 60% for xenon gas detectors (Arenson, 1995).

Plug-In Detector Modules

In modern CT scanners the entire array of detectors consists of groupings of detectors. Each grouping is known as a *detector module*, and each detector module "plugs" into a mother board unit of the detection system. The use of plug-in detector modules helps to maintain the integrity of the CT detector system through easy testing and replacement procedures.

Multislice Detectors

One major problem with single-slice, single-row detectors is related to the length of time needed to acquire data. The dual-slice, dual-row detector system was introduced to increase the volume coverage speed and thus decrease the time for data collection.

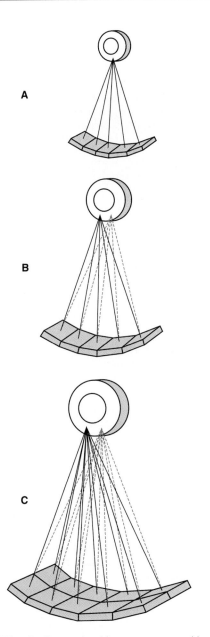

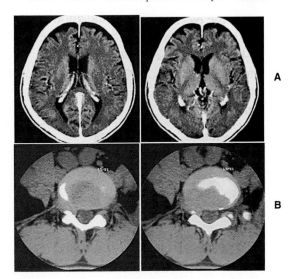

FIG. 5-28. Two contiguous slices acquired simultaneously for the brain (**A**) and spine (**B**). The brain images are contiguous 10-mm slices and the spine images are contiguous 2.5-mm slices. (Courtesy Elscint; Hackensack, NJ.)

FIG. 5-27.   A, Conventional beam geometry with single focal spot, single fan beam, and single-detector arc array. **B,** Twin-beam geometry from Elscint's dynamic focal spot system. **C,** Dual-row, dual-detector system.

Dual-Slice, Dual-Row Detectors

In 1992, Elscint introduced the first dual-slice volume CT scanner. The configuration of the dual-row detector system results in faster volume coverage compared with single-row CT systems (Fig. 5-27). This technology uses a dual-row, solid-state detector array coupled with a special x-ray tube based on a double-dynamic focus system. Fig. 5-27 also shows the conventional beam geometry (single focal spot, single fan beam, and single detector arc array) and

the beam geometry that arises as a result of the dynamic focal spot system. The dynamic focal spot is where the position of the focal spot is switched by a computer-controlled electron-optic system during each scan to double the sampling density and total number of measurements. Twin-beam technology results in the simultaneous scan of two contiguous slices with excellent resolution (Fig. 5-28) because the fan beam ray density and detector sampling are doubled twice, once for each of the two contiguous slices.

Multislice, Multirow Detectors

The goal of multislice multirow detectors is to increase the volume coverage speed performance of both single-slice and dual-slice CT scanners. The multislice, multirow detector consists of one detector with rows of detector elements (Fig. 5-29). A detector with *n* rows will be *n* times faster than its single-row counterpart. Multislice, multirow detectors are solid-state detectors that can acquire four slices per 360-degree rotation. In addition, these detectors influence the thickness of the slices.

DETECTOR ELECTRONICS
Function

The *data acquisition system* (DAS) refers to the detector electronics positioned between the detector array and the computer (Fig. 5-30). Because the

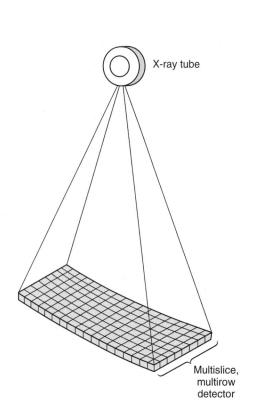

FIG. 5-29. The basic structure of a multislice multirow detector used in multislice volume CT scanners.

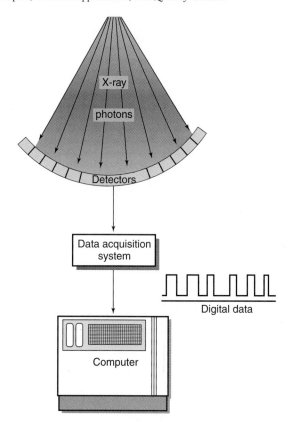

FIG. 5-30. Position of the data acquisition system in CT.

DAS is located between the detectors and the computer, it performs three major functions: (1) it measures the transmitted radiation beam, (2) it encodes these measurements into binary data, and (3) it transmits the binary data to the computer.

Components

The detector measures the transmitted x-rays from the patient and converts them into electrical energy. This electrical signal is so weak that it must be amplified by the preamplifier before it can be analyzed further (Fig. 5-31).

The transmission measurement data must be changed into attenuation and thickness data. This process (logarithmic conversion) can be expressed as follows:

Attenuation = log of transmission · thickness

$$(5-3)$$

or

$$\mu_1 + \mu_2 + \mu_3 \ldots \mu_n = \ln I_0 / I \cdot I / x$$

where μ is the linear attenuation coefficient, I_0 is the original intensity, I is the transmitted intensity, and x is the thickness of the object.

Logarithmic conversion is performed by the logarithmic amplifier, and these signals are subsequently directed to the ADC. The ADC divides the electrical signals into multiple parts—the more parts, the more accurate the ADC. These parts are measured in bits: a 1-bit ADC divides the signal into two digital values (2^1), a 2-bit ADC generates four digital values (2^2), and a 12-bit ADC results in 4096 (2^{12}) digital values. These values help determine the gray-scale resolution of the image. Modern CT scanners use 16-bit ADCs.

The final step performed by the DAS is data transmission to the computer. CT manufacturers have introduced optoelectronic data transmission schemes for this purpose because of the continuous rotation of the tube or detector arc and vast amount of data generated. *Optoelectronics* refers to the use of lens and light diodes to facilitate data transmission (Fig. 5-32). Several optical transmitters send the data to the optical receiver array so that at least one transmitter and one receiver are always in optical contact. These receivers and transmitters are light-emitting diodes capable of very high rates of data transmission; 50 million bits per second is common.

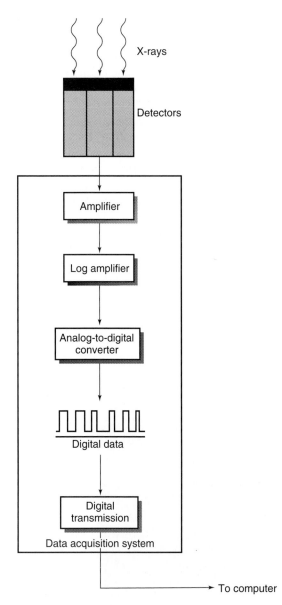

FIG. 5-31. Essential components of the data acquisition system in CT.

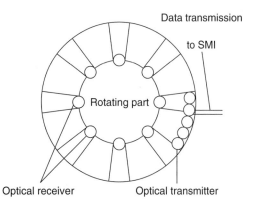

FIG. 5-32. Optoelectric data transmission. Optical transmitters on the gantry send data to the optical receiver array. At least one transmitter and one receiver are always in optical contact.

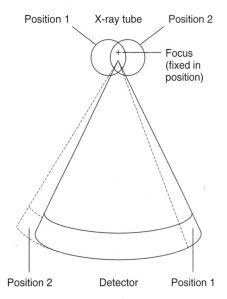

FIG. 5-33. Schematic representation of the concept of a quarter-shifted detector arc.

DATA ACQUISITION AND SAMPLING

During data acquisition, the radiation beam transmitted through the patient falls on the detectors. Each detector then measures, or samples, its beam intensity incident on it. If enough samples are not obtained, artifacts such as streaking (an aliasing artifact) appear on the reconstructed image. To solve this problem, the following methods have been devised to increase the number of samples available for image reconstruction and thus improve the quality of the image:

- Slice thickness: The imaging of thin slices helps reduce streaking artifacts related to sampling.

- Closely packed detectors: When the detectors are closely packed, more detectors are available for data acquisition, which ensures more samples per view and an increase in the total measurements taken per scan.
- Quarter-shifted detector arc: In conventional CT systems, the fan beam is composed of the same number of beams and detectors, and the spacing of the beams often causes sampling errors. These errors can be minimized if the detector arc is shifted by one-quarter detector space (Fig. 5-33). The goal of detector shifting is to provide two

sets of data that can be individually reconstructed or combined to provide a doubly fine sampling grid (Fig. 5-34) so more data are available for image reconstruction. In the Siemens Somatom Plus scanner, for example, this shifting is accomplished by the flying focal spot (dual focal spot x-ray tube)

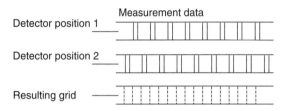

FIG. 5-34. Quarter shifting the detector arc provides a sampling grid twice as fine as a conventional sampling grid.

(Fig. 5-35). "During the normal rotation of the x-ray tube around the system axis, the focus is held in position for a pre-defined, very short period of time by an electromagnetic deflection device and then allowed to 'fly back' to its original position for the next projection. This process continues throughout the scanning operation" (Siemens Medical Systems, 1999). The same detector is used more than once to provide a large number of discrete measurements, which eliminates the aliasing artifact. This process is referred to as the *multifan measurement technique* (Siemens Medical Systems, 1999).

- The double-dynamic focus system (see Fig. 5-27) used by Elscint in their CT twin scanner is another method of increasing detector sampling during data acquisition in one used by Elscint in their CT twin scanner.

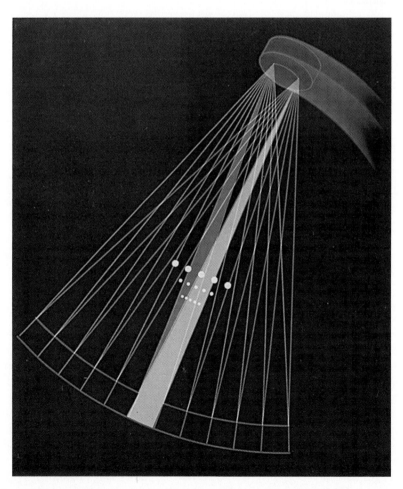

FIG. 5-35. The basic principle of the flying focal spot, a characteristic of the Siemens Somatom Plus CT scanner. (Courtesy Siemens Medical Systems; Iselin, NJ.)

REFERENCES

Arenson J: Data collection strategies: gantries and dectectors. In Goldman LW and Fowlkes JB, eds: Medical CT and ultrasound: current technology and applications, Maryland, 1995, American Association of Physicists in Medicine, pp 329-347.

Brunnett CJ et al: *CT design considerations and specifications*, Cleveland, Ohio, 1990, Picker International.

Fox SH: CT tube technology. In Goldman LW, Fowlkes JB, eds: *Medical CT and ultrasound: current technology and applications*, College Park, Md, 1995, American Association of Physicists in Medicine, pp 349-357.

Hahn G et al: Developing an ultrafast radiation detector for CT scanning, *Resear Innovat* 1:15-22, 1997.

Homberg R, Koppel R: An x-ray tube assembly with rotating-anode spiral groove bearing of the second generation, *Electromedica* 66(2):65-66, 1997.

Hupke R, Hahn D, Tschammler A: Low-dose CT imaging with the new UFC detector, *Electromedica* 66(2): 56-57, 1997.

Parker DL, Stanley JH: Glossary. In Newton TH, Potts DG, eds: *Radiology of the skull and brain: technical aspects of computed tomography*, St Louis, 1981, Mosby.

Seeram E: *Computed tomography technology*, Philadelphia, 1982, WB Saunders.

Siemens Medical Systems: *The technology and performance of the Somatom Plus*, Iselin, NJ, 1999, Siemens.

Villafana T: Physics and instrumentation: CT and MRI. In Lee SH, Rao KCVG, eds: *Cranial computed tomography*, New York, 1987, McGraw-Hill.

BIBLIOGRAPHY

Barnes GT, Lakshminarayanan AV: Computed tomography: physical principles and image quality considerations. In Lee JT et al, eds: *Computed tomography with MRI correlation*, ed 2, New York, 1989, Raven Press.

Bushong S: *Radiologic science for technologists*, ed 6, St Louis, 1997, Mosby.

Robb RA, Morin RL: Principles and instrumentation for dynamic computed tomography. In Marcus ML et al, eds: *Cardiac imaging—a comparison to Braunwald's heart disease*, Philadelphia, 1991, WB Saunders.

6

Image Reconstruction

BASIC PRINCIPLES

The basic principles related to the image reconstruction process include algorithms, the Fourier transform, convolution, and interpolation. The sequence of events after signals leave the CT detectors is shown in Fig. 6-1.

Algorithms

The algorithm is now common in radiology because computers are used in many imaging and nonimaging applications. The word *algorithm* is derived from the name of the Persian scholar, Abu Ja'Far Mohammed ibn Mûsâ Alkowârîzmî, whose textbook on arithmetic (c. 825 CE) significantly influenced mathematics for many years (Knuth, 1977). According to Knuth, an algorithm is "a set of rules or directions for getting a specific output from a specific input. The distinguishing feature of an algorithm is that all vagueness must be eliminated; the rules must describe operations that are so simple and well defined, they can be executed by a machine. Furthermore, an algorithm must always terminate after a finite number of steps."

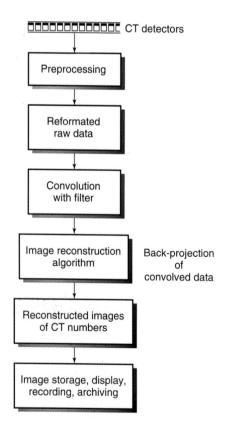

FIG. 6-1. Sequence of events after signals leave the detectors. The image reconstruction algorithms deal with the mathematics of the CT process.

The solutions to mathematical problems in computed tomography (CT) require computer programs, or reconstruction algorithms, to reconstruct the image.

Fourier Transform

The Fourier transform was developed by the mathematician Baron Jean-Baptiste-Joseph Fourier in 1807 and is widely used in science and engineering. The Fourier transform is a useful analytic tool in mathematics, astronomy, chemistry, physics, medicine, and radiology. In radiology, the Fourier transform is used to reconstruct images of a patient's anatomy in CT and also in magnetic resonance imaging (MRI).

To understand the Fourier transform, Bracewell (1989) presented an analogy with the act of hearing. Incoming sound waves that enter the ear are separated into different signals and intensities. These signals arrive at the brain and are rearranged to produce a perception of the original sound. Bracewell defined the Fourier transform as "a function that describes the amplitude and phases of each sinusoid, which corresponds to a specific frequency. (Amplitude describes the height of the sinusoid; phase specifies the starting point in the sinusoid's cycle.)" In other words, the Fourier transform is a mathematical function that converts a signal in the spatial domain to a signal in the frequency domain.

The Fourier transform divides a waveform (sinusoid) into a series of sine and cosine functions of different frequencies and amplitudes. These components can then be separated. In imaging, when a beam of x-rays passes through the patient, an image profile denoted by $f(x)$ is obtained. This can be expressed mathematically in the form of the Fourier series as follows:

$$f(x) = a_0/2 + (a_1 \cos x + b_1 \sin x) + (a_2 \cos 2x + b_2 \sin 2x) + (a_3 \cos 3x + b_3 \sin 3x) + \ldots + (a_n \cos nx + b_n \sin nx)$$

The constants—a_0, a_1, b_1, and so on—are called *Fourier coefficients* (Gibson, 1981) and can easily be calculated. Use of these Fourier coefficients makes it possible to reconstruct an image in CT.

Convolution

Convolution is a digital image processing technique to modify images through a filter function. "The process involves multiplication of overlapping portions of the filter function and the detector response curve selectively to produce a third function which is used for image reconstruction" (Berland, 1987). (This will become clear in the discussion of the filtered back-projection algorithm.)

where Y_3 is the unknown value of Y (at X_3) and Y_2 and Y_1 (at X_2 and X_1) are the nearest known values between which the interpolation is made."

Gibson, 1981

Interpolation

Interpolation is used in CT in the image reconstruction process and the determination of slices in spiral/ helical CT imaging. Interpolation is a mathematical technique to estimate the value of a function from known values on either side of the function.

"For example, if the speed of an engine controlled by a lever increases from 40 to 50 revolutions per second when the lever is pulled down by 4 cm, one can interpolate from this information and assume that moving it 2 cm gives 45 revolutions per second. This is the simplest method of interpolation, called *linear interpolation*. If known values of one variable, Y, are plotted against the other variable, X, an estimate of an unknown value of Y can be made by drawing a straight line between the two nearest known values.

The mathematical formula for linear interpolation is

$$Y_3 = Y_1 + (X_3 - X_1) (Y_2 - Y_1)/(X_2 - X_1)$$

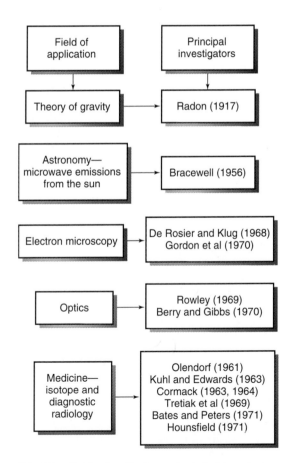

FIG. 6-2. Fields of application and principal investigators of image reconstruction techniques.

IMAGE RECONSTRUCTION FROM PROJECTIONS
Historical Perspective

The history of reconstruction techniques dates to 1917 when Radon developed mathematical solutions to the problem of image reconstruction from a set of its projections. He applied these techniques to gravitational problems. These techniques were later used to solve problems in astronomy and optics, but they were not applied to medicine until 1961 (Fig. 6-2).

In his initial work, Hounsfield's images were noisy as a result of his chosen reconstruction technique. Special algorithms (convolution back-projection algorithms) were soon introduced. These algorithms were developed by Ramachandran and Lakshminarayanan (1971) and later used by Shepp and Logan (1974) to improve image quality and processing time.

The Problem in CT

Consider an object, O, represented by an *x-y* coordinate system (Fig. 6-3). The spatial distribution of all attenuation coefficients, μ, is given by $\mu(x,y)$, which varies between points in the object. Suppose a pencil beam of x-rays passes through the object along a straight path (*arrow*), and the intensity of the transmitted beam that falls on the CT detector is I. Then a projection is given by the line integral[*] of $\mu(x,y)$:

$$I = I_0 \exp\left[-\sum_{Source}^{Detector} \mu(x,y)\right] \quad (6\text{-}1)$$

By taking the negative logarithm, Equation 6-1 can be linearized to generate integral equations of the form

$$T_\theta(x) = \ln \frac{I}{I_0} \quad (6\text{-}2)$$

$$\ln \frac{I_0}{I} = \sum_{Source}^{Detector} \mu(x,y) \quad (6\text{-}3)$$

---

[*] A *line integral* is the integral (summation of values that are infinitesimally close to each other multiplied by the infinitesimal distance separating the values) of a two-dimensional or three-dimensional object along the point of a line (Parker and Stanley, 1981).

where $T_\theta(x)$ is the x-ray transmission at angle θ, which is a measure of the total absorption along the straight line in Fig. 6-3. $T_\theta(x)$ is referred to as the *ray sum*, which is the integral of $\mu(x,y)$ along the ray.

The computational problem in CT is to find $\mu(x,y)$ from the ray sums for a sufficiently large number of beams of known locations that pass through the object, O. The beam geometries discussed in Chapter 5 ensure that every point in the object is scanned successively by a large set of ray sums $T_\theta(x)$.

A set of ray sums is referred to as a *projection* (Fig. 6-4), which can be generated as shown in Fig. 6-4, as the x-ray tube and detector scan the object simultaneously. The ray AA' is equal to $x \cos \theta + y \sin \theta = d$. The projection is given by $P(\theta,d)$:

$$P(\theta,d) = \int_{AA'} f(x,y)ds \qquad (6\text{-}4)$$

where ds is the differential along the path length s.

To understand the meaning of a projection, consider the following case in which a beam of intensity I_{in} enters an object of thickness x:

$$I_{in} \rightarrow \boxed{\mu} \rightarrow I_{out}$$
$$\leftarrow x \rightarrow$$

The beam is attenuated according to Lambert-Beer's law, as follows:

$$I_{out} = I_{in}e^{-\mu x} \qquad (6\text{-}5)$$

Because x, I_{in}, I_{out}, and e are known, μ can be calculated:

$$\mu = \frac{1}{x} \cdot \log \frac{I_{in}}{I_{out}}$$

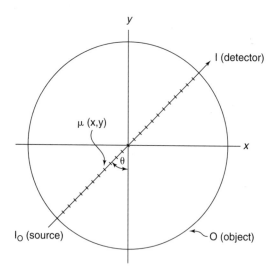

FIG. 6-3. The total distribution of attenuation coefficients in the object O is $\mu(x,y)$. The problem in CT is to calculate $\mu(x,y)$ from a set of projections specified by the angle Θ. I_0 and I represent beam intensities from the source and at the detector, respectively. (From Seeram E: *Computed tomography technology*, Philadelphia, 1994, WB Saunders.)

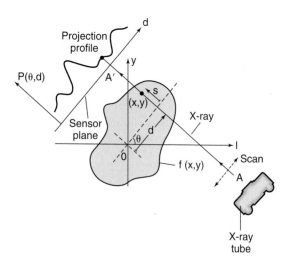

FIG. 6-4. Projection profile obtained when a parallel beam of x-rays scans the object represented by $f(x,y)$. (D is the distance of the ray $AA\{p\}$ from the origin 0).

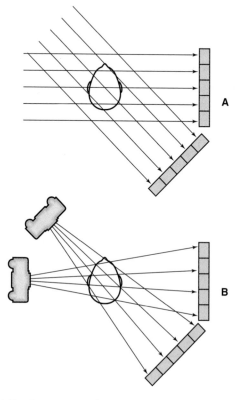

FIG. 6-5. Beam geometries used in CT to generate projection data. **A,** Parallel beam geometry used in the first CT scanners. **B,** Fan beam geometry was introduced to acquire the projection data faster than parallel beam geometries.

The following case represents the situation in the patient:

$$I_{in} \rightarrow \boxed{\mu_1 \mid \mu_2 \mid \mu_3 \mid \cdots \mid \mu_n} \rightarrow I_{out}$$

From x-ray tube $\quad \leftarrow X_1 \rightarrow \leftarrow X_2 \rightarrow \leftarrow X_3 \rightarrow \qquad \leftarrow X_n \rightarrow \quad$ To the detector

$$I_{out} = I_{in}e^{-(\mu_1 x_1 + \mu_2 x_2 + \mu_3 x_3 + \cdots \mu_n x_n)} \qquad \text{(6-6)}$$

Because $x_1 = x_2 = x_3 \cdots = x_n$,

$$1/x \log I_{in}/I_{out} = \mu_1 + \mu_2 + \mu_3 \cdots + \mu_n \qquad \text{(6-7)}$$

The problem in CT is to calculate all values for the μ terms for a large set of projections. Projections can be obtained through both parallel and fan beam geometries (Fig. 6-5). Hounsfield's original CT scanner employed parallel beam projections acquired through a 180-degree rotation.

RECONSTRUCTION ALGORITHMS

Image reconstruction from projections involves several algorithms to calculate all the μ terms in Equation 6-7 from a set of projection data. The algorithms applicable to CT include back-projection, iterative methods, and analytic methods.

Back-Projection

Back-projection is a simple procedure and does not require much understanding of mathematics. Back-projection, also called the "summation method" or "linear superposition method," was first used by Oldendorf (1961) and Kuhl and Edwards (1963). Back-projection can be best explained with a graphic or numeric approach.

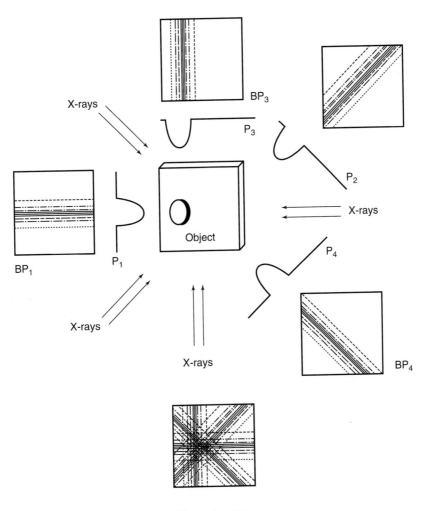

Reconstruction

FIG. 6-6. Graphic representation of the back-projection reconstruction technique.

Consider four beams of x-rays that pass through an unknown object to produce four projections, P_1, P_2, P_3, P_4 (Fig. 6-6). The problem involves the use of these profiles to reconstruct an image of the unknown object (black dot) in the box. The projected data sets are back-projected (i.e., linearly smeared) to form the corresponding images $BP1$, $BP2$, $BP3$, and $BP4$. The reconstruction involves summing these back-projected images to form an image of the object.

The problem with the back-projection technique is that it does not produce a sharp image of the object and therefore is not used in clinical CT. The most striking artifact of back-projection is the typical star pattern that occurs because points outside a high-density object receive some of the back-projected intensity of that object (Curry, Dowdey, and Murry, 1990).

Back-projection can also be explained with the following 2 × 2 matrix:

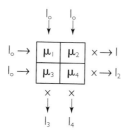

Four separate equations can be generated for the four unknowns, μ_1, μ_2, μ_3, and μ_4:

$$I_1 = I_0 e^{-(\mu_1 + \mu_2)x}$$
$$I_2 = I_0 e^{-(\mu_3 + \mu_4)x}$$
$$I_3 = I_0 e^{-(\mu_1 + \mu_3)x}$$
$$I_4 = I_0 e^{-(\mu_2 + \mu_4)x}$$

These equations can be quickly solved by a computer.

A numerical example might help to give some insight into the calculations involved. Consider an object divided into four squares (2 × 2 matrix with four pixels), as shown here.

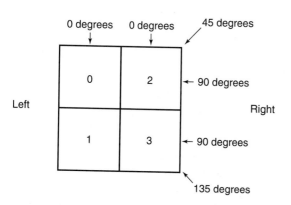

Four projections are collected at four different known locations: 0, 45, 90, and 135 degrees.

Start. Collect data for four projections: 0, 45, 90, and 135 degrees.

1. The ray sum for the 0-degree projection on the left side is 1 (0 + 1).
2. The ray sum for the 0-degree projection on the right side is 5 (2 + 3).
3. The ray sums for the 45-degree projection are 0, 3 (2 + 1), and 3.
4. The ray sum for the 90-degree projection on the upper row is 2 (2 + 0).
5. The ray sum for the 90-degree projection on the lower row is 4 (3 + 1).
6. The ray sums for the 135-degree projection are 2, 3 (3 + 0), and 1.

These projection data—1, 5, 0, 3, 3, 2, 4, 2, 3, and 1—are then used systematically as defined by the algorithm to reconstruct the original image.

1. First guess: Place the data from the 0-degree projections into the matrix to obtain the first guess:

I (0 + 1)	5 (2 + 3)
I (0 + 1)	5 (2 + 3)

2. Second guess: Add the data from the 45-degree projections to the value of each square in the first guess:

I (0 + 1)	8 (5 + 3)
4 (1 + 3)	8 (5 + 3)

3. Third guess: Add the data from the 90-degree projections to the value of each square in the second guess:

3 (1 + 2)	10 (8 + 2)
8 (4 + 4)	12 (8 + 4)

4. Fourth guess: Add the data from the 135-degree projections to the value of each square in the third guess:

6 (3 + 3)	12 (10 + 2)
9 (8 + 1)	15 (12 + 3)

The next step is to obtain the original matrix, as follows:

1. Subtract a constant value 6 (obtained by summing the values in the original matrix— $0 + 1 + 2 + 3 = 6$) from each square in the fourth guess:

0 (6 − 6)	6 (12 − 6)
3 (9 − 6)	9 (15 − 6)

2. Now reduce the preceding matrix to a simple ratio. By using the obvious common divisor, 3, the following is obtained:

0 (0 / 3)	2 (6 / 3)
1 (3 / 3)	3 (9 / 3)

This is the original 2 × 2 matrix.

Iterative Algorithms

Another approach to image reconstruction is based on iterative techniques. "An iterative reconstruction starts with an assumption (for example, that all points in the matrix have the same value) and compares this assumption with measured values, makes corrections to bring the two into agreement, and then repeats this process over and over until the assumed and measured values are the same or within acceptable limits" (Curry, Dowdey, and Murry, 1990).

Techniques include the simultaneous iterative reconstruction technique, iterative least-squares technique, and algebraic reconstruction technique (ART) (Brooks and Di Chiro, 1976; Gordon and Herman, 1974). These techniques differ in the application of corrections to subsequent iterations. The algebraic reconstruction technique was used by Hounsfield in the first EMI brain scanner (Hounsfield, 1972) and is detailed here.

Consider the following numeric illustration (Seeram, 1994):

Original projection data sets
(horizontal ray sums)

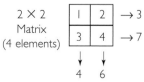

Original projection data sets
(vertical ray sums)

1. Initial estimate: Compute the average of four elements and assign it to each pixel; that is, $1 + 2 + 3 + 4 = 10$; $10 / 4 = 2.5$

New projection data sets
(horizontal ray sums)

2.5	2.5	→ 5
2.5	2.5	→ 5

2. First correction for error (original horizontal ray sums minus the new horizontal ray sums divided by 2) = $(3 - 5) / 2$ and $(7 - 5) / 2 = -2 / 2$ and $2 / 2 = -1.0$ and 1.0:

(2.5 − 1) 1.5	(2.5 − 1) 1.5
(2.5 + 1) 3.5	(2.5 + 1) 3.5

3. Second estimate:

1.5	1.5
3.5	3.5

↓ 5   ↓ 5

new project data sets
(vertical ray sums)

4. Second correction for error (original vertical ray sums minus new vertical ray sums divided by 2) = $(4 - 5) / 2$ and $(6 - 5) / 2 = -1.0 / 2$ and $+1.0 / 2 = -0.5$ and $+0.5$:

(1.5 − 0.5) 1	(1.5 + 0.5) 2
(3.5 − 0.5) 3	(3.5 + 0.5) 4

The final matrix solution is thus

1	2
3	4

Today these techniques are not used incommercial scanners because of the following limitations:

1. It is difficult to obtain accurate ray sums because of quantum noise and patient motion.
2. The procedure takes too long to generate the reconstructed image because the iteration can be done only after all projection data sets have been obtained.
3. To produce a "true" image, there should be more projection data sets than pixels. Therefore diagonal projection data sets are taken to eliminate ambiguity.

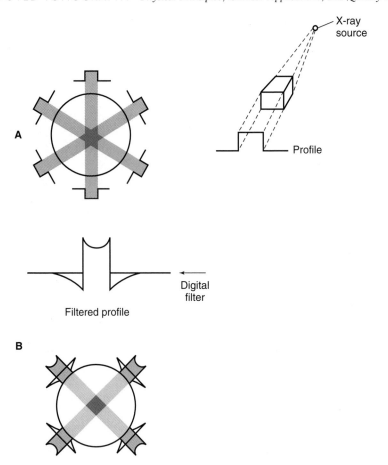

FIG. 6-7. Back-projection and filtered back-projection techniques used in CT. **A,** Back-projection results in an unsharp image. **B,** Filtered back-projection uses a digital filter (a convolution filter) to remove this blurring, which produces a sharp image.

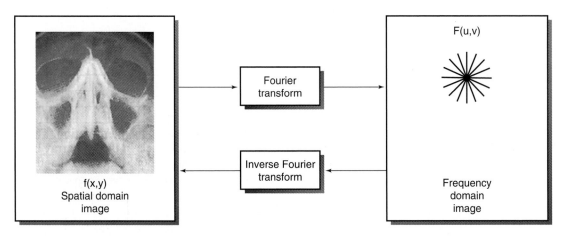

FIG. 6-8. Radiograph of an image represented in the spatial domain by the function *f(x,y)*. This can be transformed to an image in the frequency domain *F(u,v)* using the Fourier transform. In addition, *F(u,v)* can be retransformed into *f(x,y)* using the inverse Fourier transform.

Analytic Reconstruction Algorithms

Analytic reconstruction algorithms were developed to overcome the limitations of back-projection and iterative algorithms and are used in modern CT scanners. Two analytic reconstruction algorithms are the Fourier reconstruction algorithm and filtered back-projection.

Filtered Back-Projection

Filtered back-projection is also referred to as the *convolution method* (Fig. 6-7). The projection profile is filtered or convolved to remove the typical star-like blurring that is characteristic of the simple back-projection technique.

The steps in the filtered back-projection method (Fig. 6-7, B) are as follows:

1. All projection profiles are obtained.
2. The logarithm of the data is obtained.
3. The logarithmic values are multiplied by a digital filter, or convolution filter, to generate a set of filtered profiles.
4. The filtered profiles are then back-projected.
5. The filtered projections are summed and the negative and positive components are therefore canceled, which produces an image free of blurring.

Fourier Reconstruction

The Fourier reconstruction process is used in MRI but not in modern CT scanners because it requires more complicated mathematics than the filtered back projection algorithm.

A radiograph can be considered an image in the spatial domain; that is, shades of gray represent various parts of the anatomy (e.g., bone is white and air is black) in space. With the Fourier transform, this spatial domain image—the radiograph represented by the function $f(x,y)$— can be transformed into a frequency domain image represented by the function $F(u,v)$. This frequency domain image consists of a range of high to low frequencies. In addition, this image can be retransformed into a spatial domain image with the inverse Fourier transform (Fig. 6-8).

There are several advantages to this transformation process. First, the image in the frequency domain can be manipulated (e.g., edge enhancement or smoothing) by changing the amplitudes of the frequency components. Second, a computer can perform those manipulations (digital image processing). Third, frequency information can be used to measure image quality through the point spread function, line spread function, and modulation transfer function (Huang, 1999).

The Fourier slice theorem states that the Fourier transform of the projection of an object at angle Θ is equal to a slice of the Fourier transform of the object along angle Θ (Fig. 6-9) (Parker, 1991).

The Fourier reconstruction consists of the following steps (Fig. 6-10):

1. The object to be scanned is represented by the function $f(x,y)$.
2. Projection data are obtained from the object. A projection data set for at least a 180-degree rotation is required for adequate reconstruction. These projections represent a spatial domain image.
3. Each projection is transformed into the frequency domain using the Fourier transform. This image must be converted into a clinically useful image.
4. Because CT scanners use a fast Fourier transform developed specifically for digital implementation, the frequency domain image must be placed on a rectangular grid (Fig. 6-10). This is accomplished by interpolation. The fast Fourier transform requires that the pixels in the grid array be 2, 4, 8, 16, 32, 64, 128, 256, 512, 1024, and so on.
5. Finally, the interpolated image is transformed into a spatial domain image of the object through an inverse Fourier transform operation.

The Fourier reconstruction technique does not use any filtering because interpolation produces a similar result. Also, the 2D interpolation process may introduce artifacts if it is not conducted accurately and therefore is not used in CT.

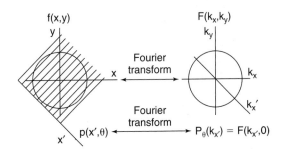

FIG. 6-9. The projection slice theorem forms the basis of Fourier reconstruction mathematics. The Fourier transform of the projection with respect to x', $P_\theta (k_x)$ is equal to a slice of the Fourier transform $F(k_x,k_y)$ in the Θ direction.

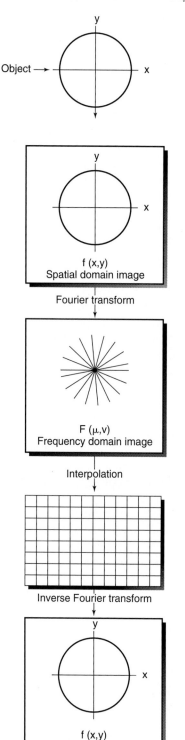

FIG. 6-10. Steps involved in Fourier reconstruction.

TYPES OF DATA

Fig. 6-11 shows the data evolution from acquisition, reconstruction, and image display. Four data types are measurement data, raw data, filtered raw data or convolved data, and image data or reconstructed data.

Measurement Data

Measurement data, or scan data, arise from the detectors. This data set is subject to preprocessing to correct the measurement data before the image reconstruction algorithm is applied. Such corrections are necessary because of errors in the measurement data from beam hardening, adjustments for bad detector readings, or scattered radiation. If these errors are not corrected, they will cause poor image quality and generate image artifacts.

Raw Data

Raw data are the result of preprocessed scan data and are subjected to the image reconstruction algorithm used by the scanner. These data can be stored and subsequently retrieved as needed.

Convolved Data

The image reconstruction algorithm used by current CT scanners is the filtered back projection algorithm, which includes both filtering and back projection. Raw data must first be filtered using a mathematical filter, or kernel. This process is also referred to as the *convolution technique*. Convolution improves image quality through the removal of blur (Fig. 6-12). Fig. 6-12, A, shows the degree of blurring present in an image before convolution. Fig. 6-12, B, demonstrates image sharpening after convolution. Convolution kernels can only be applied to the raw data.

Image Data

Image data, or reconstructed data, are convolved data that have been back-projected into the image matrix to create CT images displayed on a monitor. Various digital filters are available to suppress noise and improve detail (Fig. 6-13). Fig. 6-13 shows the relationship between image noise and image detail of a standard algorithm, a smoothing algorithm, and an edge enhancement algorithm.

The standard algorithm is usually used before the previous algorithms, especially when a balance between image noise and image detail is mandatory. Smoothing algorithms (Fig. 6-14) reduce image noise and show good soft tissue anatomy; they are used in examinations where soft tissue discrimination is important to visualize very low contrast structures. Edge enhancement algorithms emphasize the edges of structures and improve detail but create image noise (see Fig. 6-14). They are used

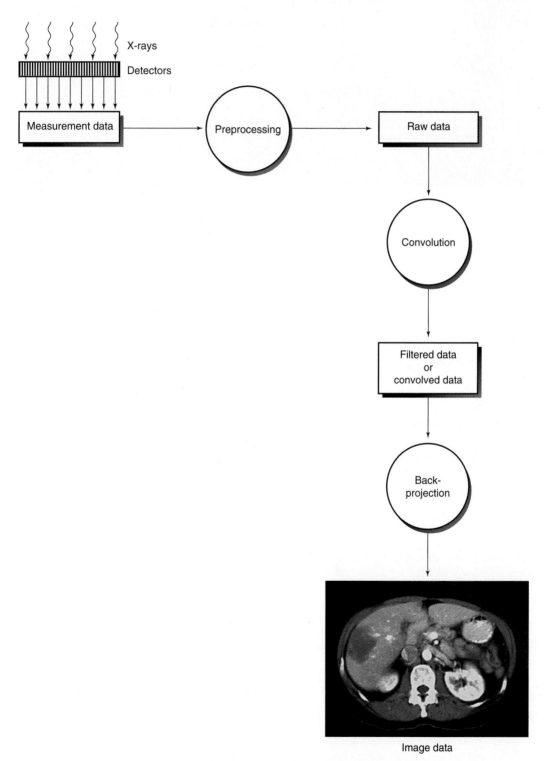

Image data

FIG. 6-11. The evolution of data in CT, from acquisition to image display on a monitor.

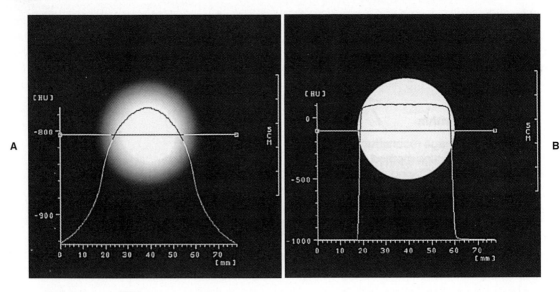

FIG. 6-12. The effect of convolution on image quality in CT. **A,** The image is back-projected without convolution. **B,** The data set has been convolved before back-projection. (Courtesy Siemens Medical Systems; Iselin, NJ.)

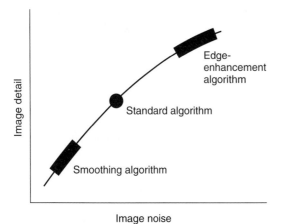

FIG. 6-13. The relationship between image detail and image noise for three digital filters in CT. Although edge enhancement algorithms provide good detail compared with smoothing algorithms, they also result in more noise. Smoothing algorithms reduce the image noise at the expense of detail but show good soft tissue structures.

in examinations in which fine detail is important, such as inner ear, bone structures, thin slice, and fine pulmonary examinations.

IMAGE RECONSTRUCTION IN SINGLE-SLICE SPIRAL/HELICAL CT

The image reconstruction algorithms previously described apply to single-slice conventional CT. In single-slice volume CT (spiral/helical CT), the same filtered back-projection algorithm is used with an additional consideration. Because the patient moves continuously through the gantry for a 360-degree rotation, the reconstructed image will be blurred and therefore interpolation is necessary before the filtered back projection is used. A planar section must first be computed from the volume data set using interpolation, after which images are generated with various interpolation algorithms

IMAGE RECONSTRUCTION IN MULTISLICE SPIRAL/HELICAL CT

A notable difference between single-slice volume CT and multislice volume CT is that the latter uses multiple detector rows that cover a larger volume at an increased speed and therefore require new algorithms. In general, multislice volume CT algorithms allow for the reconstruction of variable slice thicknesses and address the problems of increased volume coverage and speed of the patient couch. This is made possible by spiral/helical scanning with interlaced sampling, longitudinal interpolation, and fan beam reconstruction with the filtered back projection algorithm.

COMPARISON OF RECONSTRUCTION ALGORITHMS

Analytic methods, filtered back-projection, and the Fourier reconstruction are faster and generate more accurate images than those obtained with it-

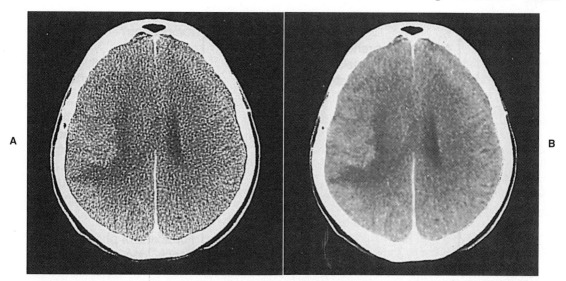

FIG. 6-14. The effect of two digital filters on the appearance of the CT image. **A,** An edge enhancement filter is used and more image noise is apparent. **B,** A smoothing digital filter is used and results in reduced image noise and good soft tissue discrimination. (Courtesy Siemens Medical Systems; Iselin, NJ.)

erative algorithms. Of the analytic methods, the filtered back projection algorithm is used in modern CT scanners including current state-of-the-art multislice volume CT scanners

3D ALGORITHMS

The applications of 3D imaging are rapidly increasing (Udupa, 1999; Calhoun et al, 1999). Three-dimensional imaging uses 3D surface and volumetric reconstruction. The algorithms for 3D imaging are based on those used in computer graphics and visual perception science. An algorithm for surface display (Fig. 6-15) is based on at least two processes, preprocessing and display, and consists of the following operations: interpolation, segmentation, surface formation, and projection (Udapa, 1999; Calhoun et al, 1999). 3D algorithms allow the user to "interactively visualize, manipulate, and measure large 3D objects on general purpose workstations" (Udapa and Odhner, 1991).

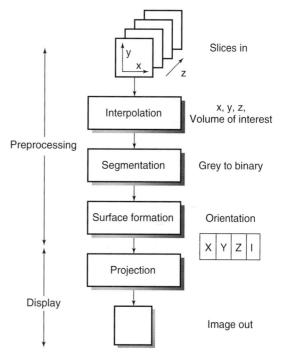

FIG. 6-15. Algorithm for surface display of 3D images from a CT scanner.

REFERENCES

Berland LL: *Practical CT: technology and techniques*, New York, 1987, Raven Press.

Bracewell R: The Fourier transform, *Sci Am* 260:86-95, 1989.

Brooks RA, Di Chiro G: Principles of computer assisted tomography (CAT) in radiographic and radioisotopic imaging, *Phys Med Biol* 21:689-732, 1976.

Calhoun PS et al: Three-dimensional volume rendering of spiral CT data: theory and method, *Radiographics* 19:745-764, 1999.

Curry TS III, Dowdey JE, Murry RC, Jr: *Christensen's physics of diagnostic radiology,* ed 4, Philadelphia, 1990, Lea & Febiger.

Gibson C, ed: *The Facts on File dictionary of mathematics*, New York, 1981, Facts on File.

Gordon R, Herman GT: Three-dimensional reconstruction from projections: a review of algorithms, *Int Rev Cytol* 38:111-123, 1974.

Hounsfield GH: *A method of and apparatus for examination of a body by radiation such as x or gamma radiation*, London, British Patent Office, Patent No. 1283915, 1972.

Huang HK: *PACS: Basic principles and applications*, New York, 1999, Wiley-Liss.

Knuth DE: Algorithms, *Sci Am* 236:63-80, 1977.

Kuhl DE, Edwards RQ: Image separation radioisotope scanning, *Radiology* 80:653-661, 1963.

Oldendorf WH: Isolated flying spot detection radiodensity discontinuities displaying the internal structural pattern of a complex object, *IEEE Trans Biomed Eng* BME 8:68-72, 1961.

Parker DL, Stanley JH: Glossary. In Newton TH, Potts DG, eds: *Radiology of the skull and brain: technical aspects of computed tomography*, St Louis, 1981, Mosby.

Ramachandran GN, Lakshminarayanan AV: Three-dimensional reconstructions from radiographs and electron micrographs: application of convolution instead of Fourier transforms, *Proc Natl Acad Sci USA* 68:2236-2240, 1971.

Seeram E: *Computed tomography technology*, Philadelphia, 1994, WB Saunders.

Shepp LA, Logan BF: The Fourier reconstruction of a head section, *IEEE Trans Nucl Sci* 21:21-43, 1974.

Udupa JK, Odhner D: Fast visualization, manipulation, and analysis of binary volumetric objects, *IEEE Comput Graph Appl* 11:53-62, 1991.

Udupa JK: Three-dimensional visualization and analysis methodologies: a current perspective, *Radiographics* 19:783-803, 1999.

BIBLIOGRAPHY

Cho ZH, Ahn IS: Computer algorithms for the tomographic image reconstruction with x-ray transmission scans, *Comput Biomed Res* 8:8-25, 1975.

Fishman EK et al: Three-dimensional imaging, *Radiology* 181:321-337, 1991.

Gabor HT: *Image reconstruction from projections*, New York, 1980, Academic Press.

Kalender WA et al: Single-breath-hold spiral volumetric CT by continuous patient translation and scanner rotation, *Radiology* 173:414, 1989.

Parker JA: *Image reconstruction in radiology*, Boca Raton, Fla, 1991, CRC Press.

Strong AB et al: Applications of three-dimensional display techniques in medical imaging, *J Biomed Eng* 12:233-238, 1990.

Instrumentation

CT SCANNER

The basic equipment configuration for CT is shown in Fig. 7-1. Three major systems are the imaging system, computer system, and image display, recording, storage, and communication system (Fig. 7-2).

The three major systems are housed in separate rooms, as follows:

1. The imaging system is located in the scanner room.
2. The computer system is located in the computer room.
3. The display, recording, and storage system is located in the operator's room.

The purpose of the imaging system is to produce x-rays, shape and filter the x-ray beam to pass through only a defined cross-section of the patient, detect and measure the radiation passing through the cross-section, and convert the transmitted photons into digital information. The major components of the imaging system are the x-ray tube and generator, collimators, filter, detectors, and detector electronics. The x-ray tube and generator are responsible for x-ray production. The radiation beam that emanates from the tube is filtered through a specially designed filter that protects the patient from low-energy rays and ensures beam uniformity at the detectors. The collimators help define the slice thickness and restrict the x-ray beam to the cross-section of interest. The detectors capture the x-ray photons and convert them into electrical signals (analog information); the detector electronics, or data acquisition system (DAS), converts this information into digital data.

The computer system receives the digital data from the DAS and processes it to reconstruct an image of the cross-sectional anatomy. In addition, the computer system performs image manipulation and various image processing operations such as windowing, image enhancement, image enlargement and measurements, multiplanar reconstruction, 3D imaging, and quantitative measurements.

The computer system generally includes input-output devices, central processing units, array processors, interface devices, back-projector processors, storage devices, and communications hardware. The computer system also includes software that allows each hardware component to perform specific tasks. For example, the software enables scanning procedures to be created and activated from an input device and extensive image display and analysis functions such as image pan and zoom, image annotation, multiple image display, windowing, reverse video, image rotation, collage and sagittal-coronal display.

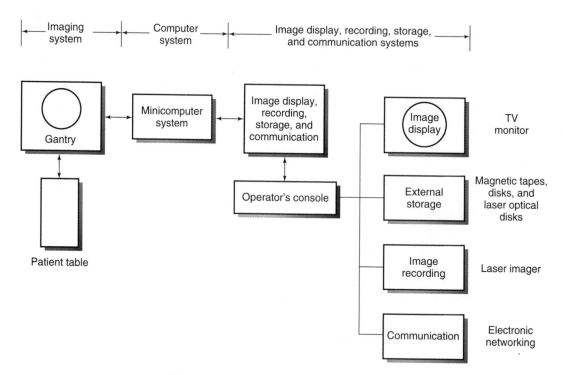

FIG. 7-1.   Basic equipment configuration for CT.

The purpose of the image display, recording, storage, and communication system is as follows:

1. To display the output digital image from the computer in a form meaningful to the observer or diagnostician.
2. To provide a hard copy of the image on a recording medium that provides for a permanent copy of the reconstructed image and accommodates the preference of the radiologist during diagnostic interpretation. Although most radiologists still prefer to make a diagnosis from x-ray films, they may have to make their primary diagnosis from a display monitor in filmless departments.
3. To facilitate the storage and retrieval of digital data to address the problems of film storage and archiving and the environmental concerns of film manufacturing, consumption, and disposal.
4. To communicate images, diagnostic reports, and patient demographic data in an electronic communications network environment.

Currently, CT images are displayed on cathode ray tubes, recorded on x-ray film, and stored on magnetic tapes and disks or optical disks.

IMAGING SYSTEM

The imaging system comprises several components housed in the gantry that work together to acquire an image from the patient. The gantry and patient couch are often referred to as the *scanner* (see Fig. 7-2).

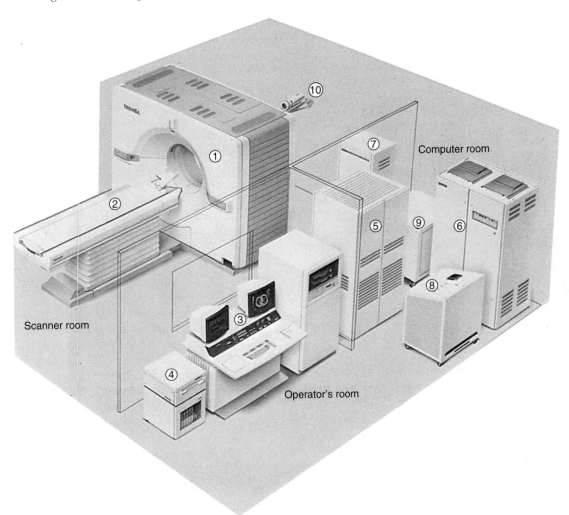

FIG. 7-2. Components of a CT imaging system. *1*, Gantry; *2*, patient couch; *3*, integrated console; *4*, optical disk system including cassette storage; *5*, high-speed processor system; *6*, x-ray high-voltage generator; *7*, couch control unit; *8*, system transformer I; *9*, system transformer II; *10*, patient observation system. (Courtesy Toshiba America Medical Systems; Tustin, Calif.)

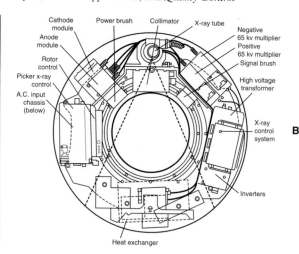

FIG. 7-3. A, The gantry houses imaging components such as the x-ray tube and generator, slip rings, collimators, detectors, and detector electronics. **B,** Cross-sectional diagram of the imaging components. (Courtesy Picker International; Cleveland, Ohio.)

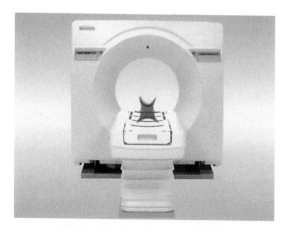

FIG. 7-4. The gantry aperture is the opening in the gantry in which the patient is positioned for the examination. The diameter of the aperture shown is 700 mm. (Courtesy Shimadzu Medical Systems; Seattle, Wash.)

Gantry

The gantry is a mounted framework that surrounds the patient in a vertical plane. It contains a rotating scan frame onto which the x-ray generator, x-ray tube, and other components are mounted.

The height and width are chosen to reduce the gantry size. For example, the dimensions of the Picker PQ-6000 scanner are 196 × 86 × 226 cm. The scanner weighs 1161 kg.

The gantry houses imaging components (Fig. 7-3) such as the slip rings, x-ray tube, high-tension generator, collimators, detectors, and DAS.

The x-ray tubes of slip-ring scanners require high instantaneous power and therefore have larger anodes with a typical diameter of 5 inches or more. Scanners may incorporate an on-board oil-to-air heat exchanger to assist in cooling the x-ray tube during operation.

The generator in the gantry is usually a small, solid-state, high-frequency generator mounted on the rotating scan frames and operated between 5 and 50 kHz. Because it is located close to the x-ray tube, only a short high-tension cable is required to couple the x-ray tube and generator. This design eliminates external x-ray control cabinets and long high-tension cables typical of some CT imaging systems.

The power ratings of generators range from 30 kilowatts to 60 kilowatts (kW), depending on the scanner. These ratings enable a large selection of exposure techniques (generally 80, 100, 120, 130, and 140 kV, and 30, 50, 65, 100, 125, 150, 175, and 200 mA).

Gantry cooling is a prime consideration because the ambient air temperature affects several components. In the past, air conditioners were placed in the gantry. Modern cooling systems circulate ambient air from the scanner room throughout the gantry. For example, the Picker PQ-6000 CT scanner uses large, low-pressure blowers and filters. The circular duct in the front covers of the gantry directs the cool air to the detector modules and gantry electronics and then exits through the top cover.

Two important features of the gantry are the gantry aperture and gantry tilting range. The gantry aperture is the opening in which the patient is positioned during the scanning procedure (Fig. 7-4). The technologist can approach the patient from both the front and back of the gantry. Most scanners have a 70-cm aperture that facilitates patient positioning and helps provide access to patients in emergency situations.

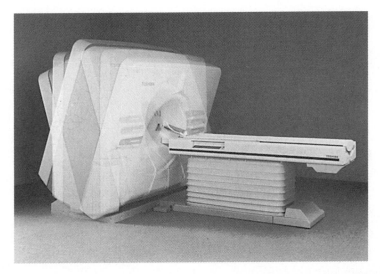

FIG. 7-5. Tilting range of the gantry. (Courtesy Toshiba America Medical Systems; Tustin, Calif.)

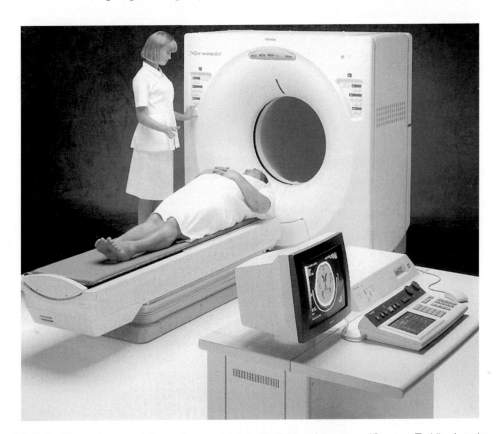

FIG. 7-6. The patient couch is a major component of a CT imaging system. (Courtesy Toshiba America Medical Systems; Tustin, Calif.)

The CT gantry must be capable of tilting (Fig. 7-5) to accommodate all patients and clinical examinations. The degree of tilt varies between systems, but ±12 to ±30 degrees is standard. The gantry also includes a set of laser beams to aid patient positioning. (Additional gantry characteristics are listed in the Appendix.)

Patient Couch

The patient couch, or patient table, provides a platform on which the patient lies during the examination (Fig. 7-6). The couch should be strong and rigid to support the weight of the patient. Additionally, it should provide for safety and comfort of the patient during the examination.

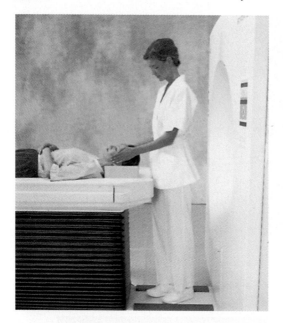

FIG. 7-7. A design feature of the gantry and table of a CT scanner that facilitates both access to and positioning of the patient. (Courtesy Siemens Medical Systems; Iselin, NJ.)

COUCH MOVEMENT CHARACTERISTICS OF THE PICKER PQ-6000 CT IMAGING SYSTEM

With its substantial capacity, the PQ-6000 offers an unsurpassed patient-positioning system. The PQ-6000 couch provides optimal clinical versatility. It supports a vast array of patient sizes within a flexible vertical adjustment range that also serves the special needs of pediatric, geriatric, and wheelchair patients.

- 450 lbs (204 kg) distributed weight limit at 0.25 mm accuracy for slice reproducibility and z-axis precision
- Easy patient access through a table height adjustment from 56 to 103 cm
- Accommodates a scannable range of 162 cm for precision volume scanning, permitting head-to-thigh patient coverage
- Total table travel: 180 cm
- Continuous table feed at various speeds for dynamic volume scanning speeds: elevation 25 mm/sec (average), lateral 25, 50, and 100 mm/sec
- Control modes: computer, electromechanical, free floating (via foot or table-mounted tape switches)

Courtesy Picker International; Cleveland, Ohio.

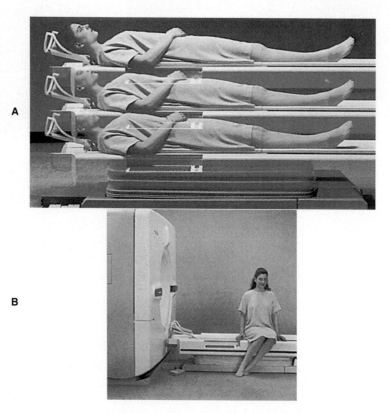

FIG. 7-8. The vertical movement of the couch can provide a range of heights (**A**) and allow the patient to mount and dismount the table with little effort (**B**). (Courtesy Toshiba America Medical Systems; Tustin, Calif.)

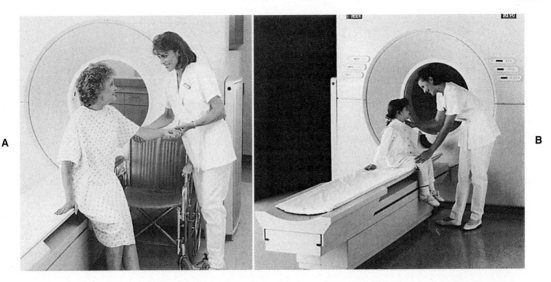

FIG. 7-9. The CT scanner should allow for easy handling of patients in wheelchairs (**A**) and pediatric patients (**B**). (Courtesy Picker International; Cleveland, Ohio.)

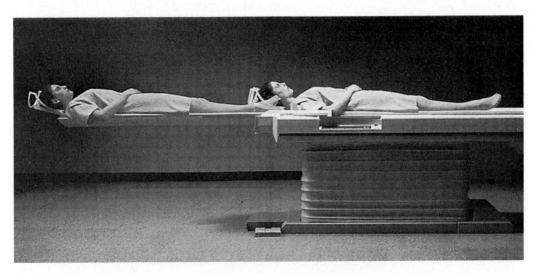

FIG. 7-10. Longitudinal or horizontal movement of the CT couch (*top*) should allow the patient to be scanned from head to thigh without repositioning. (Courtesy Toshiba America Medical Systems; Tustin, Calif.)

The couch consists of a support referred to as the *couch top*, which rests on a pedestal. The couch top is usually made of carbon fiber composites because they have low absorption and excellent vibration damping features and meet the strength requirements necessary to take images of heavy patients. The technologist has ample room between the gantry and table for patient access and positioning (Fig. 7-7). The pedestal houses the mechanical and electrical components that facilitate vertical and horizontal couch movements. The vertical movement should provide a range of heights to make it easy for patients to mount and dismount the table (Fig. 7-8). This feature is especially useful in the examination of geriatric, trauma, and pediatric patients (Fig. 7-9). Horizontal or longitudinal couch movements should enable the patient to be scanned from head to thighs without repositioning (Fig. 7-10).

The box on p. 116 lists the couch movement characteristics for one CT system.

CT COMPUTER AND IMAGE PROCESSING SYSTEM
Processing Architectures and Hardware

The computer system in CT belongs to the class of minicomputers (see Chapter 2). The two most important characteristics of the CT computer system are a large storage capacity and fast and efficient processing of various kinds of data.

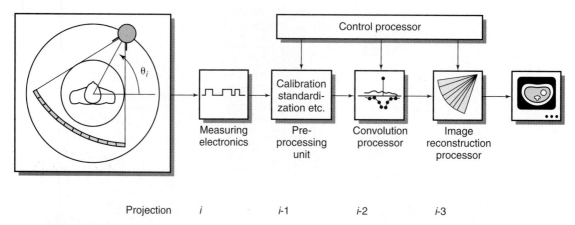

FIG. 7-11. Computer configuration of the Siemens Somatom whole-body CT scanner with pipeline processing. The reconstruction steps of preprocessing, convolution, and basic projection are assigned to separate processors. (From Dümmling K: 10 years of computed tomography: a retrospective view, *Electromedica* 52:13-28, 1984.)

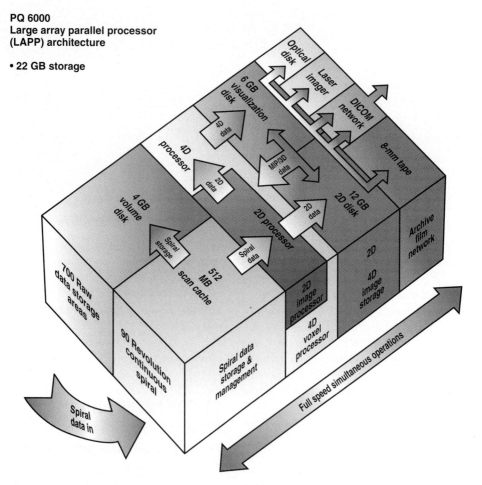

FIG. 7-12. The Picker PQ 6000 CT Imaging System is based on a large array parallel processor (LAPP) architecture. (Courtesy Picker International; Cleveland, Ohio.)

Various computer architectures for CT have been developed to accommodate fast image reconstruction and other image processing functions such as image manipulation and visualization. For example, although some CT scanners use pipeline processing architectures (Fig. 7-11), others use parallel and distributed processing architectures. The basis for these architectures depends on the way that the computer assigns various tasks (e.g., preprocessing raw data, convolution, back projection, and visualization tasks such as 3D imaging, CT angiography, and virtual reality imaging) to the numerous processors in its electronic circuits.

An important component of computer processing architectures for CT and MRI is the array processor, which is a dedicated electronic circuit capable of the high-speed calculations needed in CT.

The large array parallel processor (LAPP) architecture, a customized parallel-pipelined architecture, is used in one state-of-the-art scanner (Fig. 7-12). The LAPP architecture features four key elements: speed, power, flexibility, and expandability. To accommodate these elements, the LAPP architecture consists of the following:

- Multiple dedicated processors (voxel processor) and storage to accommodate high-speed data acquisition such as spiral/helical imaging and 2D, 3D, and 4D image reconstruction, storage, display, and recording
- Dedicated image storage and independent manipulation of data including raw spiral/helical data. The LAPP architecture can accommodate 22 gigabytes (GB) of storage capacities. Table 7-1 illustrates storage capacities for the system disk, spiral disk, visualization disk, standard 8-mm tape, and the optional optical disk for the Picker PQ 6000 CT imaging system.
- The Digital Imaging and Communications in Medicine (DICOM) network is the stan-

TABLE 7-1

Storage Capacities for the Picker PQ-6000 CT Imaging System

	STANDARD CONFIGURATION	SPIRAL-ENHANCED CONFIGURATION
Total online capacity		
Capacity	22.5 gigabytes (GB)	22.5 GB
System disk		
Capacity	12.0 GB	8 GB
Storage: uncompressed images (512²)	15,000 (7.5 days**)	10,000 (5 days)
Storage: compressed images (512²)	30,000 (15 days)	20,000 (10 days)
Spiral disk		
Scan cache	512 megabytes (MB)	512 MB
Cache storage	94 revolutions	94 revolutions
Standard volume disk	4.0 GB	8.0 GB
Standard volume disk storage	700 revolutions	1400 revolutions
Optional total storage	1400 revolutions	N/A
Visualization disk		
Capacity	6.0 GB	6.0 GB
Storage: uncompressed images (512²)	8800	8800
Standard 8-mm tape		
Capacity	2.2 GB	2.2 GB
Storage: uncompressed images (512²)	4000 (2 days)	4000 (2 days)
Storage: compressed images (512²)	8000 (4 days)	8000 (4 days)
Optional optical disk		
Storage:		
Uncompressed images (512²)	350/side	350/side
	700/platter	700/platter
Compressed images (512²)	700/side	700/side
	1400/platter	1400/platter

*Image disk space can be customized to include image archiving, scan data archiving, and other features.
**Assuming 2000 images/day in an average day.
(Courtesy Picker International; Cleveland, Ohio.)

dard for connectivity in radiology. It allows multimodality and multivendor equipment to connect electronically to facilitate data and image communications.

CT Software

The operator must be able to communicate with the system to enable scanning, which may be activated through keyboard commands or a touch screen (Fig. 7-13). In the case of the touch screen, the operator can select prestored protocols, modify protocol parameters, or select the sharp, smooth, or standard algorithm, depending on the CT examination.

Scanner Control and Image Reconstruction

Image Display and Manipulation. A wide range of image display and manipulation techniques is afforded by the CT software.

Operating Systems. Operating systems are programs that control the hardware components and the overall operation of the computer; they also enable the computer to run other programs. The operating system consists of a major program called the *supervisor,* which resides in primary memory and controls all other portions of the operating system. CT computers often use interleaved processing techniques such as multitasking, multiprocessing, and multiprogramming, which allow computers to process several programs almost si-

multaneously and thus increase the number of jobs the computer can handle at any given time. In addition, the system runs rapidly and efficiently. The operating system used in some CT systems is UNIX compatible and facilitates multiuser and multitasking capabilities.

IMAGE DISPLAY, STORAGE, RECORDING, AND COMMUNICATIONS

Image Display

A display device for CT is generally a black-and-white or color monitor (Fig. 7-14). Whereas images are usually displayed in gray scale, nonimage data such as text fields, patient data, and option selections can be displayed in color.

The image display system includes such features as the display matrix, pixel size, bit depth, CT value scale, image monitor and the number of lines, selectable window width and window center, single and double windows, and highlighting.

Image Storage

Data are stored in digital form to preserve the wide dynamic range of images, including the capability for image processing and intensity transformations, and to decrease the possibility of lost records and reduce the space needed for archiving.

Digital images are stored in 2D pixel arrays; each pixel point is represented by a number of bits that determine how many gray levels can be repre-

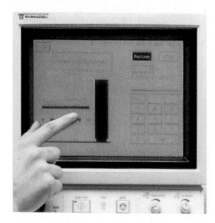

FIG. 7-13. The touch screen enables the operator to communicate with the CT system without keyboard commands. (Courtesy Shimadzu Medical Systems; Seattle, Wash.)

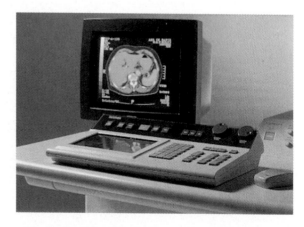

FIG. 7-14. The CT display monitor shows an image and text windows. (Courtesy Toshiba America Medical Systems; Tustin, Calif.)

sented by a particular pixel. A typical CT image has a matrix size of 512 × 512 × 8 bytes (12 bits). In this case, each has a gray level range of 512 (2^8) to 4096 (2^{12}).

A CT image of 512 × 512 × 2 bytes (16 bits) would require 0.5 megabytes (MB) of storage. If the CT examination contains about 50 images, then 25 MB of storage are needed. If 50 examinations are performed in 1 day, 1.25 GB of storage are needed (Frost et al, 1992).

Storage devices for CT include magnetic tape and disks, digital videotape, optical disks, and optical tape (Figs. 7-15 to 7-17).

Other considerations in CT image storage are the type, storage capacity, and typical number of images that can be stored on each device. Table 7-1 gives these considerations for the Picker PQ 6000 CT imaging system.

Laser Recording System

The requirements for hard copy recording of CT images are stringent because these images are used for diagnostic interpretation. The requirements are (1) broad gray-scale contrast resolution to enable the perception of subtle differences in tissue con-

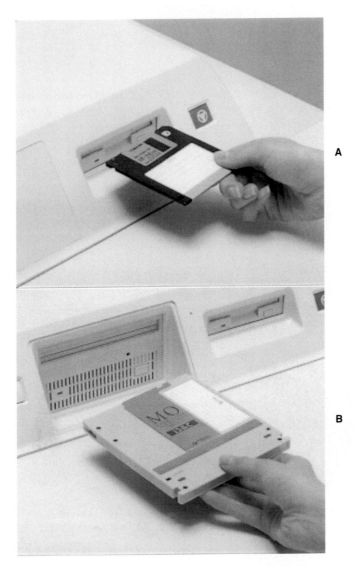

FIG. 7-15. Two magnetic storage devices used in CT: a microfloppy disk (**A**) and an optical disk (**B**). (Courtesy Toshiba America Medical Systems; Tustin, Calif.)

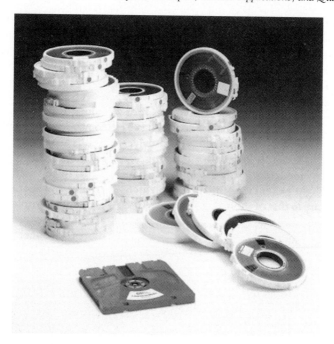

FIG. 7-16.   Optical disk for CT image storage. A single disk can hold the equivalent of 70 magnetic tapes. (From Alexander J, Krumme HJ: Somatom Plus: new perspectives in computerized tomography, *Electromedica* 56:50-56, 1988.)

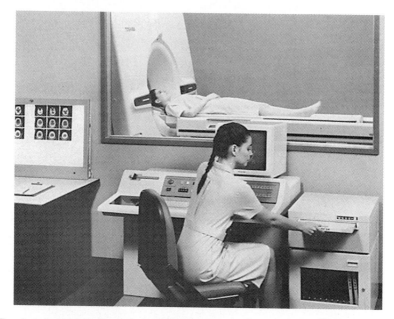

FIG. 7-17.   A technologist loads an optical disk into an optical disk unit. The Xpeed Toshiba CT scanner 5-GB optical disk can hold about 15,000 images. (Courtesy Toshiba America Medical Systems; Tustin, Calif.)

trast and (2) high spatial resolution to detect boundaries of different tissues (Lee et al, 1988).

Laser electronic image recording systems meet these requirements. Whereas multiformat video cameras were popular in the past, laser cameras, or laser imagers, are now used for the hard copy recording of digital images in digital radiography and fluoroscopy and MRI.

A laser imager, or laser printer (Fig. 7-18) is an expensive and sophisticated piece of electronic equipment. The laser and recording materials are important to the CT technologist because the film must match the spectral emission (wavelength) of the laser light.

Two types of lasers are available for film recording in CT: solid-state laser diodes and gas lasers such as helium-neon (He-Ne), helium, cadmium, argon, carbon dioxide, and nitrogen. The He-Ne laser is the simplest and most reliable gas laser. The solid-state laser typical of the 3M laser imaging systems has a wavelength of 820 nanometers (nm), but the He-Ne laser has a wavelength of 633 nm. Both systems use infrared-sensitive films (820 nm) and He-Ne laser films sensitive to the 633-nm wavelength beam.

The steps in laser-printing a film (Fig. 7-19) are as follows:

1. When the appropriate command from the operator is received, an unexposed film is transported to the exposure region of the printer.

2. In the exposure region, the film is scanned systematically, line by line. The laser receives its signal from the computer to produce a latent image.

3. Depending on the printer, the laser-scanned film is sent to a receiving magazine or a chemical processor attached to the printer for development.

4. The result is a laser-printed film ready for viewing.

Communications

Communications refers to electronic networking or connectivity using a local-area or wide-area network. Connectivity ensures the transfer of data and images from multivendor and multimodality equipment using the DICOM standard.

CT CONTROL CONSOLE

CT control consoles have evolved into the integrated type (Fig. 7-20; see also Fig. 7-14). The multimedia concept allows the operator full con-

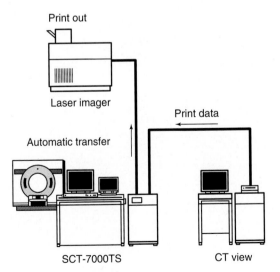

FIG. 7-18. The laser imager prints out images received from the CT scanner console and CT workstation (CT view). (Courtesy Shimadzu Medical Systems; Seattle, Wash.)

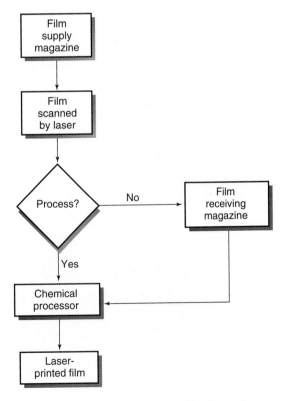

FIG. 7-19. Steps in printing a film with a laser printer.

trol of the physical system (e.g., gantry control) and allows for real-time processing such as multiplanar reformatting, 3D manipulation, zoom, and pan. The integrated console controls the entire system and enables the operation of various functions.

In general, an integrated console consists the following components:

- Floating keyboard: The floating keyboard can be positioned to facilitate use (Fig. 7-21). Important components include alphanumeric and special function keys, the trackball or mouse, and window controls.
- Touch panel: The touch panel (see Fig. 7-13) allows system parameters such as scan setup and control parameters to be actuated without typed keyboard commands.

- Window controls: Window controls include the window width and window level controls, which alter picture contrast. *Window width* refers to the range of CT numbers. *Window level* is the center of the range.
- Video display monitor: CT images are displayed on a monitor for viewing and manipulation by the operator before the final image is recorded and stored.
- Floppy disk drive: CT control consoles usually feature floppy disk drives.
- Control functions: Various automated functions such as autoarchive, autowindow, and autovoice are featured on CT control consoles. They allow the technologist to devote more time to the scanning procedure and the needs of the patient.

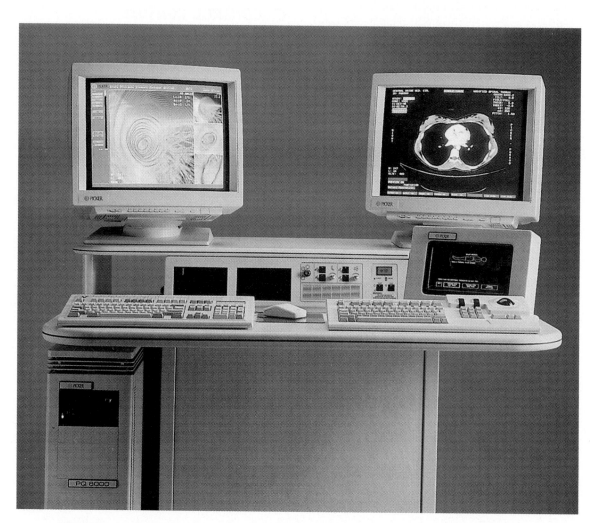

FIG. 7-20. Integrated control console of the Picker PQ-6000 CT scanner for both data acquisition (*right console*) and image visualization (*left console*). (Courtesy Picker International; Cleveland, Ohio.)

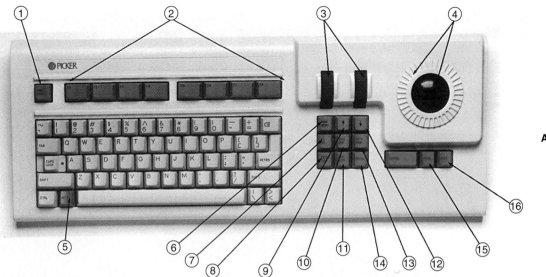

A

Keyboard Controls

(1) **Previous page:** Takes the specific display, function or task back one level.

(2) **Function keys:** Eight soft function keys are used to access and initiate various display functions. The command code for the eight soft keys is displayed and updated on the menu bar of the monitor.

(3) **Window controls:** Gray scale controls to set window width and level.

(4) **Trackball/theta ring:** X, Y, and Z axes can be controlled to position the movable cursor or for various display functions such as image reformatting.

(5) **Help:** The HELP key is always active to explain the current function.

(6) **Main menu:** Returns to the main menu. Various submenus can then be selected.

(7) **Patient directory:** Displays patient directory to select a study for display.

(8) **Enter text:** Activates keyboard to enter patient information.

(9) **Up arrow:** Moves up a directory or menu.

(10) **Save display:** Current image with any graphics is saved on disk as a "stack" or stored image.

(11) **Display keys:** "Masks" menu bar legends appearing on the display for filming.

(12) **Down arrow:** Moves down a directory or menu.

(13) **Data page:** Displays data page for current image.

(14) **Prevu:** Displays images as they are reconstructed.

(15) **Prior:** Prior image in study or prior page in menu is displayed.

(16) **Next:** Next image in study or next page in menu is displayed.

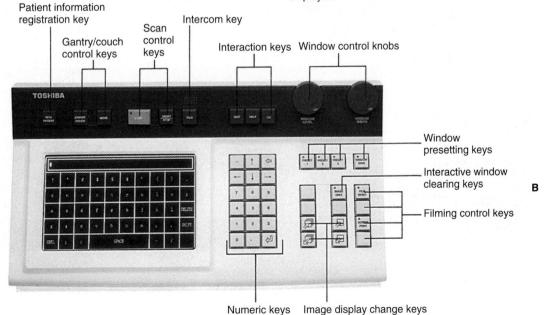

B

FIG. 7-21. Major features of two keyboards. (**A,** Courtesy Picker International; Cleveland, Ohio; **B,** Courtesy Toshiba America Medical Systems; Tustin, Calif.)

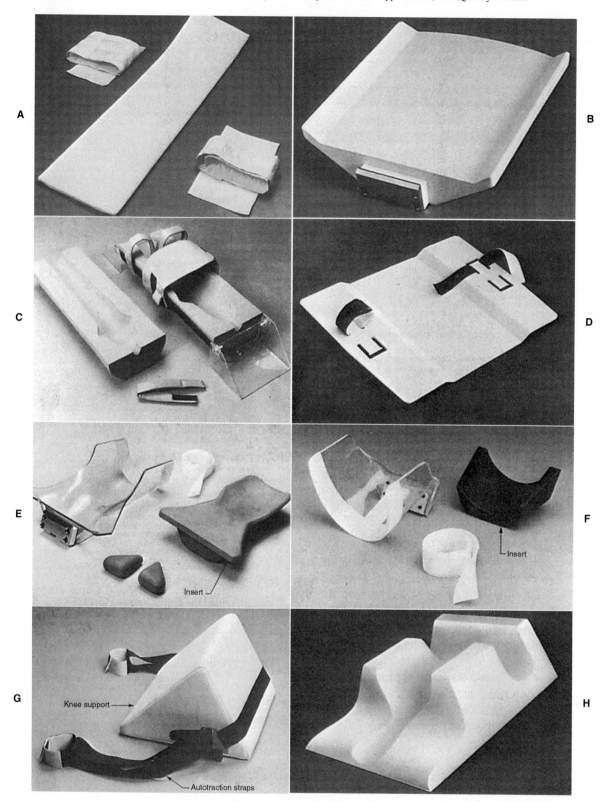

FIG. 7-22. Several accessories for CT scanners. **A,** Table mattress; **B,** table extender; **C,** pediatric cradle; **D,** arm support for procedures such as intravenous injections; **E,** axial head holder; **F,** coronal head holder; **G,** knee support with autotraction straps; **H,** head pillow with hand rest. (Courtesy Elscint; Hackensack, NJ.)

OPTIONS AND ACCESSORIES FOR CT SYSTEMS

Options

CT hardware options include optical disks, optical cartridge tape, remote diagnostic stations, independent workstations, and laser cameras.

Software options include packages for bone mineral analysis, dynamic scan, 3D image reconstruction, volumetric multiplanar reformatting, evaluation of regional cerebral blood flow (xenon CT), perfusion CT, dental CT, and networking.

Accessories

Accessories support and provide excellent immobilization of the patient to enhance the overall efficiency of the CT examination. These accessories include pediatric cradles, arm and leg supports, table mattresses, side rails, table extenders, knee supports, head pillows with hand rests, axial and coronal head holders, and autotraction straps (Fig. 7-22).

OTHER CONSIDERATIONS

Modular Design Concept

The modular design concept is intended to simplify the upgrading of scanners. The hardware modular design concept features detector modules, analog-to-digital conversion cards, tubes, genera-

tors and subassemblies, memory boards, array processors, back-projectors, display camera interfaces, and network interface boards (Fig. 7-23). Software modules allow for the easy modification, updating, and revision of software packages to meet the demands of the clinical environment.

Operating Modes of the Scanner

A modern CT scanner can operate in a variety of modes to meet the requirements of various clinical examinations. Operating modes include a routine scan mode and a rapid or dynamic scan mode. Various spiral/helical scan modes such as overlap scan, skip scan, and tilt scan are available to suit the needs of the examination (Fig. 7-24).

Room Layout for CT Equipment

The room layout for CT scanners varies among institutions and depends on the particular type of scanner. The typical room layout (Fig. 7-25) includes at least three sections or rooms to house different components of the scanner, as follows:

1. The scanning room houses the gantry and patient couch. This room should be large enough to accommodate gurneys and emergency equipment.
2. The computer room generally houses the host computer and other peripheral computing equipment.

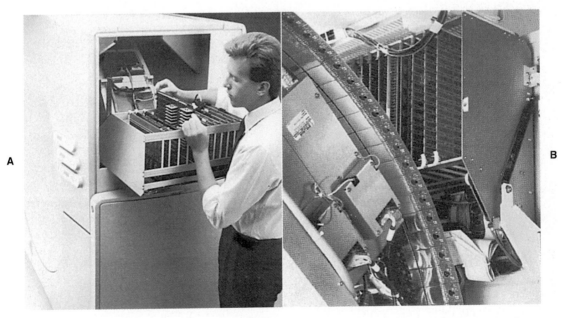

FIG. 7-23. Hardware modules for modern CT scanners. **A,** Electronic circuit boards; **B,** detector modules. (Courtesy Picker International; Cleveland, Ohio.)

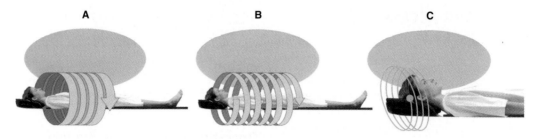

FIG. 7-24.   Three scan modes for spiral/helical CT scanning. Each scan mode includes Overlap Scan, which is useful to make high quality 3D images. Skip Scan can be used to scan a wide area in a short amount of time. Tilt Scan is used with various gantry tilts. **A,** High-quality 3D images: overlap scan; **B,** Short time/wide range scan: skip scan; **C,** According to head OM line: tilt scan. (Courtesy Shimadzu Medical Systems; Seattle, Wash.)

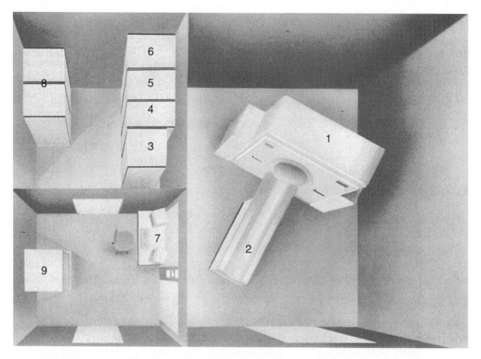

FIG. 7-25.   Typical room layout for CT scanning equipment: *1,* Scanner gantry; *2,* patient couch; *3-6 and 8,* computer and x-ray control cabinets; *7,* operator's console; *9,* multiformat camera. (Courtesy Siemens Medical Systems; Iselin, NJ.)

3. The control room houses the control console and film recording equipment.

An alternative room layout uses only the scanning room and control room (Fig. 7-26).

Equipment Specifications

The acquisition of a CT scanner is an interesting experience and the CT technologist should take advantage of the opportunity to participate in such an activity. The CT department or purchasing committee generally informs the vendor of the necessary equipment specifications. In addition, vendors will have equipment specifications available for review. (Specifications are listed in the Appendix.)

In general, the major technical specifications and features of a CT scanner to be considered are as follows:

1. The x-ray generator: both physical and operating parameters
2. The x-ray tube and detectors: heat storage capacity and cooling rates of the tube; the type, quantum detection, and conversion efficiencies of detectors

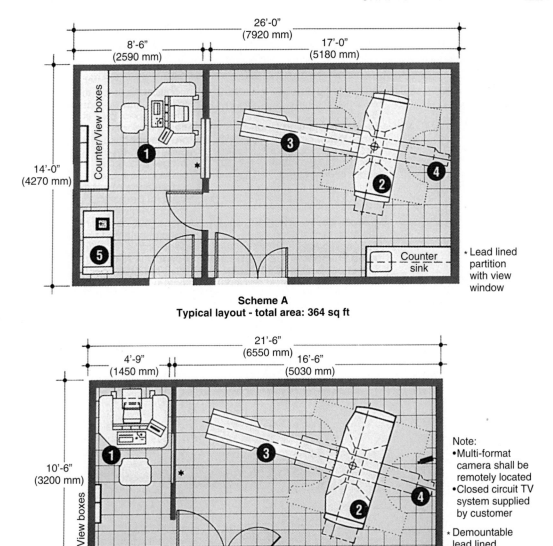

Scheme A
Typical layout - total area: 364 sq ft

Scheme B
Minimum room layout - total area: 226 sq ft
(Laser imager remotely located)

FIG. 7-26. Two schemes for an alternative room layout for the Picker PQ-2000 CT scanner. (Courtesy Picker International; Cleveland, Ohio.)

3. Scanning gantry: aperture size, tilting range, and laser positioning aids and controls
4. Patient couch: movement characteristics and strength of the couch top
5. Operator's console: characteristics of the display monitor, keyboard, and touch panel control; general ergonomics, film recording, and storage considerations
6. Physician's console: hardware and software

7. Computer hardware: the main CPU and storage
8. Computer software: image reconstruction, display, visualization and analysis packages
9. Workstations: both hardware and software
10. Laser imagers
11. Accessories
12. Quality control equipment

REFERENCES

Alexander J, Krumme HJ: Somatom Plus: new perspectives in computerized tomography, *Electromedica* 56:50-56, 1988.

Frost MM et al: Image archival technologies, *Radiographics* 12:339-343, 1992.

Fugita K et al: Advanced computer architecture for CT, *Radiology* S:63, 1992.

Lee KR et al: Hard copy recordings of analog and digital images, *Invest Radiol* 23:933-939, 1988.

Picker International: *PQ-6000 CT imaging system,* Cleveland, Ohio, 1999, Picker International.

Siemens Medical Systems: *Somatom Plus product data,* Iselin, NJ, 1999, Siemens Medical Systems.

8

Image Manipulation

CHAPTER *Outline*

IMAGE MANIPULATION

Definition

Image manipulation belongs to the domain of digital image processing. Glen et al (1981) have defined image manipulation as "those techniques (operations) or processes which modify an image or group of images to enhance the visibility of useful information while suppressing 'noise' or non-useful information." Image manipulation operations do not produce any additional information. As a result, "the information content in the processed image is always less than or equal to that in the original image" (Glen et al, 1981).

Techniques

Image manipulation techniques fall into two categories: linear and nonlinear. Whereas linear techniques include such processes as image smoothing and enhancement, nonlinear techniques concern gray scale manipulation, in which the gray scale of the image can be modified with different algorithms. This chapter discusses nonlinear techniques.

The algorithm of interest is based on a point processing technique referred to as *gray level mapping*. (It is also referred to as "contrast enhancement," "contrast stretching," "histogram modification," "histogram stretching," or "windowing.") Windowing is the most common image processing technique in CT.

WINDOWING

Windowing refers to a method by which the CT image gray scale can be manipulated using the CT numbers of the image (Seeram, 1994). The operator (the viewer) can alter these numbers to provide an optimum demonstration of the different structures (Fig. 8-1). Fig. 8-1 shows the head, chest, and abdomen. Through the manipulation of CT numbers of the various tissues, the picture can be changed to show soft tissues such as the brain and dense structures such as bone.

The picture contrast is easily changed with two control mechanisms: the window width and window level.

Window Width and Window Level

The absorption measurement range in CT (expressed in Hounsfield units, or HU) is referred to as the *window width* (WW). It determines the maximal number of shades of gray that can be displayed on the CT monitor. The *window level* (WL) is the center or midpoint of the range of CT numbers and can be positioned anywhere on the WW (Fig. 8-2).

When the WW and WL are changed, the image can be enhanced to suit the needs of the viewer. "Specifically, a large window width indicates that there is a relatively long gray scale or a large block of CT numbers that will be assigned some value of gray. Thus, the transition zone between the lower CT numbers portrayed as black and the higher CT numbers portrayed as white will be large. A narrow window width implies that the transition from black to white will take place over a relatively few CT numbers" (Morgan, 1983).

Manipulating WW and WL

In Fig. 8-3, *A*, the CT numbers range from +1000 for bone to −1000 for air. In this case, the WW is 2000; that is, there are 1000 CT numbers above 0 and another 1000 numbers below 0. The midpoint of the range (WL) is 0; this is referred to as a *refer-*

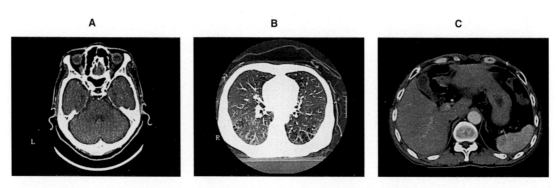

FIG. 8-1. Different structures and regions of the body can be optimized for viewing through windowing, in which the image gray scale is manipulated using the range of CT numbers that comprise the image. **A,** Brain; **B,** lung; **C,** abdomen. (Courtesy Toshiba America Medical Systems; Tustin, Calif.)

ence point because it represents water. Air, which is assigned a CT number of −1000, is also considered a reference point.

In Fig. 8-3, *B*, the WW is 200 and the WL is 0. At this setting, all CT numbers greater than +100 appear white and those less than −100 appear black, whereas those between +100 and −100 appear as shades of gray.

In Fig. 8-3, *C*, the WW is 200 and the WL is +40. CT numbers lower than −60 appear black, those greater than +140 appear white, and those between +140 and −60 appear as shades of gray.

In Fig. 8-3, *D*, the WW is 400 and the WL is 0. All CT numbers greater than +200 appear

white, those below −200 appear black, and those between +200 and −200 appear as shades of gray. If the entire range of CT numbers (the entire WW) is displayed, rather than a portion of the range, "small differences in attenuation between soft tissues will be obscured" (Zatz, 1980).

The CT number range varies between scanners. Whereas the range for some CT scanners varies from −1000 to +3095 HU (4095 CT numbers), the range for other scanners is −2048 to +6143 HU (8191 CT numbers). The tissue gray scale is stretched out with white at one end, black at the other, and shades of gray in between. The gray scale changes as the WW is expanded or nar-

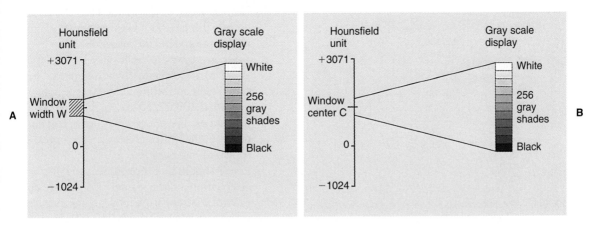

FIG. 8-2. The concept of window width (**A**) and window level (**B**) in CT windowing. (Courtesy Siemens Medical Systems; Iselin, NJ.)

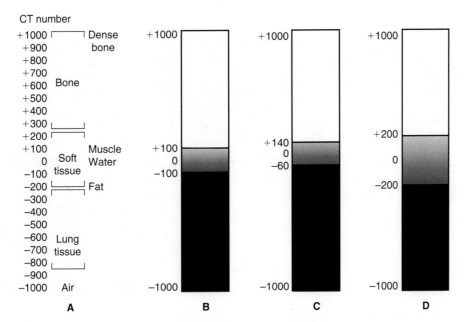

FIG. 8-3. Graphic illustration of the effect of different window width and window level settings on the appearance of the CT image.

rowed. For bone structures, the WW must include the higher CT numbers on the scale. For structures that contain air, the WW moves toward the lower CT numbers on the scale. Similarly, the WL can fall anywhere on the scale, depending on the structures of interest (Fig. 8-4). An example of the ef-

CT number

```
+1000 ┌─────┐ Dense
 +900        bone   (M + W/2)
 +800
 +700
 +600  Bone           Window      Window
 +500               level (M)     width (W)
 +400
 +300  └─────┘
 +200  ┌─────┐        (M − W/2)
 +100          Muscle
    0   Soft    Water
 −100  tissue
 −200  └──────┘ Fat
 −300
 −400
 −500
 −600  Lung
 −700  tissue
 −800  └──────┘
 −900
−1000   Air
```

FIG. 8-4. The relationship between window level (WL) and window width (WW). These windows can be moved along the scale to optimize views of particular structures.

fect of WW and WL adjustment on the appearance of the CT image is shown for the thorax (Fig. 8-5).

In his discussion of the proper use of WW and WL in clinical CT, Berland (1987) noted the following:

1. Wide windows (400 to 2000 HU) should be used to encompass tissues of greatly differing attenuation within the image. For example, body scans are usually filmed at 350 to 600 HU to encompass the attenuation numbers of fat, fluid, and muscle. Lung and bone are filmed at 1000 to 2000 HU to include air spaces and vessels for lungs and cortex and marrow for bone.

2. Narrow windows (50 to 350 HU) should be used to display soft tissues within structures that contain different tissues of similar densities. For example, brain may be displayed at 80 to 150 HU to show differences between gray and white matter. Liver may be viewed at 100 to 250 HU to highlight liver metastases. The effect of both wide and narrow window widths on image appearance is shown in Fig. 8-6.

3. Levels should be centered near the average attenuation of the tissues of interest. For example, attenuation body scans may be viewed at a level of 0 to 60 HU because fat has attenuation numbers from −60 to

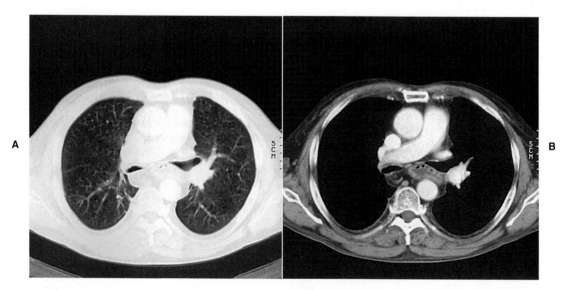

FIG. 8-5. The effect of window width and window level adjustments on image appearance. **A,** A lung window width of 1500 HU and a window level of −530 HU are used. **B,** A soft-tissue window width of 500 HU and a window level of +40 HU are used. (Courtesy Siemens Medical Systems; Iselin, NJ.)

−100 HU whereas the attenuation numbers of muscle and organs may range from 60 to 150 HU with intravenous contrast. Lung is viewed at a level of −600 to –750 HU.

Effect of WW on Image Contrast

In general, the viewer can alter the contrast of the CT image by changing the WW (Fig. 8-7). When the WW is large (wide WW), the three different structures—the lung, liver (soft tissues), and pelvis (bone)—have the same gray tone (*bottom of diagram*). With a narrow WW, there is very sharp contrast to the point where the lungs appear black, bone appears white, and the liver is shown as gray tones. Finally, image contrast is optimized with the use of a medium WW (*middle of diagram*).

The following conclusions may be drawn from the effect of WW settings of 10, 150, 300, and 500 on images of the brain with a fixed WL (+50) (Fig. 8-8):

1. As the WW increases, the contrast decreases.
2. As the WW decreases, the contrast becomes greater. The image appears totally black and white with a WW of 10 (Fig. 8-8, A).
3. Contrast is optimized with medium WW settings and is best when the image is recorded with a WW of 150 for the posterior fossa structures (Fig. 8-8, B).

Effect of WL on Image Display

The WL is the CT number in the middle of the WW and represents the medium gray scale (Fig. 8-9). When the WL is centered on the lungs (lower CT numbers), the image display is optimized for that structure and the liver (soft tissue) and pelvis (bone) are displayed as white. On the other hand, when the WL is centered on the pelvis (higher CT numbers), the image display is optimized for the pelvis and the lungs and liver appear black. Finally, with the WL centered on the liver (middle CT numbers), the pelvis appears white and the liver is optimized for viewing.

The effects of different WL settings (with fixed WW) on the display of images of the head are shown in Fig. 8-10. As the WL increases from +50 to +200, the picture changes from white (Fig. 8-10, A) to black (Fig. 8-10, D). As the WL moves toward the higher CT numbers (generally white), more CT numbers with lower values (generally black) are displayed.

Preset Windows

Preset windows are available on scanners to optimize windowing. For example, a double (dual) window display will facilitate the simultaneous display of two different density ranges. Both windows have different window widths and window levels (Fig. 8-11). Whereas a single window setting

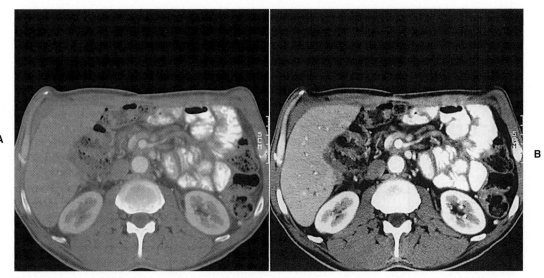

FIG. 8-6. The effect of a wide window width (**A**) and a narrow window width (**B**) on the appearance of the CT image. (Courtesy Siemens Medical Systems; Iselin, NJ.)

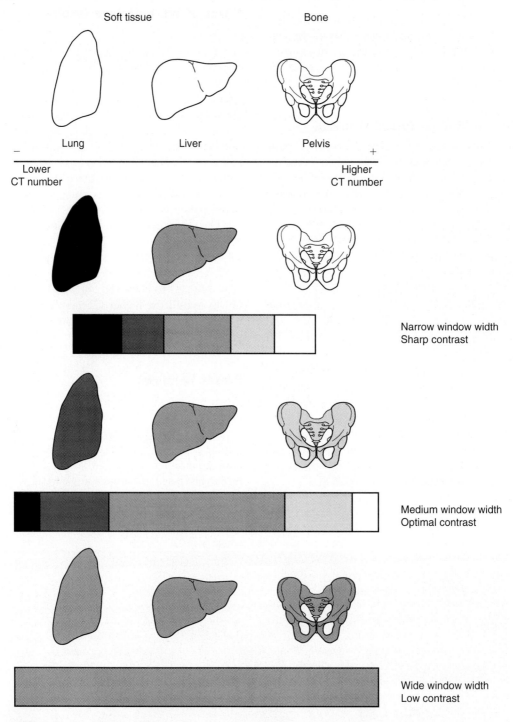

FIG. 8-7. The effect of window width on the appearance of different organs with widely varying CT numbers.

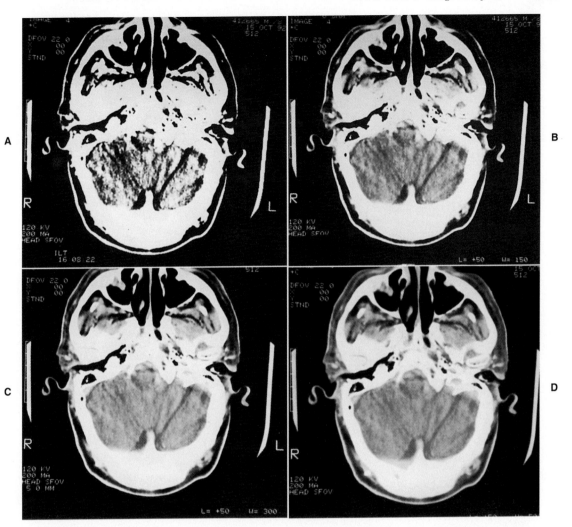

FIG. 8-8. Effect of different window width (WW) settings on image contrast with a fixed window level setting. As WW increases, contrast decreases. **A,** WW = 10; **B,** WW = 150; **C,** WW = 300; **D,** WW = 500.

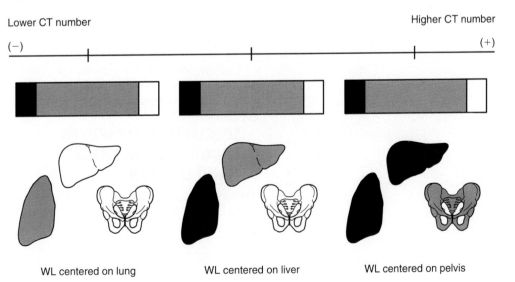

FIG. 8-9. The effect of window level (WL) on gray tone appearance of different organs.

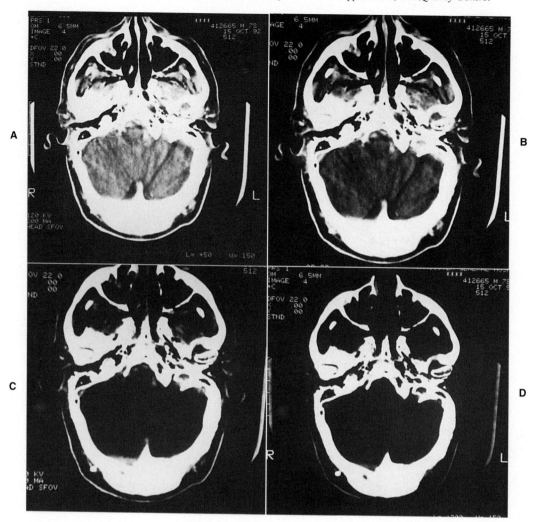

FIG. 8-10. Effect of different window level (WL) settings on image display with a fixed window width (WW). Essentially, the image changes from white to black as the WL is increased. **A,** WL = +50. **B,** WL = +100. **C,** WL = +150. **D,** WL = +200.

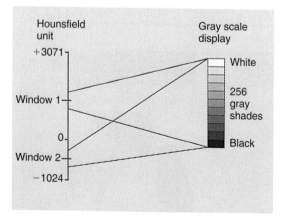

FIG. 8-11. The fundamental principles of the double (dual) window setting. (Courtesy Siemens Medical Systems, Iselin, NJ.)

displays one anatomic region, a double (or dual) window display provides well-defined contours to separate two different anatomic areas (Fig. 8-12).

SPECIALIZED COMPUTER PROGRAMS FOR IMAGE MANIPULATION

Various programs are available for image manipulation in CT, such as multiplanar reconstruction, quantitative CT (osteo-CT), 3D imaging, xenon CT, and radiation therapy treatment planning. In addition, other programs provide graphic aids such as region of interest (ROI), arrows, grids, histogram, and annotation.

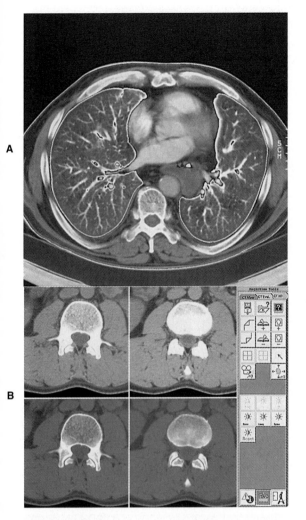

FIG. 8-12. **A,** A double (dual) window display with a WW and WL of 750 HU and −730 HU, respectively, using a WW and WL of 500 HU and 35 HU, respectively. **B,** Dual windows allow the observer to view bone and soft tissue windows of the same images simultaneously. (Courtesy Siemens Medical Systems; Iselin, NJ.)

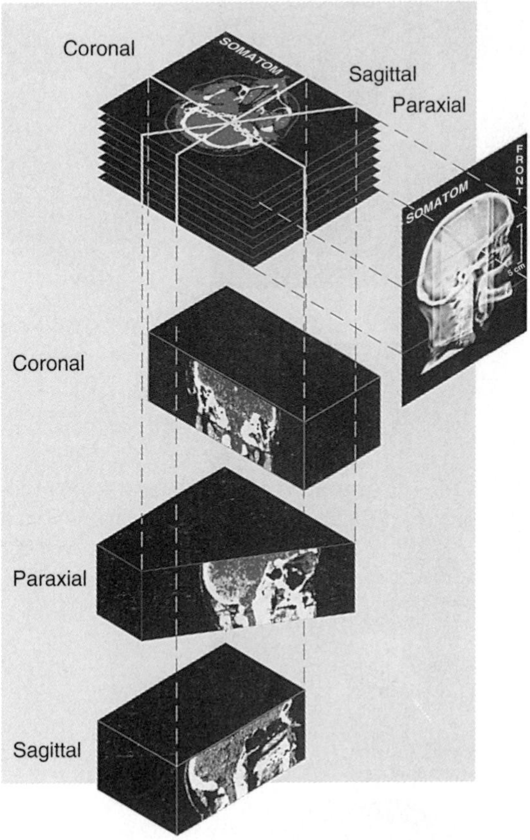

FIG. 8-13. Multiplanar reconstruction involves the use of a computer program to reformat sagittal, paraxial, and coronal views from a stack of contiguous transverse axial images. (Courtesy Siemens Medical Systems; Iselin, NJ.)

Multiplanar Reconstruction

Multiplanar reconstruction, sometimes referred to as *image reformatting* or *image reformation*, is a computer program to create coronal, sagittal, and paraxial images from a stack of contiguous transverse axial scans (Fig. 8-13).

Whereas the sagittal image defines a plane that passes through an anatomic region from anterior to posterior and divides the body into right and left sections, the coronal image defines a plane that passes through the body region from right to left (or left to right), dividing the region into anterior and posterior sections. The paraxial image, on the other hand, defines a plane that cuts through the coronal and sagittal planes in the longitudinal direction of an anatomic region.

Irregular, oblique, and other views can also be generated. The irregular view (e.g., linear or curved) can be reconstructed from a stack of contiguous transverse images (Fig. 8-14). The oblique view can be reconstructed with at least three arbitrarily definable points in different transverse images (Fig. 8-15).

In the conceptual framework to generate these images (Fig. 8-16), the voxel on the left represents the information contained and stored in a specific volume of tissue. In reformatting, the computer program uses any set of points to build an image of

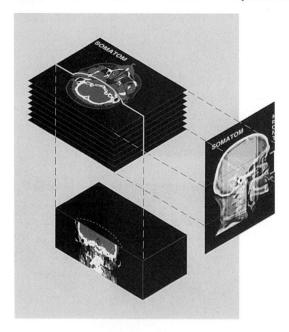

FIG. 8-14. Irregular views can be created through multiplanar reconstruction techniques using the images from a stack of contiguous transaxial slices. (Courtesy Siemens Medical Systems; Iselin, NJ.)

the selected plane. Mackay (1984) has noted the following:

Suppose in the figure that the first image computed and stored was the left-hand face of the cube, followed by the plane parallel to it with the number 2, after which the third set of projections would be collected to form the parallel plane containing the number 3, and so on. All the points in the cube would gradually be accumulated and stored in the computer, and it is convenient to think of the position of the storage of a number as corresponding to the position of a point in the cube. Any of the original planes could be displayed by "calling up" the number representing the points in that plane and producing a proportional brightness on the oscilloscope screen at the corresponding position. On the screen instead could be displayed the

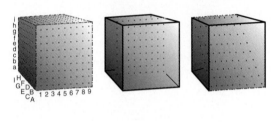

| Stored point information | One orthogonal reconstruction | Tilted reconstruction |

FIG. 8-16. A conceptual framework for generating reformatted images in CT.

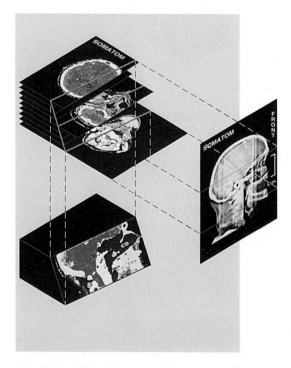

FIG. 8-15. Oblique views can be reconstructed by multiplanar reconstruction techniques using definable points in different transaxial slices. (Courtesy Siemens Medical Systems; Iselin, NJ.)

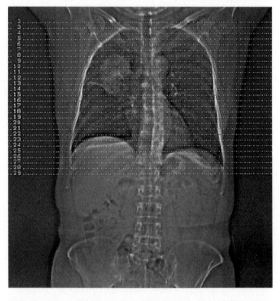

FIG. 8-17. Pre-scan localization image produced when the patient moves continuously through the gantry while the x-ray tube and detectors remain in a fixed position. (Courtesy Siemens Medical Systems; Iselin, NJ.)

dots shown at the center section [of Fig. 8-16]. On the lower left of the screen would be displayed the point designated (1, B, a), which came from the first section, for example. Next to it would be displayed a point from the bottom of the second section and in one increment from the right side, and so on. By sequentially calling up all the points located inward one increment from the right face of the cube one can display a section through the subject perpendicular to all the planes that were originally scanned. In the display one can instead move to the left one increment from each successive step inward to a new line on the television screen; this results in the display of a plane at an angle through the body as shown in the right-hand part of the figure. It should be clear that from this array of computed data one can display any section through the volume. Often the sections across a subject are more widely spaced than are the lines across the section in making the original projections, in which case the resolution in a tilted display will not be the same up and down as across the image.

There are both advantages and disadvantages to reformatted images (see box below). Major advantages include the following:

1. To enable the visualization of specific structures such as the optic nerves and lesions in relation to surrounding structures.
2. To determine the true extent of lesions or fractures and to help localize lesions and intraarticular bone fragments or foreign bodies (Fishman et al, 1992).

One major disadvantage of multiplanar reconstruction relates to image quality. Image detail is not as good as that obtained in transaxial images. The reformatted image quality depends on the quality of the axial images, and it is therefore important that the patient does not move or breathe during the scanning procedure. In addition, the plane thickness affects image detail and thus thick planes result in blurring and loss of structural detail.

Quantitative CT

Quantitative CT (QCT) is the most sensitive of all x-ray techniques for the measurement of the mineral content of trabecular bone in osteoporosis (Goodsitt and Johnson, 1992). This measurement is the bone mineral density (BMD).

QCT involves at least seven steps, as follows:

1. A prescan localization image is obtained (Fig. 8-17). This is sometimes referred to as a *scout view* (General Electric), *topogram* (Siemens), or *pilot scan* (Picker). The image is obtained as the patient moves through the gantry aperture while the x-ray tube and detector remain stationary. The computer then builds an image that resembles a conventional radiographic image.
2. The slices are selected from the prescan localization image, and the midvertebral planes are examined.
3. Transverse axial images are obtained. At this time, a reference phantom (Fig. 8-18, A) that contains water and bone-equivalent parts, is positioned and scanned with the patient (Fig. 8-18, B).
4. An automatic contour tracing (Nagel et al, 1987) of trabecular and cortical regions of interest (ROI) is obtained (Fig. 8-19).
5. The computer calculates the mean values of the ROI.

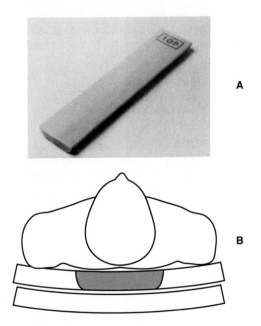

FIG. 8-18. Reference phantom (**A**) and its position in relation to the patient (**B**) for quantitative CT.

REFORMATTED IMAGES

Advantages
- Enables visualization of specific structures in relation to surrounding structures
- Determines extent of lesions or fractures
- Helps to localize lesions, bone fragments, or foreign bodies

Disadvantages
- Loss of image detail

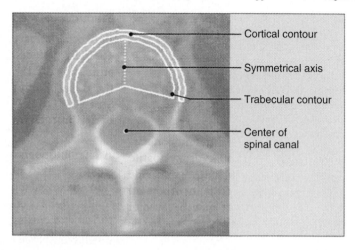

- Cortical contour
- Symmetrical axis
- Trabecular contour
- Center of spinal canal

FIG. 8-19.   Automatic contour tracing of trabecular and cortical regions of interest. (From Nagel W et al: Recent clinical results on the use of QCT in diagnosis of osteoporosis, *Electromedica* 55:104-110, 1987.)

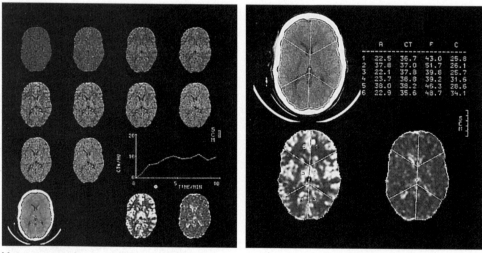

Measurement of regional CBF with XENON CT   Evaluation of the XENON CT measurement

FIG. 8-20.   Images from a xenon CT study (CBF, cerebral blood flow). (Courtesy Siemens Medical Systems; Iselin, NJ.)

6. The ROI values are converted to BMD values.
7. An image graphics output is obtained, which shows the BMD values plotted as a function of age. The bone mineral content is then determined and compared with normal values (Kalender et al, 1989).

Xenon CT

The use of xenon gas in CT is possible with inhalation equipment. Its high atomic number, high-fat solubility, and ability to cross the blood-brain barrier make xenon an ideal gas for regional cerebral blood flow imaging and the study of brain function (Fig. 8-20). As pointed out by Berland (1987), "Xenon contrast inhalation studies have demonstrated a wide variety of cerebral disorders, but the technique is particularly useful in evaluating regional perfusion in cerebrovascular disease and in studying brain metabolism. It may find a significant clinical role in dementia, degenerative and sleep disorders, migraines, and epilepsy."

3D Imaging

Special software gathers information from the transaxial scan data to display 3D images on a 2D television screen (Fig. 8-21).

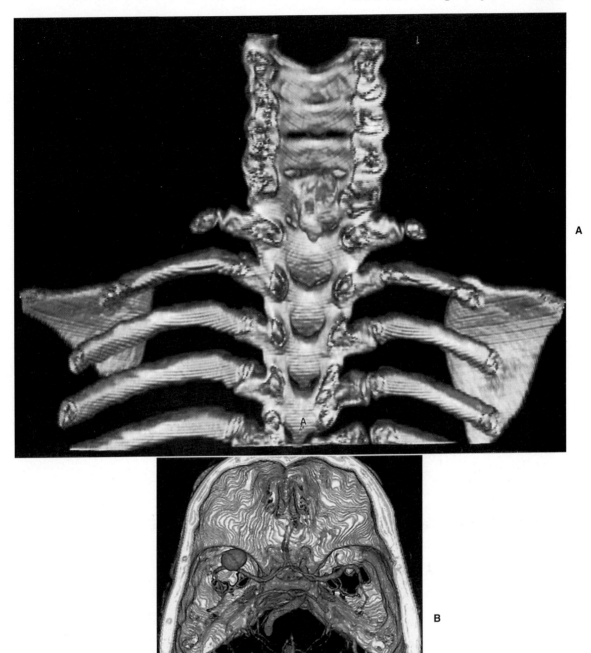

FIG. 8-21. Examples of 3D images. (Courtesy Vital Images; Minneapolis, Minn.)   *Continued*

C

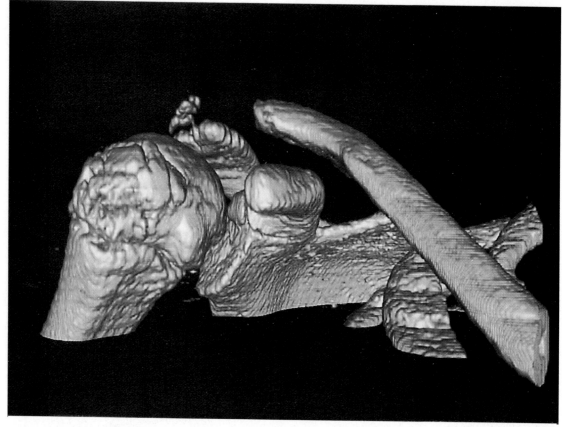

FIG. 8-21, cont'd. Examples of 3D images.

Radiation Therapy Treatment Planning

CT is used in radiation treatment planning (RTP) according to the following protocol:

1. Patients are first examined by conventional CT, during which they are placed in exactly the same position as they would be on the radiation treatment planning couch or table.
2. The scan data go to the CT computer.
3. The processed data are stored on magnetic tapes.
4. The magnetic tape data are fed into the RTP computer.
5. Images are subsequently displayed and used in plans for radiation beam positions and depth dose calculations. Isodose curves are also superimposed on the image, and the appropriate treatment plan is determined.
6. In the final step, the patient receives the radiation treatment.

In RTP, CT numbers are used to calculate physical and electron densities, which are then used in the dose computations.

VISUALIZATION TOOLS

Visualization tools such as windowing are computer programs that provide the observer-diagnostician with additional information to facilitate diagnosis. Visualization tools range from basic to advanced.

Basic Tools

Basic visualization tools are basic computer programs integrated into the CT system with the following capabilities (Fig. 8-22):

1. Multiple imaging and multiple windows (Fig. 8-22, A)
2. Image magnification (Fig. 8-22, B)
3. Evaluation of geometric characteristics such as distances and angles (Fig. 8-22, C)
4. Superimposition of coordinates on the image to provide a reference for biopsies (Fig. 8-22, D)
5. Highlighting, in which the pixels in certain regions of the image can be made to appear brighter (Fig. 8-22, E)

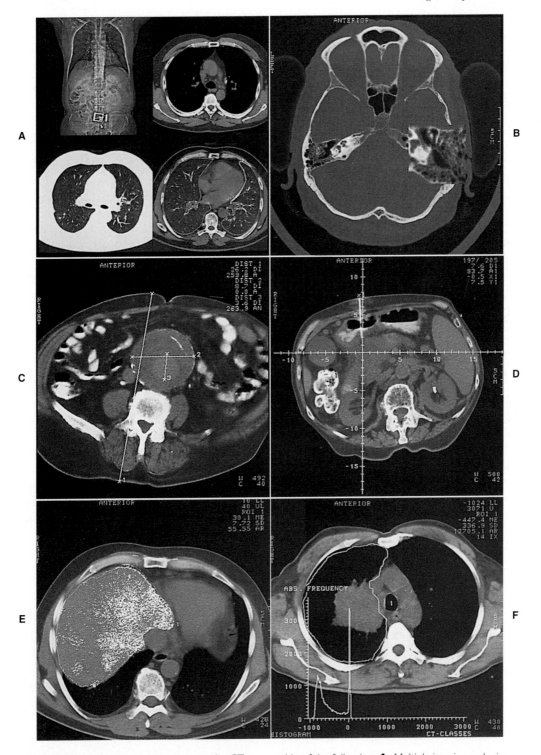

FIG. 8-22. Other computer programs for CT are capable of the following: **A,** Multiple imaging and windows; **B,** image magnification; **C,** measurement of distances; **D,** superimposition of coordinates on the image; **E,** highlights; and **F,** histogram. (Courtesy Siemens Medical Systems; Iselin, NJ.)

6. CT histogram, which is a plot of the pixel values as a function of the frequency with which each value occurs. This can be done for the entire image or a portion of the image, as defined by the ROI (Fig. 8-22, F).
7. ROI statistics, which allow for statistical calculations such as the mean and standard deviation within the ROI
8. ROI transfer, whereby the ROI can be transferred from slice to slice
9. Split imaging, in which an image can be split into two detailed thin slices, and fused imaging, in which two contiguous thin slices can be fused into a single thick slice

Optional software packages are also available for dental CT applications, dynamic CT, networking, workstations, and 3D imaging.

Advanced Tools

Advanced visualization tools require powerful computer workstations (Fig. 8-23) with advanced image processing capabilities and increased memory to handle the vast amount of data used in various visualization techniques. Currently, a wide variety of advanced visualization tools are commercially available, as follows:

- 3D visualization tools allow the user to render various 3D images from the axial data set. 3D rendering falls into three categories: surface shaded display (surface rendering), volume rendering, and maximum intensity projection (MIP).
- Computed tomography angiography (CTA) is a relatively new technique based on volume scanning principles. CTA is an application of 3D imaging and is becoming more popular in the examination of the circulatory system. Examples of CTA visualization tools include 4D angio (Picker International; Cleveland, Ohio), vessel tracking, skull removal, and multiple target volume.
- In 4D angio, the fourth dimension is opacity instead of time. 4D angio is based on volume rendering technology. Changes in the opacity values of various tissues enable the observer to simultaneously visualize bone, soft tissues, and vascular structures and therefore both foreground and background structures are visible (Fig. 8-24). Fig. 8-24 shows a comparison of the conventional MIP and 4D angio images of the liver, kidney, and superior mesenteric vein. 4D angio is useful and is preferred over conventional MIP

techniques for the visualization of aortic aneurysms, renal arteries, stents, and carotid bifurcation. Target Volume MIP (TVMIP) allows the user to render only a selected volume of data and does not require segmentation techniques.

- The vessel tracking tool allows the user to produce a set of MPR images (batches) including curved MPR images for the entire vessel. The skull removal tool facilitates the subtraction of bones of the skull from the CTA image and allows the observer to visualize very detailed images of the vessels and soft tissues. Fig. 8-25 shows clinical examples of TVMIP, vessel tracking, curved MPR, and skull removal.
- Multiplanar reconstruction tools display all types of MPR images from the axial data set in the axial, coronal, sagittal, and oblique planes.
- Interactive visualization tools offer the following features in any 3D rendering mode: window/level adjustment, volume of interest adjustment, scan information display, movie creation and playback, split screen presentation, zoom, and measurements.
- Cine visualization tools allow the user to view a large set of images very quickly.

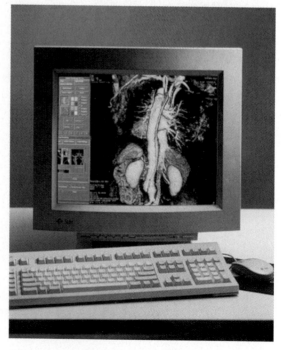

FIG. 8-23. An example of a workstation for advanced image processing. (Courtesy General Electric Medical Systems, Milwaukee, Wis.)

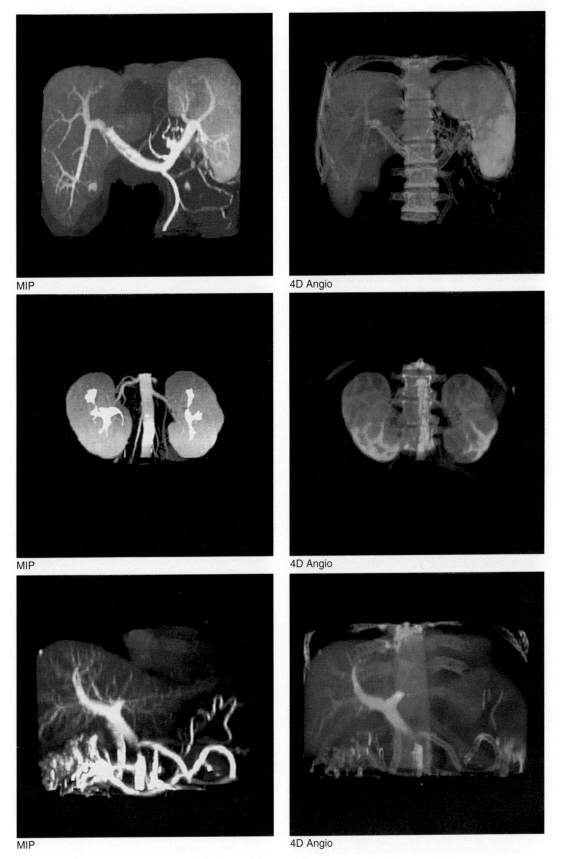

MIP
4D Angio

MIP
4D Angio

MIP
4D Angio

FIG. 8-24. A comparison of the appearance of conventional MIP and 4D angio CT images. (Courtesy Picker International; Cleveland, Ohio.)

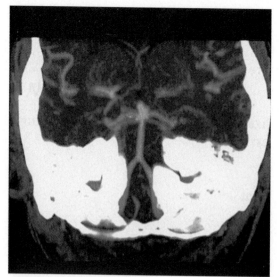

TVMIP

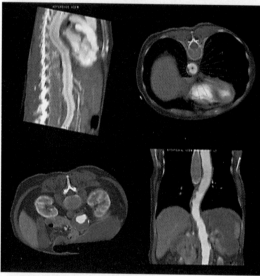

Vessel tracking

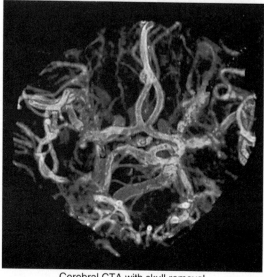

Cerebral CTA with skull removal

- Advanced quantitative measurement tools facilitate measurements such as distances, angles, areas, mean, standard deviation, minimum and maximum voxel values, density value in Hounsfield units, density histogram for a particular region of interest, and volume of 3D objects.
- Multimodality image fusion tools allow the user to combine images from a wide variety of imaging modalities such as CT, MRI, PET, and SPECT to facilitate diagnosis of tumor localization and quantification, surgical planning, and oncology planning (Fig. 8-26). In Fig. 8-26, two such images from CT and SPECT examinations are shown for the brain and abdomen.
- Virtual reality visualization tools include Voyager (Picker International; Cleveland, Ohio) and 3D Navigator. These tools create 3D and 4D images of tubular structures such as the colon and bronchi and allow the user to "fly through" the images of hollow organs in a technique referred to as CT *virtual endoscopy*, which is gaining widespread attention in radiologic imaging.

ADVANCED VISUALIZATION AND ANALYSIS WORKSTATIONS
Hardware Components

Hardware components include the central processing unit, various processors, data and image storage devices. The host computer of an advanced visualization and analysis workstation can be a Sun SPARC (Sun Microsystems) or a Silicon Graphics platform with varying amounts of random access memory (RAM) depending on the cost of the system. The operating system of both platforms is the UNIX multitasking system, which provides optimum speed and system response. In addition, these workstations feature various microprocessors to improve data processing (Fig. 8-27).

The monitor of the workstation must provide good image quality. These monitors are usually cathode ray tubes (CRTs) or flat panel displays with at least $2.5 \times 2K$ pixel resolution. Display monitors must be capable of a wide range of display

FIG. 8-25. Clinical examples of TVMIP, vessel tracking, curved MPR, and skull removal. (Courtesy Picker International; Cleveland, Ohio.)

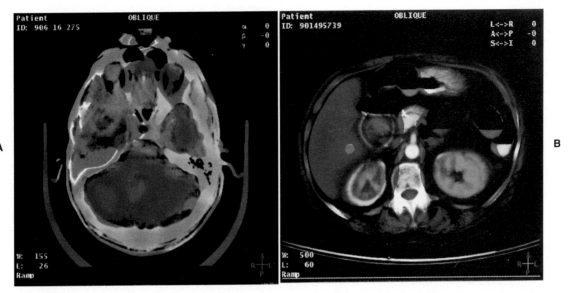

FIG. 8-26. Examples of image fusion from CT and SPECT examinations of the skull (**A**) and abdomen (**B**). (Courtesy Picker International; Cleveland, Ohio.)

formats, as shown in Fig. 8-27, A. If the monitor is used for image interpretation, it must be capable of a spatial resolution of ≥ 2.5 line pairs/mm and have a contrast resolution of ≥ 8 bits/pixel (American College of Radiology, 1998).

The keyboard is a full alphanumeric keyboard with function, archiving, and display keys. Additionally, a mouse can be used to communicate with the computer (Fig. 8-28).

Data and image storage devices include hard disks and 8-mm magnetic tape. The storage capacity of these media varies depending on the system. Typical image storage capacities are provided in Table 8-1.

Connectivity

Connectivity, or networking, is an important feature of current workstations because of the current trend toward filmless radiology departments through the implementation of picture archiving and communication systems, radiology information systems, and hospital information systems (see Chapter 2).

The transfer of data and images to and from the CT scanner and workstations is an essential component of connectivity (Fig. 8-29). Such transfer must comply with industry standards for electronic communications between different imaging modalities and devices from multiple vendors. One such standard is the Digital Imaging and

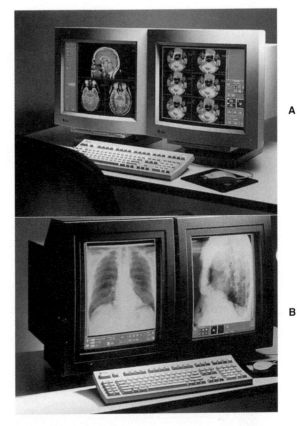

FIG. 8-27. Examples of display formats from the monitors of two advanced visualization workstations used in CT and MRI. (Courtesy General Electric Medical Systems, Milwaukee, Wis.)

TABLE 8-1

Image Storage Capacities for the Voxel Q, an Advanced Visualization System

STANDARD IMAGE DISK	VOXEL Q
Capacity	2.0 gigabytes (GB)
Storage: uncompressed images (256^2)	9.360
Storage: uncompressed images (512^2)	2.340
OPTIONAL IMAGE DISK	VOXEL Q
Additional capacity 2.0 GB	4.0 GB total
Total storage : uncompressed images (256^2)	23,760
Total storage : uncompressed images (512^2)	5940
Additional capacity 6.0 GB	6.0 GB total
Total storage : uncompressed images (256^2)	38,160
Total storage : uncompressedi Images (512^2)	9540
ULTRASPARC STANDARD IMAGE DISK	VOXEL Q
Capacity	GB
Storage: uncompressed images (256^2)	81,120
Storage: uncompressed images (512^2)	20,280
STANDARD 8-MM TAPE	
Capacity	2.2 GB
Storage : uncompressed images (512^2)	4000

(Courtesy Picker International; Cleveland, Ohio.)

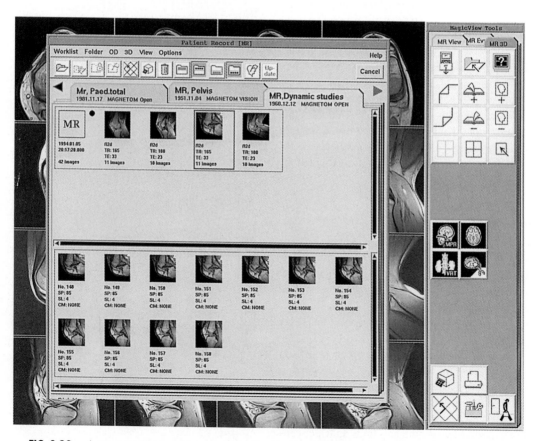

FIG. 8-28.   A mouse can be used to communicate with the computer by clicking on various icons and/or images displayed on the monitor. (Courtesy Siemens Medical Systems; Iselin, NJ.)

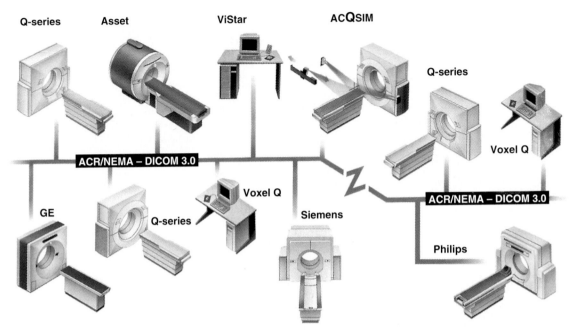

FIG. 8-29. Connectivity ensures that all types of imaging devices and modalities can be physically linked for the sole purpose of communication using various network topologies and the DICOM standard. (Courtesy Picker International; Cleveland, Ohio.)

Communications in Medicine (DICOM), and workstations for CT, MRI, and other imaging modalities, must be DICOM compliant. Other features of workstations are presented in the Appendix for a visualization and multislice CT workstation.

REFERENCES

American College of Radiology: *Standards 1998*, Reston, Va, 1998, The College.

Berland LL: *Practical CT: technology and techniques*, New York, 1987, Raven Press.

Fishman EK et al: The role of CT with multiplanar reconstruction, *Appl Radiol* 2:36-41, 1992.

Glen W et al: Image manipulation and pattern recognition. In Newton TH, Potts DG, eds: *Radiology of the skull and brain: technical aspects of computed tomography*, St Louis, 1981, Mosby.

Goodsitt MM, Johnson RH: Precision in quantitative CT: impact of x-ray dose and matrix size, *Med Phys* 19:1025-1035, 1992.

Kalender W et al: Automated evaluation of CT images in the diagnosis of osteoporosis, *Electromedica* 57: 20-24, 1989.

Mackay RS: *Medical images and displays*, New York, 1984, John Wiley & Sons.

Morgan CL: *Basic principles of computed tomography*, Baltimore, 1983, University Park Press.

Nagel W et al: Recent clinical results on the use of quantitative computed tomography in the diagnosis of osteoporosis, *Electromedica* 55:104-110, 1987.

Seeram E: Computed tomography technology, Philadelphia, 1994, WB Saunders.

Zatz LM: Basic principles of computed tomography scanning. In Newton TH, Potts DG, eds: *Radiology of the skull and brain: technical aspects of computed tomography*, St Louis, 1984, Mosby.

Electron Beam
Computed Tomography

IMAGING MOVING ORGANS

A major problem with conventional CT scanners is associated with taking images of moving organs such as the heart, as well as motion that results from breathing. Motion of any type gives rise to poor image quality such as blurring and hence poor spatial resolution. In an attempt to solve this problem, methods were devised to obtain sharp images of the heart and reduce the scan time. Dynamic CT and gated CT techniques were developed for imaging the heart. In dynamic CT, multiple 1- to 5-seconds scans are taken in rapid sequence, usually in conjunction with the bolus administration of contrast medium, to study the heart, lungs, and circulation. Although this technique has proved more useful than static CT (single scans with an effective scan time of 1 to 5 seconds), persistent problems include high radiation dose and poor image quality caused by noise.

Gated CT, a technique in which the heartbeat is synchronized with the scan views using the information from an electrocardiogram (ECG), has attempted to reduce the motion problem caused by the beating heart. As pointed out by Robb and Ritman (1979):

Gated CT scanning based on the electrocardiogram cannot be used for stop-action synchronous volume imaging of the myocardium or for angiographic imaging of vascular anatomy or circulatory function. This is because the beat-to-beat myocardial geometry and the transient dynamic distribution pattern and concentration of contrast material during and following its injection vary continuously and non-reproducibly. Moreover, the pharmacologic effect of contrast material alters the hemodynamic status considerably so that beat-to-beat constancy of the heartbeat cannot be achieved during or for a considerable period after the injection of contrast material particularly into the coronary arteries.

Spiral/helical CT based on slip-ring technology is available to take an image of a volume of tissue in a single breath hold. Spiral CT scanners offer continuous volume acquisition and good resolution studies; however, short acquisition times in the order of 0.1 seconds or less are needed to take an image of moving organs such as the beating heart without artifacts due to motion.

These limitations have been overcome by the electron beam CT (EBCT) scanner, a high-speed CT system designed specifically to image the beating heart. EBCT has also been referred to as *cine CT*, *fifth-generation CT*, *scanning electron beam CT*, and *ultrafast CT*.

ELECTRON BEAM CT SCANNER
Evolution

The principles and operation of the EBCT scanner were first described by Douglas Boyd and colleagues (1979) as a result of research done at the University of California at San Francisco during the late 1970s. In 1983, Imatron developed Boyd's high-speed CT scanner for imaging the heart and circulation (Boyd and Lipton, 1983). At that time, the machine was referred to by such names as the *cardiovascular computed tomography* (CVCT) scanner and the *cine CT* scanner. Today, the machine is known as the *EBCT scanner* (McCollough, 1995). It is expected that more of these machines will be distributed worldwide in the near future. (Siemens Medical Systems will distribute the EBCT scanner under the name "Evolution.")

The overall goal of the EBCT scanner is to produce high-resolution images of moving organs (e.g., the heart) that are free of artifacts caused by motion. In this respect, the scanner can be used for imaging the heart and other body parts in both adults and children. The scanner performs this task well because its design enables it to acquire CT data 10 times faster than conventional CT scanners.

Principles and Instrumentation

The design configuration of the EBCT scanner (Fig. 9-1) is different from that of conventional CT systems in the following respects:

1. The EBCT scanner is based on electron beam technology and no x-ray tube is used.
2. There is no mechanical motion of the components.
3. The acquisition geometry of the EBCT scanner is fundamentally different compared with those of conventional systems.

The basic configuration of an EBCT scanner is shown in Fig. 9-1. At one end of the scanner is an electron gun that generates a 130-kV electron beam. This beam is accelerated, focused, and deflected at a prescribed angle by electromagnetic coils to strike one of the four adjacent tungsten target rings. These stationary rings with a 90-cm radius span an arc of 210 degrees. The electron beam is steered along the rings (Fig. 9-2), which can be used individually or in any sequence. As a result, heat dissipation does not pose a problem as it does in conventional CT systems.

When the electron beam collides with the tungsten target, x-rays are produced. Collimators

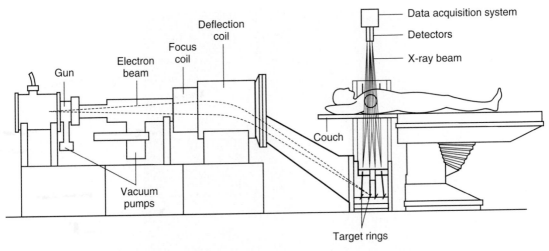

FIG. 9-1. Basic configuration of the EBCT scanner, also referred to as the *ultrafast CT scanner* and marketed by Siemens Medical Systems as the "Evolution" CT Scanner based on electron beam technology. (Courtesy Siemens Medical Systems; Iselin, NJ.)

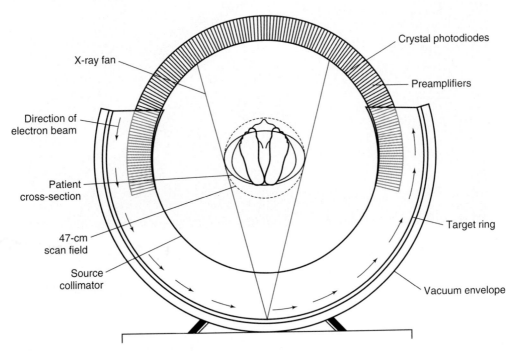

FIG. 9-2. Cross-sectional view of the EBCT scanner showing acquisition geometry. (Courtesy Siemens Medical Systems; Iselin, NJ.)

shape the x-rays into a fan beam that passes through the patient, who is positioned in a 47-cm scan field, to strike a curved, stationary array of detectors positioned opposite the target rings.

The detector array consists of two separate rings with a 67.5-cm radius holding a 216-degree arc of detectors. The first ring holds 864 detectors, each half the size of those in the second ring, which holds 432 detectors (McCollough, 1995). This arrangement allows for the acquisition of either two image slices when one target ring is used or eight image slices when all four target rings are used in sequence.

Each solid-state detector consists of a luminescent crystal and cadmium tungstate (which converts x-rays to light), coupled optically with silicon

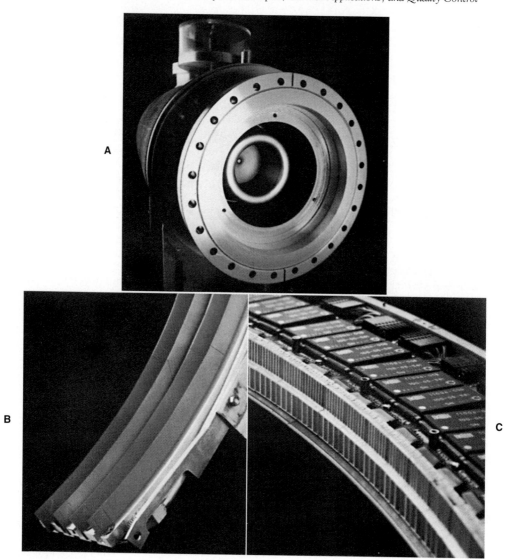

FIG. 9-3. Three major components of the EBCT scanner. **A,** Electron gun; **B,** tungsten targets; **C,** detectors. (Courtesy Siemens Medical Systems; Iselin, NJ.)

photodiodes (which convert light into current) connected to a preamplifier. The output from the detectors is sent to the data acquisition system (DAS) (Fig. 9-3).

The DAS consists of analog-to-digital converters, or digitizers, that sample and digitize the output signals from the detectors. In addition, the digitized data are stored in bulk in random access memory (RAM), which can hold data for 63 and 160 scans in the multislice and single-slice modes, respectively (McCollough, 1995). This information is subsequently sent to the computer for processing.

The computer for the EBCT scanner is capable of reconstruction speeds of 4 seconds for 256^2 images in the multislice mode and 10 to 12 seconds for 512^2 images in the single-slice mode. The reconstruction diameters vary from 9 to 47.5 cm for both modes of operation. Image reconstruction is based on the filtered back-projection algorithm used in conventional CT systems.

Whereas the computer memory can hold 1.34 gigabytes (GB) of information, disk capacity is 2375 512^2 images in the single-slice mode and 9500 256^2 images in the multislice mode. Addi-

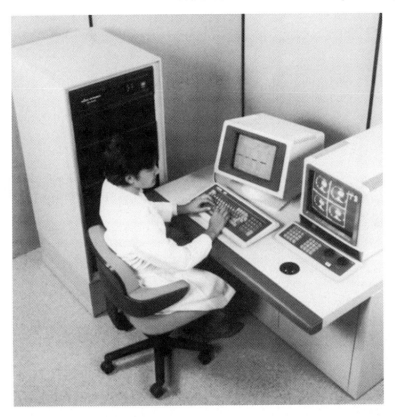

FIG. 9-4. Control console of the EBCT scanner showing keyboard, track ball, and monitors. (Courtesy Siemens Medical Systems; Iselin, NJ.)

tional external storage is available on magnetic tape and optical disk. Tape can hold 250 256^2, 125 360^2, or 63 512^2 images, but optical disks can store 15,000 256^2, 7500 360^2, or 3750 512^2 images. The computer system also allows for three image matrix sizes, 256^2, 360^2, and 512^2, with very small pixel sizes for both the single-slice and multislice operational modes.

After the images have been reconstructed, they can be displayed on a television monitor for viewing by the radiologist and technologist. Windowing can be performed on the image. Whereas the CT number range is −1000 to +3000 Hounsfield units (HU), the window level (WL) and window width (WW) ranges can vary from −1000 to +3000 HU and 1 to 4000 HU, respectively. Other display capabilities and image analysis programs include movie mode, time-density analysis, subtract image, measure distance, multiplanar reformatting with movie display, region of interest, zoom, pan, identify, save, and print

screen. Images can also be recorded on film using laser cameras. These functions can be performed by the technologist or radiologist with the keyboard and trackball, which are essential components of the control console (Fig. 9-4).

Patient Positioning

Positioning of the patient for an EBCT examination is facilitated by the patient couch and the large aperture of the gantry (Fig. 9-5). The aperture is 78 cm with a tunnel depth of 45 cm. The patient couch can be moved in various ways to facilitate the examination of difficult areas such as the posterior and anterior walls of the heart and the valves. In addition to the routine movements of up, down, in, and out of the gantry aperture, the couch can be angled from 0 to 25 degrees and can swivel through an angle of 25 degrees. Patient positioning within the scan field is also optimized with a laser positioning system.

Modes of Operation

The EBCT scanner can operate in the single-slice (SS) mode and the multislice (MS) mode (McCollough et al, 1999). These two modes can accommodate functional, flow, and anatomic stud-

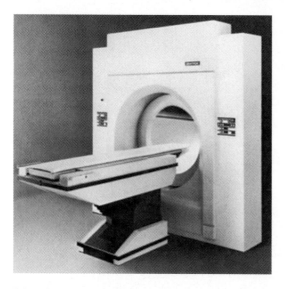

FIG. 9-5. The EBCT scanner gantry and patient couch. (Courtesy Siemens Medical Systems; Iselin, NJ.)

ies. The single-slice mode is based on scanning one of the four tungsten target rings using collimation, which will yield images with scan widths of 1.5 to 10 mm. On the other hand, the multislice mode is based on scanning all four tungsten target rings using two detector arrays to generate 2, 4, 6, or 8 scans with the patient immobilized (McCollough et al, 1999).

Additionally, the EBCT scanner can operate using four different acquisition protocols: movie mode, flow mode, step-volume scanning (SVS) mode, and continuous volume scanning (CVS) mode.

The SVS mode is similar to the "step-and-shoot" mode characteristic of conventional CT. After one slice is scanned using collimator widths of 1.5, 3, or 6 mm, the patient is positioned for the next slice with an interscan delay of about 1 second. In the CVS mode, the patient is translated through the gantry aperture continuously, a technique that is almost identical to spiral/helical CT but with a few differences. For example, to reduce artifacts from patient movement, a very short scan time in the order of 0.1 second is used in conjunction with a table displacement shorter than the scan width (McCollough et al, 1999). However, if

TABLE 9-1

Comparative Radiation Dosimetry for the EBCT and Two Conventional CT Systems

SCANNER MODE	SCAN WIDTH (mm)	SCAN INTERVAL (mm)	TIME (sec)	BODY CTDI* (cGy)	MSAD** (cGy)
ADULT BODY EXAMINATIONS					
Imatron C-100/SS (130 kVp, 250 mA)	6	6	0.4	6.9	8.4
Imatron C-100/SS (130 kVp, 250 mA)	6	10	0.4	6.9	5.0
Picker PQ 2000† (120 kVp, 200 mA)	10	10	1.0	2.9	2.9
GE HiSpeed Advantage‡ (120 kVp, 280 mA)	10	10	1.0	1.6	1.6
CARDIAC EXAMINATIONS					
Imatron C-100/SS (130 kVp, 62.5 mA)	3	3	0.1	1.0	1.2
Imatron C-100/MS (130 kVp, 31.3 mA)	8	—	0.05	0.9	0.6
Imatron C-100/MS (130 kVp, 31.3 mA)	8	80	0.05	0.9	0.7

*Radiation absorbed dose to water (0.984 cGy/R) at 6.0 position measured with ionization chamber
**MSAD = CTDI × scan width/scan interval.
†Picker International; Cleveland, Ohio.
‡General Electric Medical Systems; Milwaukee, Wis.
Modified from McCollough CH: Principles and performance of electron beam CT. In Goldman LW, Fowlkes JB, eds: *Medical CT and ultrasound, current technology and applications,* College Park, Md, 1995, American Association of Physicists in Medicine.

the distance the table moves for 0.1 second equals the scan width, the interpolation algorithm (see Chapter 13) must be used to eliminate artifacts from table movement (McCollough et al, 1999).

Imaging Performance Characteristics

McCollough (1995) compared the results obtained with EBCT and conventional systems for a number of characteristics including radiation dose, spatial and low-contrast resolution, uniformity, noise, CT number linearity, and geometrical accuracy.

Comparative dosimetry data are given in Table 9-1 for both conventional and EBCT. The dose is reported using the concepts of multiple scan average dose (MSAD) and the computed tomography dose index (CTDI). Whereas the MSAD is the average dose at the center of a series of scans, the CTDI is measured using a single ionization chamber measurement and is used to calculate the MSAD. The CTDI is the area under a single dose profile divided by the slice width (SW). When the SW equals the bed index (BI), the MSAD is numerically equal to the CTDI (Seeram, 1999).

The dose distribution within a 32-cm diameter acrylic CT phantom is shown in Fig. 9-6. Although the dose distribution is uniform at the periphery of the phantom for conventional CT (Fig. 9-6, A), it is not uniform for the EBCT scanner (Fig. 9-6, B). The dose is greatest at the edges of the phantom that are closest to the tungsten target rings and decreases to about 15% at the top of the

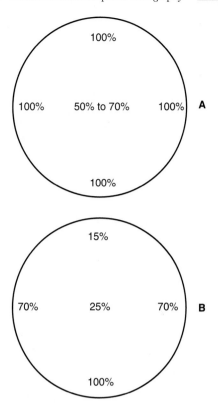

FIG. 9-6. The radiation dose distribution in conventional CT (**A**) and EBCT (**B**).

phantom. This is not the case with a conventional CT scanner.

The spatial (detail) resolution for the EBCT scanner is presented in Table 9-2. Compared with

TABLE 9-2

Spatial Resolution for the EBCT and Two Conventional CT Scanners

SCANNER/MODE	SCAN WIDTH (mm)	TIME (sec)	SPATIAL RESOLUTION* (lp/cm)
ADULT BODY EXAMINATIONS			
Imatron C-100/SS	6	0.4	5.0
(130 kVp, 200 mA)			
Picker PQ2000	10	1.0	7.9
(120 kVp, 200 mA)			
GE HiSpeed Advantage	10	1.0	6.3
(120 kVp, 280 mA)			
CARDIAC EXAMINATIONS			
Imatron C-100/SS	3	0.1	3.9
(130 kVp, 62.5 mA)			
Imatron C-100/MS	8	0.05	1.9
(130 kVp, 31.3 mA)			

*Using "normal" or "standard" reconstruction algorithm.
Modified from McCollough CH: Principles and performance of electron beam CT. In Goldman LW, Fowlkes JB, eds: *Medical CT and ultrasound, current technology and applications,* College Park, Md, 1995, American Association of Physicists in Medicine.

TABLE 9-3

Low-Contrast Resolution for the EBCT Scanner and Two Conventional CT Scanners

SCANNER/MODE	SCAN WIDTH (mm)	TIME (sec)	LOW CONTRAST RESOLUTION* (lp/cm)
ADULT BODY EXAMINATIONS			
Imatron C-100/SS	6	0.4	4.5
(130 kVp, 200 mA)			
Picker PQ2000	10	1.0	3.0
(120 kVp, 200 mA)			
GE HiSpeed Advantage	10	1.0	3.0
(120 kVp, 280 mA)			
CARDIAC EXAMINATIONS			
Imatron C-100/SS	3	0.1	20.0
(130 kVp, 62.5 mA)			
Imatron C-100/MS	8	0.05	20
(130 kVp, 31.3 mA)			

*0.6 % contrast.
Modified from McCollough CH: Principles and performance of electron beam CT. In Goldman LW, Fowlkes JB, eds: *Medical CT and ultrasound, current technology and applications*, College Park, Md, 1995, American Association of Physicists in Medicine.

TABLE 9-4

Noise for the EBCT Scanner and Two Conventional CT Scanners

SCANNER/MODE	SCAN WIDTH (mm)	TIME (sec)	NOISE (Std Dev)* (HU)
ADULT BODY EXAMINATIONS			
Imatron C-100/SS	6	0.4	19
Picker PQ2000	10	1.0	11.2
(120 kVp, 200 mA)			
GE HiSpeed Advantage	10	1.0	7.7
(120 kVp, 280 mA)			
CARDIAC EXAMINATIONS			
Imatron C-100/SS	3	0.1	47
(130 kVp, 62.5 mA)			
Imatron C-100/MS	8	0.05	35
(130 kVp, 31.3 mA)			

*Using "standard" or "normal" reconstruction algorithms.
Modified from McCollough CH: Principles and performance of electron beam CT. InGoldman LW, Fowlkes JB, eds: *Medical CT and ultrasound, current technology and applications*, College Park, Md, 1995, American Association of Physicists in Medicine.

the single-slice mode, the spatial resolution for the multislice mode is less because the detector aperture is increased by a factor of 2 (432 detector elements are used in the MS mode compared with 864 detector elements used in the SS mode) (McCollough, 1995). The low-contrast resolution is given in Table 9-3, and the noise data for both conventional and EBCT systems are given in Table 9-4.

Clinical Applications

As stated earlier, EBCT has unique applications in cardiology and other areas of the body (Figs. 9-7 to 9-9). The accompanying box summarizes its various clinical applications.

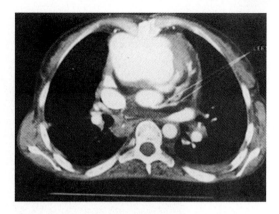

FIG. 9-7. EBCT scan of the chest with a scan time that freezes all cardiac and pulmonary motion. (Courtesy Siemens Medical Systems; Iselin, NJ.)

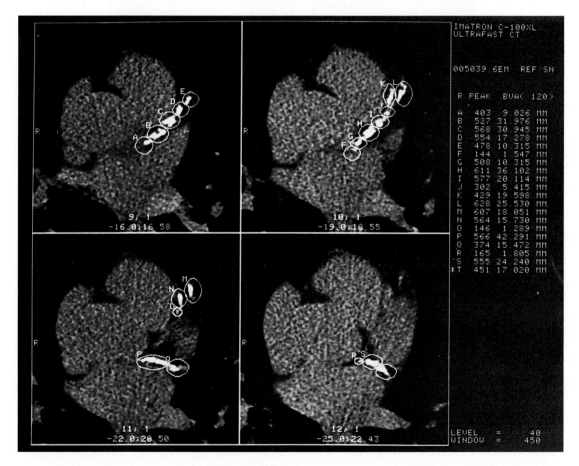

FIG. 9-8. Four levels of a noncontrast EBCT coronary artery scan showing several areas of calcification in the left anterior descending and circumflex coronary arteries. An automatic program quantifies the amount of calcification. (Courtesy Siemens Medical Systems; Iselin, NJ.)

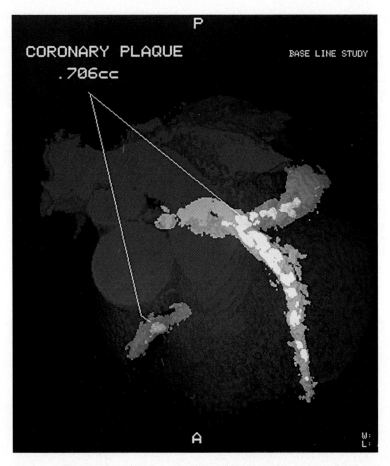

FIG. 9-9. 3D reconstruction of a coronary artery study that demonstrates the excellent slice registration of 0.1-sec ECG-triggered images. (Courtesy Siemens Medical Systems; Iselin, NJ.)

VARIOUS CLINICAL APPLICATIONS OF THE EBCT SCANNER

Left and right ventricular function	Blood flow in liver, kidneys, and brain
Valve motion	Aortic dissection
Left and right systolic volumes	Coronary artery bypass graft patency
Left and right diastolic volumes	Myocardial infarct sizing
Ejection fraction	Aneurysm
Wall motion	Myocardial mass
Cardiac wall thickening	Pericardial disease
Orthopedic joint motion	Head
Respiratory airway	Chest
Myocardial perfusion	Pulmonary nodules
Coronary arteries	Spine
Carotid arteries	Abdomen
Cardiac output	Neck
Valvular regurgitation	Pediatric studies
Arterial grafts, shunts	Trauma studies

Courtesy Siemens Medical Systems; Iselin, NJ.

REFERENCES

Boyd DP et al: A proposed dynamic cardiac 3D densitometer for early detection and evaluation of heart disease, *IEEE Trans Nucl Sci* 2724-2727, 1979.

Boyd DP, Lipton MJ: Cardiac computed tomography, *Proc IEEE* 198-307, 1983.

McCollough CH: Principles and performance of electron beam CT. In Goldman LW, Fowlkes JB, eds: *Medical CT and ultrasound, current technology and applications*, College Park, Md, 1995, American Association of Physicists in Medicine.

McCollough CH et al: Experimental determination of section sensitivity profiles and image noise in electron beam computed tomography, *Med Phys* 26(2), 1999.

Ritman EL et al: *Imaging physiological functions: experience with the dynamic spatial reconstructor*, New York, 1985, Praeger.

Robb RA, Ritman EL: High-speed synchronous volume computed tomography of the heart, *Radiology* 133:655-661, 1979.

Seeram E: Radiation dose in computed tomography, *Radiol Technol* 70:534-556, 1999.

Mobile Computed Tomography

RATIONALE

Several problems are associated with transporting patients to a fixed CT scanner: (1) the risks of transporting unstable patients, (2) the costs associated with the workload of staff who are involved in patient transportation, and (3) the maintenance of the nurse-to-patient ratio in critical care. The mobile CT scanner facilitates the performance of CT examinations at the patient's bedside.

PHYSICAL PRINCIPLES

The mobile CT scanner described in this chapter is the Tomoscan M, which is marketed by Philips Medical Systems. As of 1999, more than 100 of these units have been distributed worldwide. It is the only known mobile CT scanner in operation.

The mobile CT scanner is based on the same physical principles as fixed CT scanners (see Chapter 4). The goal of the mobile CT scanner is to produce diagnostic quality images based on x-ray attenuation data collected from the patient and measured by a set of detectors. The detectors convert the x-ray photons into electrical signals

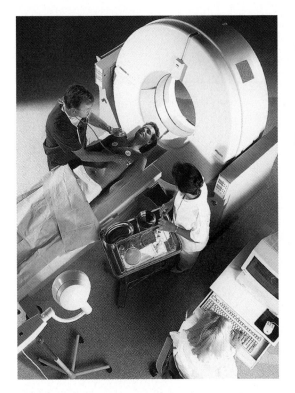

FIG. 10-1. Major components of the Tomoscan M, a mobile CT scanner: the gantry, patient table, and operator's console. (Courtesy Philips Medical Systems, Shelton, Conn.)

(analog data) that are subsequently converted into digital data by the detector electronics (analog-to-digital converters). The digital data are then sent to the computer for image reconstruction.

Image reconstruction is based on the filtered back-projection technique described in Chapter 6. Raw data are first preprocessed, sent to the array processors for convolution, and then sent to the back projector to produce the image data for display or storage.

INSTRUMENTATION

The Tomoscan M is a compact mobile CT scanner that can be transported to take images of patients who are critically ill. Each of the three major equipment components is mounted on wheels to facilitate transport of the scanner to the patient's bedside (Fig. 10-1). These components include a compact CT gantry, a patient support or table (couch), and an operator's console. The dimensions and weight of each major component are listed in Table 10-1.

General System Requirements

The general system requirements can be described in terms of site requirements (space, room, temperature, and humidity) and installation requirements (power requirements and minimum line current ratings) (see accompanying box). The scanner does not require any special electrical considerations because it can operate with single-phase alternating current (AC) power and the 120 volt wall power outlets.

In case of a power failure, the scanner is equipped with an independent battery power source that can accommodate examinations requiring up to 25 slices.

Gantry Characteristics

The mobile CT gantry (Fig. 10-2) houses the x-ray tube, generator, detectors, and detector electronics. The detector electronics play an important role in analog-to-digital conversion and digital data transmission to the minicomputer system, which is responsible for image reconstruction and image processing.

The gantry characteristics include the gantry aperture, tilt range, fan angle, maximum scan field-of-view (SFOV), and gantry translation. The gantry aperture is 60 cm and is smaller than the apertures of fixed CT scanners. The tilt range varies from +30 to −25 degrees (Fig. 10-3). The gantry can accommodate a fan angle of 48 degrees with a maximum SFOV of 46 cm. An important gantry characteristic is its ability to translate along the horizontal axis by as much as 35 cm while the patient remains immobile to accommodate examinations of the head, face, and neck (Fig. 10-4).

The x-ray tube is low-power and has an anode diameter of either 102 mm or 108 mm, depending on the type of tube, with a target angle of 12 de-

TABLE 10-1

Dimensions and Weight of the Tomoscan M Mobile CT Scanner

| COMPONENT | DIMENSIONS | | | | | | WEIGHT | |
| | (mm) | | | (inches) | | | | |
	W	L	H	W	L	H	(kg)	(lbs)
Gantry	870	1980	1860	34	78	73	460	1014
Patient table	840	2290	1020	33	90	40	240	530
Operator's console	640	760	1320	25	30	52	50	110

Courtesy Philips Medical Systems; Shelton, Conn.

INSTALLATION AND SITE REQUIREMENTS FOR THE MOBILE CT SCANNER

INSTALLATION REQUIREMENTS
Power requirements   88 to 264 VAC, single phase
Total power requirements: gantry: <2 kW peak, 0.6 kW in standby mode
                  console: 0.9 kW peak, 0.6 kW continuous
Minimum line
Current rating : 100 or 120 V line − gantry: 20A, console: 15A
          200 or 240 V line − gantry: 10A, console: 6A

SITE REQUIREMENTS
Space requirements: 19 m² (200 ft²) to operate the system
Room requirements: 2.44 m (8 ft) recommended ceiling height
Temperature range: 15° to 40° C (59° to 104° F)
Humidity range: 30% to 80% without condensation

Courtesy Philips Medical Systems; Shelton, Conn.

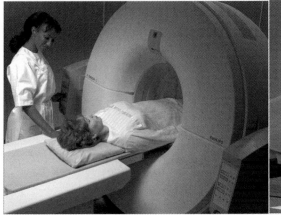
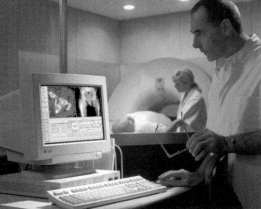

A   B

FIG. 10-2. The gantry and patient table (**A**) and operator's control console (**B**) of the Tomoscan M. (Courtesy Philips Medical Systems; Shelton, Conn.)

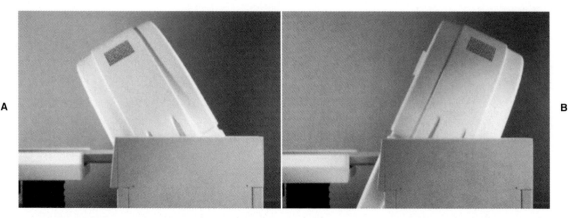

FIG. 10-3. The mobile CT scanner can be tilted +30 to −25 degrees to accommodate a range of examinations. (Courtesy Philips Medical Systems; Shelton, Conn.)

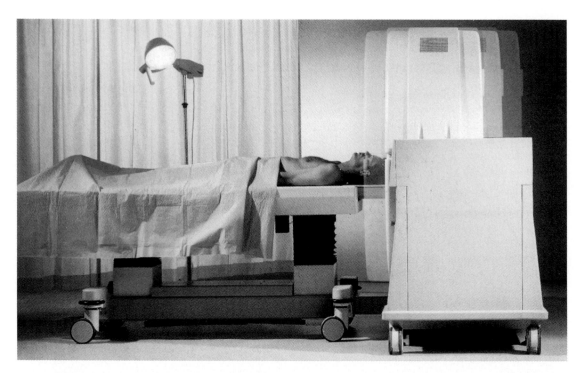

FIG. 10-4. A unique feature of the mobile CT scanner is that the gantry translates while the patient remains immobile. (Courtesy Philips Medical Systems; Shelton, Conn.)

grees. The focal spot size is 1.3 × 0.55 mm and 1.7 × 0.7 mm for anode diameters of 102 and 108 mm, respectively. This tube produces an x-ray spectrum best suited to take images of the difference in contrast between gray and white matter in the brain.

The anode heat storage capacity and cooling rate varies depending on the tube. Typical heat storage capacities are 600 kilo heat units (kHU) and 1 million heat units (MHU) with a cooling rate of 125 kHU/min and 200 kHU/min. The x-ray generator is a small, high-frequency generator with a power output of 6 kilowatts (kW), which can be increased to 18 kW with the fractional power concept. This concept ensures the use of less power and lower mA values to produce high-quality images by increased detector efficiency and dose efficiency. Whereas increased detector efficiency results in decreased power requirements, dose efficiency is made possible with a more compact beam geometry. A

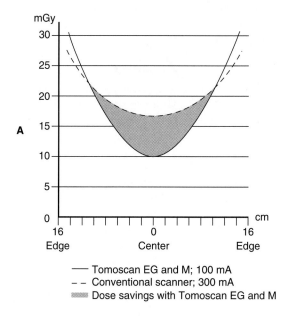

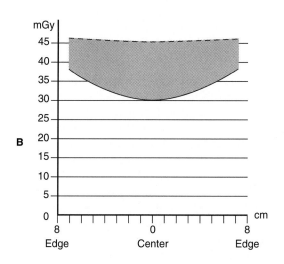

A

— Tomoscan EG and M; 100 mA
- - Conventional scanner; 300 mA
░░ Dose savings with Tomoscan EG and M

B

FIG. 10-5. A comparison of the dose distribution for two phantoms between the mobile CT scanner and a conventional CT scanner. **A,** Dose distribution in 32-cm body phantom; **B,** dose distribution in 16-cm head phantom. (Courtesy Philips Medical Systems; Shelton, Conn.)

FIG. 10-6. Several images from the mobile CT scanner using different mA values. (Courtesy Philips Medical Systems; Shelton, Conn.)

comparison of the dose distribution of the mobile CT scanner and a conventional CT scanner is shown in Fig. 10-5. For the same perceived noise level and resulting image quality, the effective patient dose is less for the mobile CT scanner using one-third of the mA of a conventional CT scanner. Examples of CT images from the mobile CT scanner are shown for different mA values (Fig. 10-6).

The mobile CT scanner is based on the third-generation CT design concept, in which the x-ray tube is coupled to an array of detectors. Both the x-ray tube and detectors rotate at the same time during data collection. The scanner employs an asymmetric geometry that combines opposing half fans of data to reduce the number of detectors. The fan data are obtained over a 360-degree rotation.

The detectors are solid state with an array of 400 elements and about 16 reference channels. The data collected by the detectors are transmitted by a radiofrequency link between the rotating and stationary parts of the gantry.

Mobile Patient Table

The patient table or support (couch) is mounted on wheels (Fig. 10-7) and can be docked with the gantry using interlocks. The table is made of carbon and epoxy over a foam core. This composition results in low attenuation of the x-ray beam as it passes through the tabletop to the detectors. The support allows for a height adjustment from 645 to 1030 mm at a speed of 15 mm/second and a longitudinal range of 1300 mm. The table top can support a maximum weight of 160 kg (350 lbs) and travels up to 100 mm/second. The table support can also provide an indexing accuracy of ±0.25 mm/second increment at 140 kg (300 lbs).

Operator's Console

An integral component of the mobile CT scanner system is the operator's console, which is mounted on wheels, is available separately as a "mobile cart," and is connected to the scanner through cables. The console is a Sun SPARC 5 (Sun Microsystems; Scottsdale, Ariz.) minicomputer workstation based on the UNIX operating system.

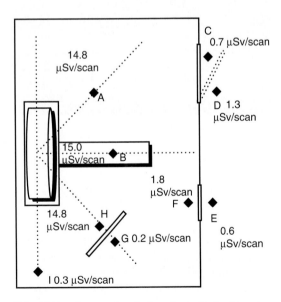

FIG. 10-7. Scattered radiation dose distribution measured in an ICU room. (From Butler WE et al: A mobile computed tomographic scanner with intraoperative and intensive care unit applications, *Neurosurgery* 42: 1304-1310, 1998.)

Major features of the workstation include a video monitor, audio system, camera interface, network facilities, and storage devices. The video monitor is a 17-inch color monitor with a display matrix of 512 × 512 and 256 gray levels. Images can be stored on the system disk or external optical disks. The system disk storage capacity is 1 gigabyte and can hold 1200 512^2 images. Optional storage devices such as a 2.3 gigabyte-8mm magnetic tape cartridge and a system disk extension are available. Images can also be recorded on film with a laser camera and then networked because the workstation is DICOM compatible (see Chapter 2).

The workstation allows the operator to select scan protocols from 100 prerecorded anatomic protocols and prestored window settings optimized from specific protocols. The operator can also perform several image processing functions such as zoom reconstruction, multiple image display, image mirroring, annotation, histogram generation, geometric processing, and so on.

SCAN PARAMETERS

Several operational scan parameters are possible with the mobile CT scanner including scan speed, exposure technique factors including scan times, slice thickness, detector sampling rate, reconstruction matrix and reconstruction time, and convolution filters. In addition, volume scanning is also possible with the mobile CT scanner.

The slice thickness selection includes 2 mm, 3 mm, 5 mm, and 10 mm, and scan speeds vary between 2, 4, and 6 seconds. X-ray exposure technique includes the use of 10, 20, 30, 40, 45, and 50 mA stations with 120 kVp or 130kVp settings and selectable scan times of 2, 4, and 6 seconds. The rate of sampling during scanning is 1440 views per second with an image reconstruction time of 5 seconds. Several convolution filters are available for brain, body, and bone examinations.

In the volumetric scan mode, a rotation time of 2 seconds is available with 25 or 35 rotations, depending on the tube. Additionally, the table speed can vary from 2, 3, 5, 10, and 20 mm/rotation during scanning. Slice thickness in this mode can be selected from 2-, 3-, 5-, 7-, and 10-mm sections.

IMAGING PERFORMANCE

The imaging performance of the mobile CT scanner can be described in terms of spatial resolution, contrast resolution, noise, and radiation dose considerations. The data are provided by Philips Medical Systems.

Spatial Resolution

Spatial resolution refers to the ability of the scanner to image fine detail, measured in line pairs/cm. The spatial resolution of the mobile CT scanner has been measured with a 2-second scan time at 40 mA and 120 kVp using a spatial resolution phantom. The spatial resolution of the mobile CT scanner has been reported to be 10 line pairs/cm.

Contrast Resolution

Contrast resolution refers to the ability of the scanner to demonstrate small differences in tissue contrast. The contrast resolution of the mobile CT scanner has been measured using a 16-cm phantom with 10-mm slice thickness at 120 mA and 120 kVp and has been reported to be 3 mm at 0.3%.

Noise

Image quality from the mobile CT scanner is also affected by noise. In CT, *noise* refers to the fluctuation of CT numbers between points in the image for a scan of uniform material such as water. The *noise level* is a percentage of contrast in CT numbers. The noise level of the mobile CT scanner is 0.3% at 120 mA.

Computed Tomography Dose Index

Manufacturers of CT scanners are now required by law to provide the computed tomography dose index (CTDI) for their scanners. For the mobile CT scanner, the CTDI per mA at 120 kVp and a slice thickness of 10 mm is specified for the head and body. The CTDI for the center and edge of a head phantom is 30.9 mGy and 38.2 mGy, respectively. The CTDI for the center and edge of a body phantom is 10.3 mGy and 32.9 mGy, respectively.

SCATTERED RADIATION CONSIDERATIONS

As in any mobile x-ray imaging procedure, scattered radiation from the mobile CT scanner concerns radiation workers and those individuals working in areas in which mobile CT examinations are performed.

In an effort to quantify the scattered radiation levels from a mobile CT scanner, Butler et al (1998) conducted measurements of exposure levels in a neurosurgery intensive care unit. Using both head and body phantoms, scattered radiation levels were measured at 1 meter from the gantry center and 45 and 90 degrees to the table axis. In addition, radiation levels were measured 2 m outside the room and 1 m behind a mobile lead shield located in the room (see Fig. 10-7). The authors report that "the scattered radiation exposure from the head phantom at 1 m along the table axis was 15.0 μSv per scan, for a 10 mm thick slice, 50 mA, 200 kVp, 4 second scan. A glass window at 2.3 m from the phantom attenuated the scatter from 1.8 to 0.6 μSv, whereas a wood door attenuated the exposure from 1.3 to 0.7 μSv. A lead shield attenuated the exposure by a factor of approximately 46. In each case, the resulting levels fell within the acceptable criteria for radiation safety and quality assurance."

CLINICAL APPLICATIONS

The scanner has been used in a wide range of clinical situations. For example, Zonneveld (1998) has demonstrated the usefulness of a mobile CT scanner to monitor the progress of surgical operations, especially in the resection of deep-seated brain tumors and pathologies and in the treatment of arteriovenous malformations, thus eliminating the need to transport these patients to fixed CT scanners. Winn and Stanley (1998) used a mobile CT scanner to eliminate the risks and costs of patient transfer to a fixed CT scanner and to maintain the nurse-to-patient ratio in the intensive care unit. Winn and Stanley (1998) also report that the mobile CT scanner helps them to improve their surgical performance and confidence because of their capability to perform preoperative, intraoperative, and postoperative scanning.

Other researchers such as Butler et al (1998), Perneczky (1998), and Koos et al (1998) also report the effectiveness of mobile CT in neurosurgery, intraoperative and perioperative CT, and image-guided neurosurgery, respectively. Additionally, Mirvis (1997) showed that mobile CT scanning can result in positive gains in a major shock trauma center. In a three-phase study involving the trauma resuscitation unit, intensive care unit, and operating room, Mirvis et al (1997) and Butler et al (1998), showed that the mobile CT scanner significantly contributes to safety, efficiency, and

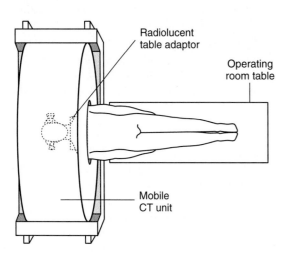

FIG. 10-8. A mobile CT scanner can be transported for use in the operating room.

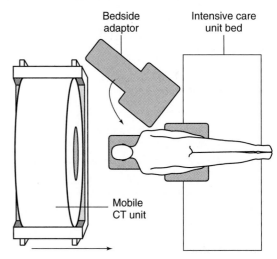

FIG. 10-9. The use of a mobile CT scanner in the intensive care unit requires a bedside adapter so the patient can be positioned in the gantry.

economy. Additionally, Butler et al (1998) showed the scanner's use in intraoperative CT (Fig. 10-8) and the neurosurgery ICU unit (Fig. 10-9).

REFERENCES

Butler WE et al: A mobile computed tomographic scanner with intraoperative and intensive care unit applications, *Neurosurgery* 42:1304-1310, 1998.

Koos WT et al: Image-guided neurosurgery with intraoperative CT, *Medicamundi* 42:26-32, 1998.

Mirvis SE et al: Mobile CT in a trauma-critical care environment: preliminary clinical experience, *Abstract Book Eighth Annual Scientific Meeting of the American Society of Emergency Radiology*, 1997.

Perneczky A: Intra- and peri-operative CT, *Medicamundi* 42:21-25, 1998.

Winn HR, Stanley RB: Intra-operative CT in neurosurgery and maxillofacial reconstruction, *Medicamundi* 42:12-14, 1998.

Zonneveld FW: Intra-operative CT: implementation of the Tomoscan M, *Medicamundi* 42:6-13, 1998.

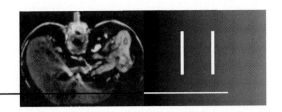

Image Quality

Essentially, five characteristics of the radiographic image determine its quality: spatial resolution, contrast resolution, noise, distortion, and artifacts (Sprawls, 1995). Each characteristic is influenced by several factors related to processing, geometry, motion, subject contrast, film contrast technique, image receptor, focal spot size, viewing conditions, and observer performance.

In CT, several factors that affect image quality have been identified and discussed in some detail (Pfeiler et al, 1976; Blumenfeld and Glover, 1981; Hanson, 1981; Morgan, 1983; Villafana, 1987; Sprawls, 1995; and Barnes and Lakshminarayanan, 1989). Kalender and Polacin (1991) also discussed image quality for CT scanning in spiral geometry.

QUALITIES
General Expression

Robb and Morin (1991) have presented a partial list of factors that influence image quality: x-ray beam characteristics, dose, transmissivity of the subject, slice thickness, scatter, efficiency of analog-to-digital conversion, pixel size, reconstruction algorithm, and display resolution.

Robb and Morin (1991) have also given an algebraic expression for image quality in CT:

$$\sigma^2(\mu) \cong kT / (td^3R) \qquad (11\text{-}1)$$

where $\sigma(\mu)$ is variance (a measure of the variability of μ about a mean) that results from noise, T is transmissivity (inverse of attenuation, taking into consideration tissue composition and distribution), t is slice thickness, d is pixel size, R is dose, and k is a factor used to convert skin dose to absorbed dose.

To improve image quality, the dose and pixel size (d) can be changed "since the transmissivity of the subject cannot generally be changed and for any scan setting the slice thickness would be fixed" (Robb and Morin, 1991).

Measurement

The quality of the CT image is determined by the factors shown in Fig. 11-1. Several methods can be used to measure some of these parameters, such as the point spread function (PSF), line spread function (LSF), contrast transfer function (CTF), and modulation transfer function (MTF). Of these, the MTF is the most commonly used descriptor of spatial resolution in CT and conventional radiography.

The PSF describes the lack of sharpness that results when a point in the object is not reproduced as a "true" point in the image. This lack of sharpness results in a blurring effect (i.e., the point spreads to form a measurable circle). The measure of the spatial resolution is the width of the point

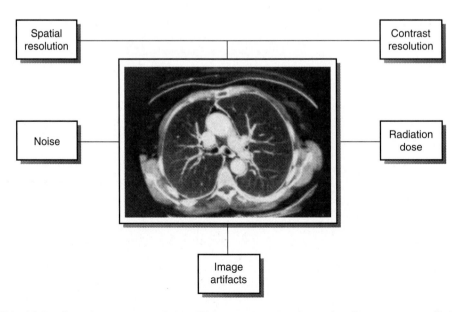

FIG. 11-1. Several parameters of the CT image determine its quality. (Photo courtesy Elscint; Hackensack, NJ.)

spread function at half its maximum value. This measure is called the *full width at half-maximum* (FWHM), which is often seen on CT data for spatial resolution.

The LSF also describes the *unsharpness* of an imaging system when a line or slit object is not reproduced as a line or slit image, but instead spreads out as a measurable distance.

The CTF, also referred to as the *contrast response function*, measures the contrast response of an imaging system. For a resolution test pattern that consists of a series of slits and spaces, the resultant contrast is the difference in density between adjacent regions of the slits. If a graph is plotted between the resultant contrast of the image slits as a function of the number of slits per unit length, the CTF can be obtained. Image contrast decreases as the number of slits per unit length decreases.

The MTF can be derived from the LSF, PSF, and the edge response function (ERF), which describes the response of an imaging system to adjacent regions of high and low densities. The MTF can be obtained with the Fourier transform of the LSF, PSF, and ERF. It measures the resolution capabilities of a system by breaking down an object into its frequency components (Fig. 11-2). Optical density expresses the image fidelity, or the faithfulness with which the object can be reproduced in the image. An MTF of 1 means that the imaging system has reproduced the object exactly, whereas an MTF of 0 indicates no transfer of object to image.

In Fig. 11-2, at 1 line pair (lp)/cm spatial frequency, the optical density is 0.88; at 2 lp/cm, the optical density is 0.59, and so on. If the spatial frequency is plotted as a function of the image fidelity, an MTF curve is obtained (Fig. 11-3). The MTF is the most common transfer function for CT scanners. In the MTF curves for two CT scanners (Fig. 11-4), scanner A can image 5.2 lp/cm at 0.1 MTF compared with scanner B, which can only image 3.5 lp/cm at 0.1 MTF. This simply

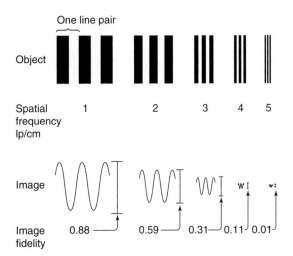

FIG. 11-2. A bar pattern (object) consists of line pairs (*lp*, one line pair equals one bar plus one space). The number of line pairs per unit length is called the *spatial frequency*. Large objects have a low spatial frequency, whereas small objects have a high spatial frequency.

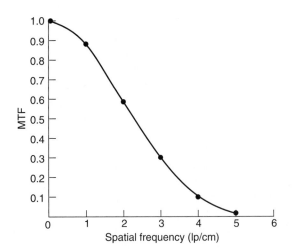

FIG. 11-3. A modulation transfer function (MTF) curve obtained from the data given in Fig. 11-2.

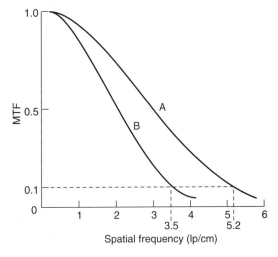

FIG. 11-4. MTF curves for two CT scanners.

means that scanner A has a better spatial resolution capability than scanner B.

What is the absolute size of an object for CT imaging? Bushong (1997) gave the answer as "equal to the reciprocal of the spatial frequency." For example, if the spatial frequency of a CT scanner is 15 lp/cm (15 lp/cm^{-1}), then the CT scanner can resolve an object 0.3 mm in size (1/15 lp/cm = 10/15 lp/mm = 0.6 mm/lp = 0.3 mm).

Finally, the noise in an image can be measured by the noise power spectrum, or Wiener spectrum (Fig. 11-5). This description can also be used to study the total noise of the system. Fig. 11-5 shows that the noise power spectrum is obtained with the Fourier transform to break down the image noise into its frequency components. Whereas the MTF expresses spatial resolution, the noise power spectrum describes contrast resolution.

Phantoms

CT manufacturers provide various phantoms for routine measurement, but other phantoms can be obtained for additional measurements. Two popular phantoms are the starburst and bar patterns typical of the Catphan phantom (Alderson Research Laboratories) and the Plexiglass phantom consisting of a series of holes of different diameters arranged in rows (American Association of Physicists in Medicine (AAPM)). Fig. 11-6 illustrates several phantoms to measure noise, spatial resolution, contrast resolution, and slice thickness.

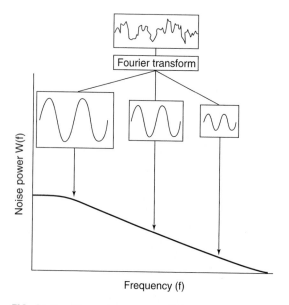

FIG. 11-5. The noise power, or Wiener, spectrum describes contrast resolution. The spectrum is obtained by breaking down image noise into its frequency components using the Fourier transform.

RESOLUTION

Resolution in CT can be discussed in terms of spatial resolution and contrast resolution. This section presents the essential characteristics of both.

Spatial Resolution

Spatial resolution describes the degree of blurring in an image. For a CT scanner, spatial resolution "is a measure of the ability to discriminate objects of varying density a small distance apart against a uniform background" (Robb and Morin, 1991).

Spatial resolution is often represented by the PSF, LSF and MTF (see Fig. 11-4). Barnes and Lakshminarayanan (1989) have used the MTF to describe the spatial resolution of a CT system, as follows:

$$MTF_{system}(f) = MTF_{geometry}(f) \cdot MTF_{algorithm}(f)$$
$$(11\text{-}2)$$

where f is the spatial frequency. Equation 11-2 shows that CT spatial resolution is generally affected by two categories of factors: geometric factors and the reconstruction algorithm.

Geometric Factors

Geometric factors refer to factors that play a role in the data acquisition process (Blumenfeld and Glover, 1981) such as focal spot size; detector aperture width; slice thickness; distance between the focus, isocenter (center of rotation of the gantry), and detector; and sampling distance. Reconstruction algorithms, however, influence spatial resolution based on their ability to smooth or enhance edges.

In CT, the effective focal spot size at the isocenter represents the size of the focal spot in the x-ray tube. If the effective focal spot size increases, details in the object are distributed over several detectors, thus decreasing the spatial resolution.

The *aperture size* refers to the width of the aperture at the detector. Generally, the objects can be resolved when the aperture size is smaller than the spacing between objects. Higher spatial resolution can be obtained for smaller aperture sizes. Both the focal spot size and detector aperture width affect resolution in terms of the effective scan beam width at the isocenter. This beam width is affected by the focus-to-isocenter and focus-to-detector distances. Smaller focal spots and smaller detector aperture widths improve spatial resolution.

Imaging small objects faithfully (i.e., with excellent spatial resolution) depends on the slice thickness, or collimation. For example, if the object size is 4 mm, a 10-mm slice thickness results in spreading the 4-mm object over the entire slice thickness and thus an incorrect CT number. This effect is called the *partial volume effect*. A slice thickness close to the object size, such as a 5-mm slice thickness, would be a significant improvement and thus increase spatial resolution.

The number of projections also influences spatial resolution. As the number of projections increases, more data are available for image

Phantom for noise, spatial homogeneity, high contrast resolution

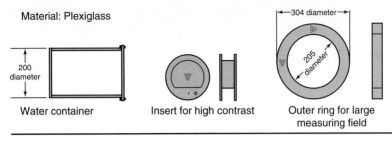

Material: Plexiglass

Water container   Insert for high contrast   Outer ring for large measuring field

Insert for high contrast

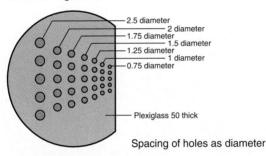

Spacing of holes as diameter

Phantom for low contrast

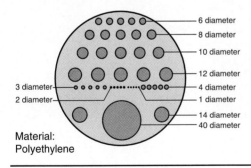

Phantom for determination of the slice thickness

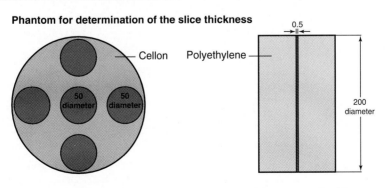

FIG. 11-6. Representations of several phantoms to measure CT image quality. (Courtesy Siemens Medical Systems; Iselin, NJ.)

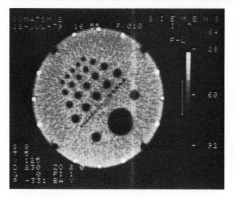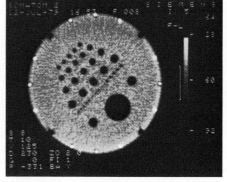

Projections:	360	Projections:	720
mAs:	230	mAs:	230
Slice thickness:	8 mm	Slice thickness:	8 mm
Zoom factor:	1.5	Zoom factor:	1.5
Convolution kernel:	1	Convolution kernel:	1
Contrast:	1.5% ≙ 30 CT units	Contrast:	1.5% ≙ 30 CT units

FIG. 11-7. Influence of the number of projections on spatial resolution. (Courtesy Siemens Medical Systems; Iselin, NJ.)

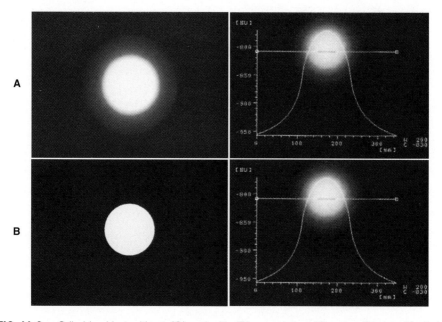

FIG. 11-8. Cylindric object without (**A**) and with (**B**) convolution. (Courtesy Siemens Medical Systems; Iselin, NJ.)

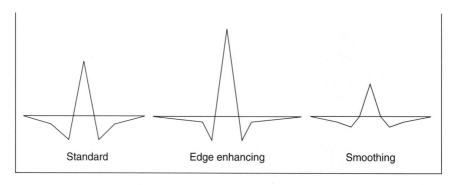

FIG. 11-9. Three convolution algorithms affect spatial resolution. (Courtesy Siemens Medical Systems; Iselin, NJ.)

reconstruction and spatial resolution improves (Fig. 11-7).

Reconstruction Algorithm

Recall from Chapter 7 that image reconstruction involves two mathematical procedures: convolution and back-projection. Essentially, if the projection profiles are back-projected without correction, blurring results (Fig. 11-8, *A*). To sharpen the image, a convolution process (basically a high-pass filter) is applied to weight the scan profiles before back-projection (Fig. 11-8, *B*). The nature and degree of the weighting depend on the convolution algorithm (Fig. 11-9).

The convolution algorithm, or kernel, affects the appearance of image structures. Convolution algorithms have been developed for each anatomic-specific application. In general, these algorithms are applied to emphasize soft tissue (standard algorithm) and bone and are known as the *soft tissue* and *bone detail* algorithms. Whereas the former is applied to the spine, pancreas, adrenal, lung nodules, or any soft tissue region, the latter is applied to bony structures such as the inner ear and dense bone.

Spatial resolution at high contrast is also called *high-contrast resolution* and can be determined from the MTF or the CT image of the phantom (Fig. 11-10). When high-contrast resolution is determined by the MTF at 0.1% (see Fig. 11-4), it is referred to as *limiting resolution* (Bushong, 1997).

(The limiting resolution for several popular CT scanners can be found in Appendix B.)

The *display resolution* is defined as the number of pixels per horizontal and vertical dimension of the matrix on the monitor screen or film sheet. Formerly, images were displayed with matrix sizes of 80 × 80, 128 × 128, and 256 × 256 (Fig. 11-11). The effect of matrix size on resolution is apparent in Fig. 11-11.

Today, CT scanners use higher matrix sizes in conjunction with selected convolution algorithms to improve display resolution. One CT scanner may use 512 × 512 reconstruction matrix with a selected pixel size between 0.06 and 1 mm. When

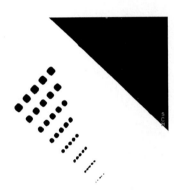

FIG. 11-10. CT image of a bore hole phantom for high-contrast resolution using an ultra high-resolution algorithm. (Courtesy Siemens Medical Systems; Iselin, NJ.)

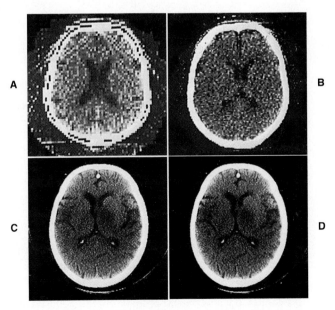

FIG. 11-11. Effect of four matrix sizes on resolution of the CT image. (From Schare P, Weckesser WE, Peter F: Problems in the display of CT images by the use of television and photography, *Electromedica* 2:62-65, 1979.)

this image is displayed, a 1024 × 1024 image matrix facilitates discrimination of the anatomic details and more sharply demarcates anatomic structures of high contrast. Another scanner may use a 1024 × 1024 reconstruction matrix and a high-resolution display (1024 × 1280) to give a 20 lp/cm resolution.

High-Resolution CT

High-resolution CT (HRCT) is a technique introduced in the mid-1980s as a result of significant improvements in the CT process and in comput-

ers. It was developed to evaluate diseases of the lung and "is currently the most accurate noninvasive tool for evaluation of lung structure" (Mayo, 1991). The technical aspects of HRCT have been described by a number of workers, most notably Mayo (1991). HRCT is "a technique that optimizes the spatial resolution of conventional scanners" (Swensen et al, 1992).

Narrow beam collimation ensures that thin slices are obtained. Slice thicknesses of 1.0, 1.5, and 2.0 mm, compared with an 8- to 10-mm slice thickness in conventional CT scanning, are common. These thin slices reduce artifacts caused by

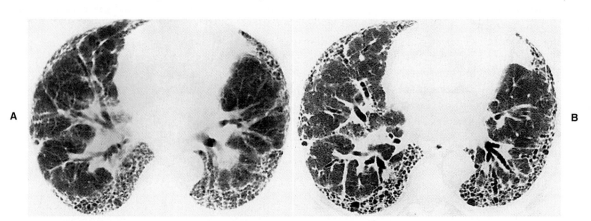

FIG. 11-12. Comparison of the degree of spatial resolution of slices with two different thicknesses. The spatial resolution of the thinner slice (**B**) taken with 1.5-mm collimation is apparent when compared with the image of the slice taken with 10-mm collimation (**A**). (From Mayo JR: High-resolution computed tomography, *Radiol Clin North Am* 29:1043-1048, 1991.)

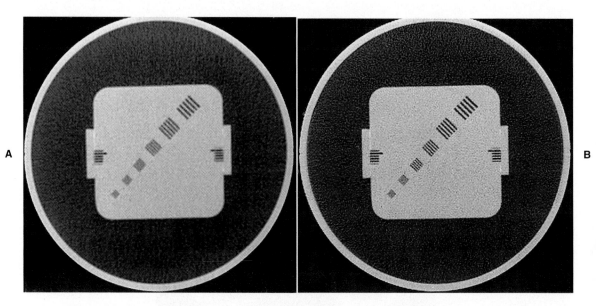

FIG. 11-13. Effect of algorithms on spatial resolution. **A,** Line pair phantom image reconstructed with a low spatial frequency algorithm. **B,** Same line pair phantom image reconstructed with a high spatial frequency algorithm. The spatial resolution is better in **B**. (From Mayo JR: High-resolution computed tomography, *Radiol Clin North Am* 29:1043-1048, 1991.)

partial volume averaging. Fig. 11-12 presents a comparison of the degree of spatial resolution afforded by two slices of different thicknesses.

The next parameter optimized for HRCT is the reconstruction algorithm. High spatial frequency algorithms have been shown to increase spatial resolution significantly but at the expense of noise (Mayo, 1991) (Fig. 11-13). According to Meziane (1992), increased noise usually does not affect the interpretation of scans, although noise can obscure subtle parenchymal changes. To reduce the noise, the low spatial frequency algorithm can be used to smooth the image, but this algorithm is not suitable for use in HRCT of the brain and abdomen, where subject contrast is not as dramatic as the lungs (Galvin et al, 1992).

Finally, HRCT requires the reduction of the pixel size to provide a further increase in spatial resolution. This is accomplished with the use of a smaller field of view (FOV).

$$\text{Pixel size} = \frac{\text{FOV}}{\text{matrix size}} \qquad (11\text{-}3)$$

For a 40-cm FOV at a matrix size of 512 × 512, the pixel size is 0.78 mm (400 mm / 512). If the FOV is reduced to 20 cm, the pixel size is 0.49 mm; for a 13-cm FOV, the pixel size is 0.25 mm. This reduction is referred to as *targeting*. By retrospective targeting or retargeting, "a subset of the scan data is again reconstructed on a smaller reconstruction grid, thereby increasing the spatial resolution" (Mayo, 1991) (Fig. 11-14).

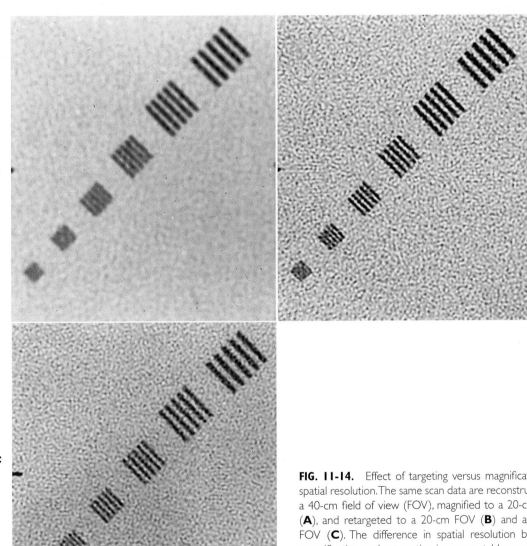

FIG. 11-14. Effect of targeting versus magnification on spatial resolution. The same scan data are reconstructed at a 40-cm field of view (FOV), magnified to a 20-cm FOV (**A**), and retargeted to a 20-cm FOV (**B**) and a 13-cm FOV (**C**). The difference in spatial resolution between magnification and retargeting is apparent. However, there is little difference between retargeting at **B** and **C**. (From Mayo JR: High-resolution computed tomography, *Radiol Clin North Am* 29:1043-1048, 1991.)

The technique factors for HRCT usually range from 120 kVp and 140 mA to 140 kVp and 200 mA, with scan times between 2 and 3 seconds (Mayo, 1991; Galvin et al, 1992; Swensen et al, 1992; and Meziane, 1992). If the technique factors, particularly mA and scan time, are increased to decrease the noise in the image, the result is a corresponding increase in the radiation dose to the patient.

Contrast Resolution

Low-contrast resolution, or tissue resolution, is the ability of an imaging system to demonstrate small changes in tissue contrast. In CT, this is sometimes referred to as the *sensitivity of the system* (Hounsfield, 1978). Contrast resolution can also be stated in terms of the ability of the CT unit to image objects 2 to 3 mm in size that vary slightly in density from the environment in which they are located (Curry et al, 1990). In this case, the term *low-contrast detectability* is used to describe the contrast resolution in CT.

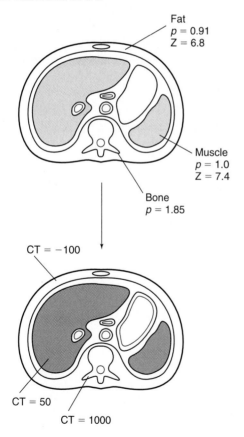

FIG. 11-15. Densities (p) and atomic numbers (Z) for three types of tissue. When they are imaged by CT, excellent low-contrast resolution is obtained. (From Bushong S: *Radiologic science for technologists,* ed 6, St Louis, 1997, Mosby.)

To understand low-contrast resolution, consider three different tissues of differing densities and atomic number (Z) (Fig. 11-15). If these tissues were imaged by conventional radiography, the obtained image would show good contrast between bone and soft tissue (muscle and fat) only. The values of the density and Z for muscle and fat are too close to be clearly distinguished by radiography and they appear as "soft tissue shadows." The contrast between bone with a Z of 13.8 and soft tissue with a Z of 7.4 is apparent because of the significant difference between the densities and Z of these two tissues.

An advantage of CT is that contrast resolution is significantly better than in conventional radiography. CT can image tissues that vary only slightly in density and atomic number. Whereas radiography can discriminate a density difference of about 10% (Curry et al, 1990), CT can detect density differences from 0.25% to 0.5%, depending on the scanner. (The low-contrast resolution for several popular CT scanners is presented in the Appendix.)

Low-contrast resolution in CT is affected by several factors including photon flux, slice thickness, patient size, sensitivity of the detector, reconstruction algorithm, image display, recording, and noise (see the box below) (Morgan, 1983).

The photon flux depends on kVp, mAs, and beam filtration. These factors affect both the quality and quantity of photons that reach the detector. In addition, the size of the patient affects the attenuation of the beam and thus the photon flux at the detector. Whereas increased technique factors (kVp and mAs) increase photon flux, increased beam filtration and patient size reduce photon flux because of its greater radiation attenuation. In CT, these factors are optimized to improve low-contrast resolution.

Slice thickness also influences low-contrast resolution. It was stated in Chapter 4 that collimation is one way CT overcomes the contrast degra-

---

FACTORS THAT AFFECT LOW-CONTRAST RESOLUTION

- Photon flux
- Slice thickness
- Patient size
- Detector sensitivity
- Reconstruction algorithm
- Image display
- Image recording
- Quantum noise

dation typical of conventional radiography because of its open beam geometry. In CT, collimation controls the slice thickness; very thin slices require very narrow collimation. This type of collimation reduces the scattered rays that intercept the detector and thus improves contrast resolution. However, as the slice thickness decreases, the technique factors must also increase.

Detector sensitivity affects contrast resolution in that CT detectors must be capable of discriminating among small differences in x-ray attenuation, which is required to measure small differences in soft tissue contrast in the order of at least 1% (Morgan, 1983).

The effect of the reconstruction algorithm on contrast resolution is dramatic. The influence of the high spatial frequency algorithm in the improvement of spatial resolution has already been discussed (see Fig. 11-13). Similarly, the low spatial frequency algorithm can be used for image smoothing, which "may enhance the perceptibility of low-contrast lesions such as metastases" (Morgan, 1983). In addition, this algorithm is useful when imaging the brain and abdomen because of subtle differences in subject contrast (Galvin et al, 1992). The size of the television screen (viewer size) and the viewing distance also affect contrast resolution. McCullough (1977) has noted that as the viewing distance increases for large screens, the ability to detect low-contrast images improves.

Finally, noise affects low-contrast resolution in CT. In this context, *noise* refers to quantum noise. If too few photons are detected, then the image appears as "noise" and low-contrast resolution is degraded. Together, noise and spatial resolution capability at low contrast are called *low-contrast resolution*. To improve both contrast and spatial resolution, the radiation dose must be increased so that more photons are available at the detector to generate stronger signals.

Contrast-Detail Diagram

The contrast-detail diagram (CDD) is a graph on which the measured contrast is plotted on the ordinate as a function of the detectable diameter of the object, which is plotted on the abscissa. From this graph, information can be obtained for both the low-contrast and high-contrast resolution of a CT scanner.

In two CDDs of the abdomen and cerebrum (Fig. 11-16), the asymptote (a straight line toward which a curve approaches but never meets) indicates the spatial resolution capability at high con-

trast. At 100% contrast (1000 ΔCT/HU) the resolution limit (the smallest diameter that can be perceived) occurs (Villafana, 1987). The resolution at low contrast can be determined from the diagram for any diameter.

"As contrast decreases, resolution falls. At low contrast levels, curves tend to flatten out (this is referred to as the noise limit)" (Villafana, 1987). The contrast-detail diagram can be determined as follows:

The matrix method is a relatively simple method to determine the CDD, in which a noise-free simulated image of a bore hole phantom is superimposed on a pure noise image. The object contrast is then determined, at which point the rows of bore holes are just barely discernible in the derived image.

This bore hole phantom contains a very large number of equidistant holes of a diameter d— between 64 and 44 holes, depending on their diameter—and a center-to-center distance of 2d. These holes are arranged in the shape of a matrix. The image of the structure can be calculated based on the point spread function, whereby any desired contrast, K_0, can be easily obtained. The result is an image, $I_0 (K_0, d)$, as would be acquired with a real phantom comprising the bore hole configuration described (e.g., a plexiglass bore hole plate).

A noise reference image, I_n, is obtained as follows: Two transaxial images are acquired from a 20-cm water phantom and then subtracted to eliminate regular structures such as vignetting. In this differential image, the standard deviation is computed over a central circular area of about 40 square centimeters (pixel noise σ) and normalized for a level of noise σ.

The preselected object contrast K_0 of the image I_0 is normalized with S_K so that the bore hole pattern is just distinguishable in the image derived from the addition of image $I = S_K$ in the reference noise image I_n. *Distinguishable* is defined as the ability to count 50% of the bore holes in this image. When this criterion is fulfilled, a reference contrast ($CT_{Ref} = S_K \times K_0$ is produced as the signal for the pixel noise. Thus the detectability of a hole with a diameter d depends solely on the signal-to-noise ration. For a pixel noise of a selected scan mode, the contrast $CT (d)$ that can just barely be discriminated is therefore produced as follows:

$$\Delta CT = \sigma \frac{\Delta CT_{Re}}{\sigma_{Ref}} \qquad (11\text{-}4)$$

If the diameter d of the holes is varied, a . . . CT can be clearly determined for which d can be

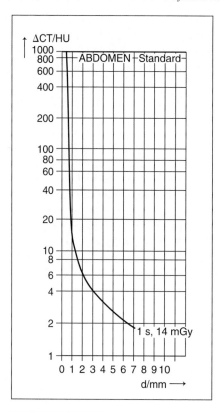
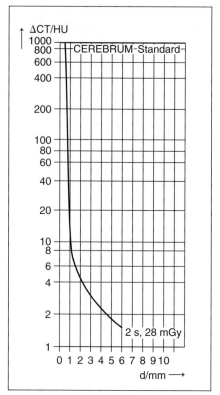
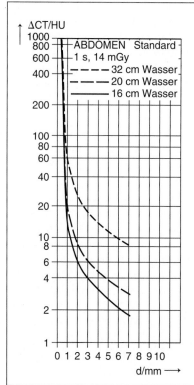
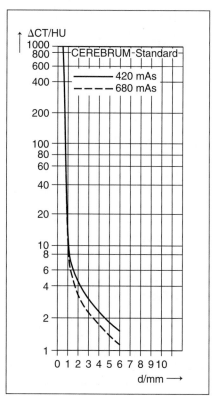

FIG. 11-16. Contrast detail diagrams for the abdomen and cerebrum. (Courtesy Siemens Medical Systems; Iselin, NJ.)

recognized as above. The CDD is then determined for the many possible combinations of contrast and bore hold diameter.

The advantage of this method is the simplicity with which any given bore hole diameter can be visualized with an exactly defined level of contrast.

With mixed contrast agent solutions, it is generally quite difficult to achieve the exact levels of contrast required for the given bore hold diameters.

A CDD can be quickly determined with the matrix method, using several image reconstructions and image superpositionals. The resulting CDD can be easily confirmed by measurements of low-contrast phantoms for various combinations of contrast and bore hole diameter (Siemens, 1989).

NOISE PROPERTIES

In CT, noise is the fluctuation of CT numbers between points in the image for a scan of uniform material such as water. Noise can be described with the standard deviation σ of the values in an image matrix (pixels) using the following expression:

$$\text{Noise } (\sigma) = \sqrt{\frac{\sum(x_i - \bar{x})^2}{n - 1}} \qquad (11\text{-}5)$$

where n is the total number of pixel values within the region, x_i is an individual pixel value, and $\bar{x}$ is the mean of the pixel values. The computed answer indicates the statistical spread in the reconstructed CT numbers.

Noise Level

The noise level can be stated as a percentage of contrast or in CT numbers. If 3 is the standard deviation for a CT unit with CT number range of ± 1000, then the noise level expressed as a percentage of contrast is as follows:

$$\text{Noise level (\%)} = \frac{3}{1000} \times 100$$
$$= 3/10$$
$$= 0.3\%$$

That is, 3 units out of 1000 represent 0.3%.

Noise can be measured by scanning a water phantom placed in the scan field and computing the mean and standard deviation for a region of interest (ROI). The pixel noise is then the standard deviation of the signals within this ROI (Fig. 11-17).

The noise levels for CT scanners vary and depend on several factors including mAs, scan time,

kVp, slice thickness, object size, and the algorithm. For example, at 210 mAs, 1-second scan, 10-mm slice, 120 kVp, and a soft detail algorithm, the noise for the Somatom Plus is 2.9 HU (Siemens, 1989).

Sources

Noise in CT is mainly related to the following: (1) number of detected photons (quantum noise), (2) matrix size (pixel size), (3) slice thickness, (4) algorithm, (5) electronic noise (detector electronics), (6) scattered radiation, and (7) object size. Brooks and Di Chiro (1976) have described an expression for noise in CT that relates to several of these factors:

$$\sigma(\mu) \; \alpha \; \left[\frac{B}{W_3 h D} \right]^{1/2} \qquad (11\text{-}6)$$

or

$$\sigma^2 \; \alpha \; \frac{1}{W^3 h D} \qquad (11\text{-}7)$$

or

$$D \; \alpha \; \frac{IE}{\sigma^2 W^3 h} \qquad (11\text{-}8)$$

where σ is the standard deviation, μ is the linear attenuation coefficient, B is the fractional attenuation of the patient, W is the width of the pixel, h is the slice thickness, D is the entrance dose, I is the intensity in mAs, and E is the beam energy in keV.

Equation 11-6 indicates the following:
1. If the width of the pixel increases, the noise decreases, but spatial resolution decreases.

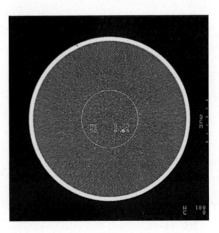

FIG. 11-17. Pixel noise with a 20-cm water phantom. The noise can be measured for the region of interest shown. (Courtesy Siemens Medical Systems; Iselin, NJ.)

TABLE 11-1

Characteristics of the American Association of Physicists in Medicine CT Phantom

MATERIAL	DENSITY (g/ml)	LINEAR ATTENUATION COEFFICIENT (cm^{-1}) AT 60 keV	APPROXIMATE CT NUMBER
Polyethylene, C_2H_4	0.94	0.185	−85
Polystyrene, C_8H_8	1.05	0.196	−10
Nylon, $C_6H_{11}NO$	1.15	0.222	100
Lexan, $C_{16}H_{14}O$	1.20	0.223	115
Plexiglas, $C_5H_8O_2$	1.19	0.229	130
Water, H_2O	1.00	0.206	0

Modified from Bushong S: *Radiologic science for technologists,* ed 6, St Louis, 1997, Mosby.

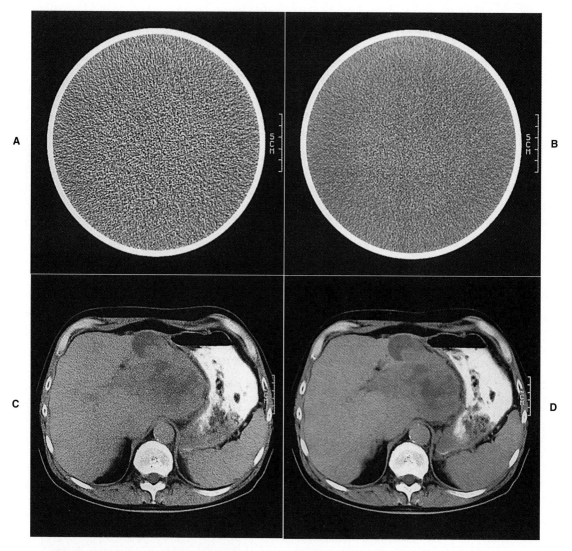

FIG. 11-18. Effect of dose on noise in a CT image. As the dose increases, the noise decreases. Phantom images are shown in **A** (less dose, more noise) and **B** (more dose, less noise), whereas patient images are shown in **D,** where the mA is increased by a factor of 4 compared with image **C,** thus reducing the noise by 50%. (Courtesy Siemens Medical Systems; Iselin, NJ.)

2. If slice thickness increases, noise decreases and spatial resolution decreases.
3. If the dose increases, noise decreases (Fig. 11-18).

A more general relationship of noise to spatial resolution and dose has been given by Riederer et al (1978) as follows:

$$\sigma^2 \; \alpha \; \frac{1}{N} \, r^3 \qquad\qquad (11\text{-}9)$$

where N is the number of detected primary protons (dose) and r is the spatial resolution.

This expression indicates that, to improve spatial resolution by a factor of 2 while keeping σ constant, the dose must be increased by a factor of 8.

LINEARITY

Linearity is another important parameter in CT image quality because it is used in the performance evaluation of the CT scanner. *Linearity* refers to the relationship of CT numbers to the linear attenuation coefficients of the object to be imaged. This can be checked by a daily calibration test, during which an appropriate phantom is scanned to ensure that the CT numbers for water and other known materials of which the phantom is made are correct. Such phantom characteristics are given in Table 11-1.

When an image of the phantom is obtained, the average CT numbers can be plotted as a function of the attenuation coefficients of the phantom materials. The relationship should be a straight line (Fig. 11-19) if the scanner is in good working order (Bushong, 1997).

CROSS-FIELD UNIFORMITY

The uniformity of CT numbers throughout the entire scan field of view is one indication that the CT scanner imaging performance is acceptable. This uniformity refers to the values of the pixels in the reconstructed image—they should be constant at any point in the image of the appropriate test phantom.

"Cross-field uniformity can be verified by inserting five regions of interest, each with an area equal to about five percent of the total phantom area, into a circular water phantom of 20 cm diameter" (Siemens, 1989) (Fig. 11-20). The maximum deviation of CT numbers at the center and the periphery should be no larger than 2 HU.

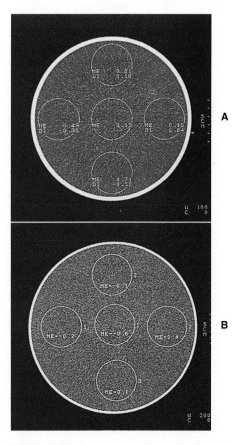

FIG. 11-20. Verification of cross-field uniformity with a 20-cm water phantom. (Courtesy Siemens Medical Systems; Iselin, NJ.)

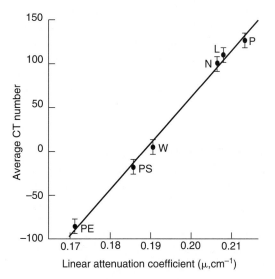

FIG. 11-19. Plot of average CT numbers as a function of linear attenuation coefficients. This indicates acceptable CT linearity if the relationship is a straight line. (From Bushong S: *Radiologic science for technologists,* ed 5, St Louis, 1993, Mosby.)

IMAGE ARTIFACTS

Artifacts can degrade image quality and affect the perceptibility of detail. This can cause serious problems for the radiologist who has to provide a diagnosis from the images obtained by the technologist. Therefore it is mandatory that the technologist understand the nature of artifacts in CT.

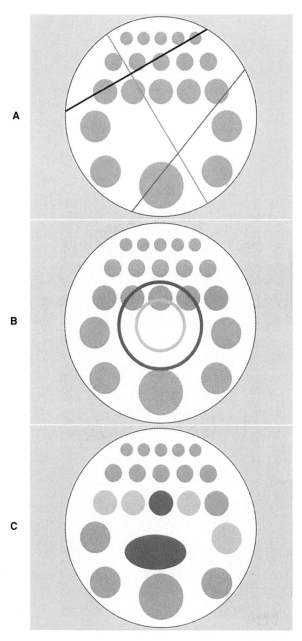

FIG. 11-21. CT artifacts as they appear as streaks (**A**), rings (**B**), and CT number distortions (**C**). (Courtesy Siemens Medical Systems, Iselin, NJ.)

Definition

In general, an *artifact* is "a distortion or error in an image that is unrelated to the subject being studied" (Morgan, 1983). For example, a pair of earrings on a patient will appear on the images of the skull during a CT examination. This appearance is an error in the image and has no relationship to the anatomy under investigation.

Specifically, a CT *image artifact* is defined as "any discrepancy between the reconstructed CT numbers in the image and the true attenuation coefficients of the object" (Hsieh, 1995). This definition is comprehensive and implies that anything that causes an incorrect measurement of transmission readings by the detectors will result in an image artifact. Because CT numbers represent gray shades in the image, incorrect measurements will produce incorrect CT numbers that do not represent the attenuation coefficients of the object. These errors result in various artifacts that affect the appearance of the CT image.

Sources

In CT, artifacts arise from a number of sources including the patient, the imaging process itself, and problems relating to the equipment such as malfunctions or imperfections.

Patients who are uncooperative and move during the examination will cause image artifacts. Built-in corrections of the data during the acquisition process include calibration procedures and preprocessing and postprocessing operations (Hsieh, 1995). Equipment problems can arise from the system electronics and mechanics and computer algorithms. Additionally, carelessness of the part of the technologist, such as improper positioning of patients in the FOV, will result in image artifacts.

Types and Causes

Artifacts in CT can be classified according to cause and appearance. In the classification of artifacts based on their appearance in the image, Hsieh (1995) identifies four major categories including streaks, shadings, rings, and bands, and "miscellaneous" factors such as the basket weave and Moire patterns (Fig. 11-21).

Streak artifacts may appear as intense straight lines across an image and may be caused by improper sampling of the data (aliasing), partial volume averaging, motion, metal, beam hardening, noise, spiral/helical scanning, and mechanical failure or imperfections. Shading artifacts often appear near objects of high densities and can be caused by beam hardening, partial volume averaging, spiral/helical scanning, scatter radiation, off-focal radiation, and incomplete projections. Rings and bands are caused by bad detector channels in third-generation CT scanners (Hsieh, 1995, 1998) (Table 11-2).

Common Artifacts and Correction Techniques

Patient Motion Artifacts

Patient motion can be voluntary or involuntary. Voluntary motion is directly controlled by the patient, such as swallowing or respiratory motion. Involuntary motion is not under the direct control of the patient, such as peristalsis and cardiac motion (Fig. 11-22). Both voluntary and involuntary motion appears as streaks that are usually tangential to high-contrast edges of the moving part. Additionally, motion artifacts can arise from movement of oral contrast in the gastrointestinal tract.

The appearance of streaks results from the inability of the reconstruction algorithm to deal with data inconsistencies in voxel attenuation arising from the edge of the moving part. The computer has difficulty in tracking the location of the voxels.

There are several methods to reduce CT artifacts from motion. For patient movements such as breathing and swallowing, it is important to im-

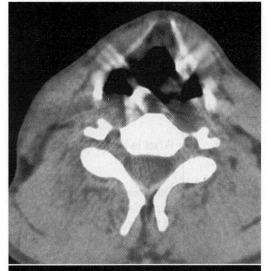
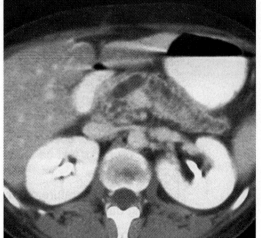
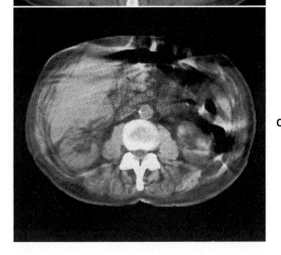

FIG. 11-22. Motion artifacts due to swallowing (**A**), peristalsis (**B**), and patient movement (**C**). (Courtesy Siemens Medical Systems; Iselin, NJ.)

TABLE 11-2

Classification of Artifacts Based on Appearance

APPEARANCE	CAUSE
Streaks	Improper sampling of data; partial volume averaging; patient motion; metal; beam hardening; noise; spiral/helical scanning; mechanical failure
Shading	Partial volume averaging; beam hardening; spiral/helical scanning; scatter radiation; off-focal radiation; incomplete projections
Rings and bands	Bad detector channels in third-generation CT scanners

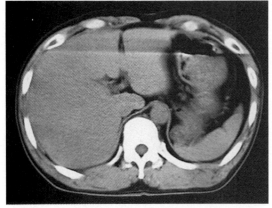

Conventional image

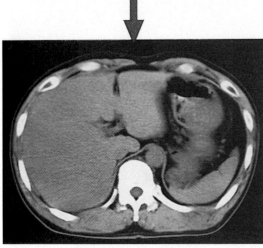

Motion artifact correction

FIG. 11-23. The use of software to correct for motion artifacts in CT. The real-time motion artifact correction (MAC) reduces artifacts that arise from air/fluid interfaces in the gastrointestinal tract. MAC reconstruction occurs during the scan. (Courtesy Shimadzu Medical Systems, Seattle, Wash.)

mobilize patients and use positioning aids to make them comfortable and to ensure that patients understand the importance of remaining still and following instructions during scanning. Another useful motion artifact reduction technique is to use short scan times for the examination. Correction of motion artifacts can also be accomplished with software. The CT manufacturer Shimadzu uses real-time motion artifact correction (MAC) software to reduce the effect of streaks on the CT image (Fig. 11-23).

Metal Artifacts

The presence of metal in the patient also causes artifacts. Metallic materials such as prosthetic devices,

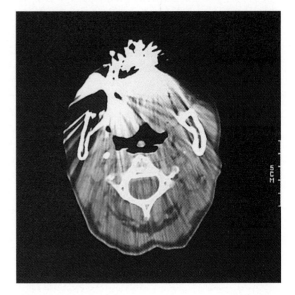

FIG. 11-24. Artifacts due to metallic implants. (Courtesy Siemens Medical Systems; Iselin, NJ.)

dental fillings, surgical clips, and electrodes give rise to streak artifacts on the image (Fig. 11-24).

The creation of these artifacts and a method of correction are illustrated in Fig. 11-25. As shown in Fig. 11-25, *A*, the metal object absorbs the radiation, which results in incomplete projection profiles. This loss of information leads to the appearance of typical star-shaped streaks.

Metal artifacts can be reduced by the removal of all external metal objects from the patient. Software such as the metal artifact reduction (MAR) program can also be used to complete the incomplete profile through interpolation (Fig. 11-25, *B*). The procedure is described by Felsenberg and colleagues (1988) as follows:

1. Acquisition and storage of the raw data
2. Reconstruction of a CT image
3. Rough tracing of the implant with a light pen by the examiner
4. Automatic definition of the boundaries of the implant within the projection data. For each projection, that is, each angular setting of the tube/detector system, the implant boundaries are automatically defined within the given ROI by the use of given threshold values.
5. Linear interpolation of the missing projection data
6. Reconstruction of the artifact-reduced image from the newly computed projection data.

Beam Hardening Artifacts

Beam hardening refers to the increase in the mean energy of the x-ray beam as it passes through the

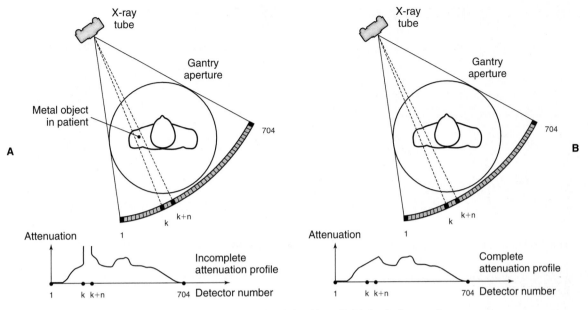

FIG. 11-25. **A,** Creation of metal artifacts. **B,** Method of correction.

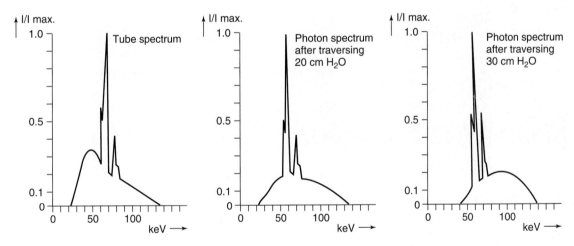

FIG. 11-26. Effect of beam hardening as the x-ray beam traverses different object sizes. (Courtesy Siemens Medical Systems; Iselin, NJ.)

patient (Fig. 11-26). As the object size increases, the mean energy shifts to the right because lower energy photons are absorbed as the beam passes through the object. As a result, the CT numbers of certain structures change, which creates artifacts (Joseph and Ruth, 1997). Additionally, beam hardening can occur when the radiation beams have different path lengths (Fig. 11-27). Fig. 11-27 shows a short and a long path length, both of which result in beam hardening. There is less beam hardening at the periphery of the object where the radiation path is short, compared with the center of the object where the radiation path is longer. Fig. 11-28 demonstrates that without beam hard-

ening correction, the relative intensity profile changes from A to A′. Specifically, this change produces beam hardening artifacts from errors in CT numbers from the periphery to the center of the FOV.

This change in CT numbers results in beam hardening artifacts, which appear as broad dark bands or streaks. This is known as the "cupping" artifact (Fig. 11-29). The CT numbers are higher at the periphery and lower at the center of the image.

Beam hardening artifacts can be reduced or eliminated with a bowtie filter that ensures the uniformity of the beam at the detectors. In addition, software can correct for the effects of beam harden-

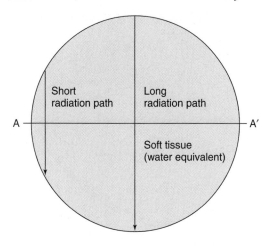

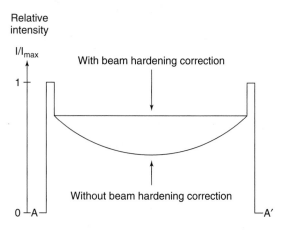

FIG. 11-27. Short and long radiation paths through an object will result in beam hardening. (Courtesy Siemens Medical Systems; Iselin, NJ.)

FIG. 11-28. The relative radiation profile as a result of beam hardening and beam hardening correction (*top curve*) results in a change in CT numbers from the periphery to the center of the image (cupping artifact). (Courtesy Siemens Medical Systems; Iselin, NJ.)

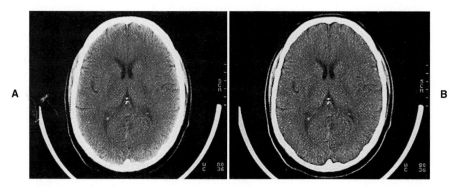

FIG. 11-29. The effect of beam hardening on the appearance of the CT image. **A,** The cupping artifact is visible. **B,** The cupping artifact is reduced through software. (Courtesy Siemens Medical Systems; Iselin, NJ.)

ing with improved appearance of soft tissue densities and constant window levels (Fig. 11-29, *B*).

Partial Volume Artifacts

CT number calculations are based on the linear attenuation coefficients for a voxel of tissue. If the voxel contains only one tissue type, the calculation will not be problematic. For example, if the tissue in the voxel is dense bone, the CT number is computed at 1000. If the voxel contains three similar tissue types in which the CT numbers are close together—for example, blood (CT number = 40), gray matter (43), and white matter (46)—then the CT number for that voxel is based on an average of the three tissues (43). This is known as *partial volume averaging.*

Partial volume averaging can lead to the partial volume effect and thus lead to partial volume artifacts (Fig. 11-30).

In Fig. 11-30, the detector on the left measures the transmission through bone only and a true CT number for bone is calculated from the transmission measurements. In the diagram on the right, the detector measures x-rays transmitted from bone and air and a CT number is calculated for the two types of materials. Mathematically, the two intensities I_1 and I_2 are measured as $I_1 + I_2$, but for accurate calculation of the CT number, it is necessary to take the logarithm (ln) of each and add them together as follows:

$$ln\ I_1 + ln\ I_2$$

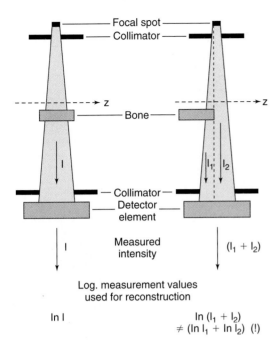

FIG. 11-30. The origin of the partial volume effect. (Courtesy Siemens Medical Systems; Iselin, NJ.)

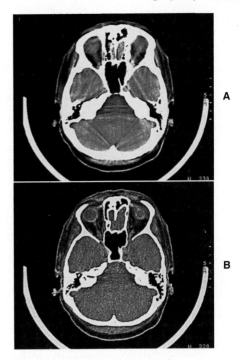

FIG. 11-31. Partial-volume artifacts appear as streaks across the petrous and occipital protuberances. (Courtesy Siemens Medical Systems; Iselin, NJ.)

If $ln\ I_1 + I_2$ is used to calculate the CT numbers, then inaccuracies occur:

$$ln\ I_1 + I_2 \neq ln\ I_1 + ln\ I_2 \qquad (11\text{-}10)$$

These inaccuracies result in partial volume artifacts in the image, which appear as bands and streaks (Fig. 11-31).

Partial volume artifacts can be reduced with thinner slice scans and computer algorithms. Hsieh (1995) recommends the first method (Fig. 11-32). With two slices, the correct CT number can be calculated from summing the logarithms of the intensities from each slice, $ln\ I_1 + ln\ I_2$ (not $ln\ I_1 + I_2$).

The volume artifact reduction (VAR) technique can also reduce partial volume artifacts (Fig. 11-33). In Fig. 11-33, an 8-mm slice containing bone and soft tissue is divided into four thin slices with a table feed between each. The raw data sets are averaged to produce a composite 8-mm slice image free of partial volume artifacts (Hupke, 1990).

Equipment-Induced Artifacts

Streak artifacts can also be created by the CT equipment itself through mechanical failure or imperfections such as poor gantry rigidity, mechanical misalignment, x-ray tube rotor wobble, and

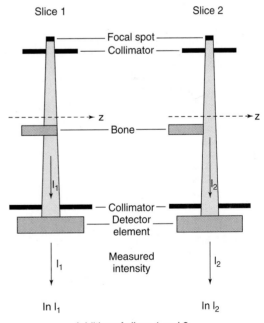

FIG. 11-32. The elimination of partial volume effect by scanning thinner slices. (Courtesy Siemens Medical Systems; Iselin, NJ.)

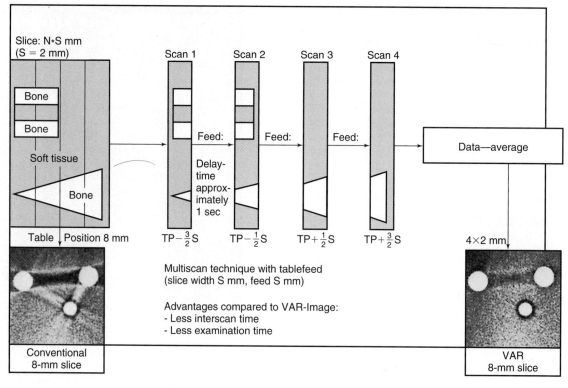

FIG. 11-33. Volume artifact reduction technique. (From Hupke R: The advantages of fast and continuously rotating CT systems. In Fuchs WA, ed: *Advances in CT,* New York, 1990, Springer-Verlag.)

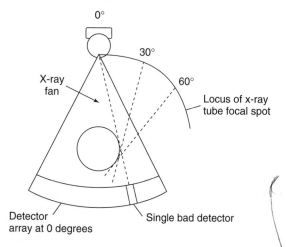

FIG. 11-34. Creation of ring artifacts on third-generation CT scanners.

of ring artifacts is described by Barnes and Lakshminarayanan (1989) as follows:

The reason for the ring is that during the rotation of the x-ray tube and detector array, the rays measured by a given detector are tangent to a circle. If a detector has an offset or gain difference of 0.1% with neighboring detectors, a circular artifact will be present in the image. Such an artifact indicates that the detector gain needs to be calibrated. A faulty detector in a fourth-generation scanner does not give rise to a noticeable artifact because each detector acquires a view and the bad data are spread evenly across the image. Also, detector-to-detector channel variations rarely create a problem in a fourth-generation scanner because the detector is calibrated by the raw radiation beam during a scan.

To correct for ring artifacts in third-generation CT scanners, the bad detector or detectors must first be located and subsequently recalibrated. Additionally, these artifacts can be eliminated with software such as the balancing algorithm, which will correct the raw data during acquisition or after scanning (Fig. 11-35).

Aliasing Artifacts. A sampling problem arises when structures and spaces cannot be distin-

poor sampling of the detector signals (Hsieh, 1995). Additionally, bad detectors can create ring artifacts.

Ring Artifacts. Ring artifacts are characteristic of third-generation CT scanners and result from one or more bad detectors that produce varying signal outputs (Fig. 11-34). The creation

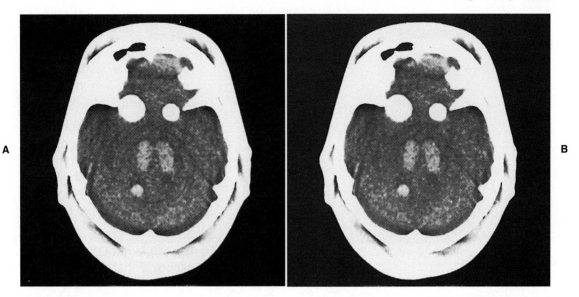

FIG. II-35. The ring artifact (**A**) and correction using the balancing algorithm (**B**). (Courtesy Siemens Medical Systems; Iselin, NJ.)

guished. The solution to this problem requires the use of the sampling theorem, which states that to faithfully reproduce object points in the patient, the sampling frequency f_A (the number of rays/cm in the fan-beam) must be at least twice the smallest object to be scanned (the number of separate object points/cm and the spacing between points). Mathematically, this can be expressed as follows:

$$f_A \geq 2f_O$$

If the above criterion, or Nyquist criterion, is not met, then aliasing artifacts (streaks) result from an insufficient number of samples available for image reconstruction (Fig. 11-36). If f_A is less than or equal to f_O, aliasing occurs. Aliasing artifacts can arise from insufficient views for image reconstruction (Fig. 11-37). Fig. 11-37 shows a torso phantom that was scanned using half the normal number of views (Hsieh, 1999).

Various methods are available to minimize aliasing artifacts. In some cases the number of views or number of ray samples per view can be increased (Fig. 11-38). A convolution filter can also be used to smooth the image and thus improve its appearance.

Noise-Induced Artifacts

Noise is influenced by the number of photons that strike the detectors as a result of poor patient positioning in the scan field-of-view (SFOV) and poor selection of exposure technique factors (kVp, mA), scan speed, and limitations of the CT scanner such as aperture size. More photons means less

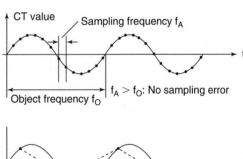

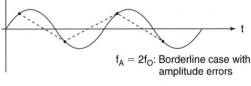

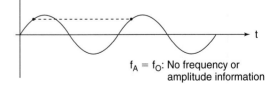

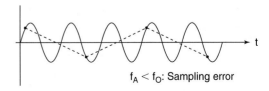

FIG. II-36. The process of sampling. (Courtesy Siemens Medical Systems; Iselin, NJ.)

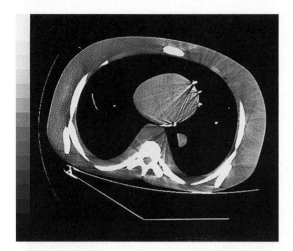

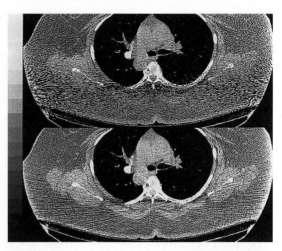

FIG. 11-37. View aliasing artifacts due to 50% of the normal number of views used to scan this torso phantom. The artifacts are apparent at the periphery of the phantom. (Courtesy Jiang Hsieh, General Electrical Medical Systems; Milwaukee, Wis.)

FIG. 11-39. **A,** Streak artifacts can arise from an increase in noise due to reduced photons at the detector. **B,** Correction of the streaks by adaptive filtering. (Courtesy Jiang Hsieh, General Electrical Medical Systems; Milwaukee, Wis.)

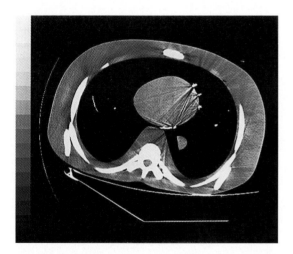

FIG. 11-38. Scanning the same torso phantom shown in Fig. 11-37 at the Nyquist criterion can reduce view aliasing artifacts. (Courtesy Jiang Hsieh, General Electrical Medical Systems; Milwaukee, Wis.)

the x-ray flux level at each projection channel. By selectively smoothing only the channels that contribute to the streaking artifacts, and by varying the degree of smoothing based on the noise level of the signal, the objectives of simultaneously reducing the streaks artifacts in the images and preserving the spatial resolution of the system are achieved" (Hsieh, 1998).

IMAGE QUALITY IN SPIRAL/HELICAL CT

CT scanning in spiral/helical geometry can also lead to streaks and shading artifacts. Kalender (1995) notes that several artifacts characteristic of conventional CT "manifest themselves in the same form" for spiral/helical CT (e.g., beam hardening and sampling artifacts). However, the effect of patient motion has been minimized in spiral/helical because of subsecond scan times, and table motion artifacts have been corrected with z-interpolation.

Partial volume artifacts are exaggerated in spiral/helical CT because of slice sensitivity profile degradation. These artifacts can be reduced with thin slices, a pitch of 1, and 180-degree algorithms. However, the image reconstruction and summing of thin slices is time consuming. Recently, Heuscher and Vembar (1999) presented a scheme to reduce partial volume artifacts using an integrating spiral interpolator (ISI). ISI "allows the user to plan and reconstruct thin-slice spiral

noise and a stronger detector signal, whereas few photons (photon starvation) results in more noise and a weaker detector signal (Fig. 11-39). Reduced photons (increased noise) will lead to streak artifacts as shown in Fig. 11-39, B.

The technologist should optimize patient positioning, scan speed, and exposure technique factors to correct streak artifacts. These artifacts can also be reduced with adaptive filtering algorithms (Fig. 11-39, B). These algorithms "dynamically adjust the amount of smoothing operation based on scans as if they were thick spiral scans but with significantly reduced partial volume artifacts. Since only the necessary clinical images are reconstructed, the reconstructions can be prospectively planned as if the scan was being performed with a collimated slice thickness several times that of the actual slice thickness used" (Heuscher and Vembar, 1999).

Artifacts can also arise from CT angiography with 3D and maximum intensity projection (MIP) displays. In the MIP images, the artifacts appear as bright and dark horizontal strips and have been called "zebra artifacts" (Hsieh, 1997). The strips result from a nonuniform distribution of noise. The zebra artifact can be reduced with improved noise uniformity in the reconstructed image through scanning or image processing.

Finally, Hsieh (1999) groups a class of artifacts he describes as *miscellaneous* ("others") such as the basket weave pattern and Moire pattern.

QUALITY CONTROL

Quality control is an integral part of equipment testing and maintenance programs in hospitals. Quality control ensures the optimal performance of the CT scanner through a series of daily, monthly, and annual tests for spatial resolution, contrast resolution, noise, slice width, kVp waveform, average CT number of water, standard deviation of CT numbers in water, and radiation scatter and leakage. These tests constitute a general quality control program for CT scanners.

REFERENCES

Barnes GT, Lakshminarayanan AV: Computed tomography: physical principles and image quality considerations. In Lee JK et al, eds: *Computed tomography with MRI correlation,* ed 2, New York, 1981, Raven Press, 1989.

Blumenfeld SM, Glover G: Spatial resolution in computed tomography. In Newton TH, Potts DG, eds: *Radiology of the skull and brain: technical aspects of computed tomography,* vol 5, St Louis, 1981, Mosby.

Bushong S: *Radiologic science for technologists,* ed 6, St Louis, 1997, Mosby.

Curry TS et al: *Christensen's physics of diagnostic radiology,* ed 4, Philadelphia, 1990, Lea & Febiger.

Felsenberg D et al: Reduction of metal artifacts in computed tomography—clinical experience and results, *Electromedica* 56:97-104, 1988.

Galvin JR et al: High-resolution computed tomography and diffuse lung disease, *Curr Prob Diagn Radiol* 21:39-51, 1992.

Hanson KM: Noise and contrast and discrimination in computed tomography. In Newton TH, Potts DG, eds: *Radiology of the skull and brain: technical aspects of computed tomography,* vol 5, St Louis, 1981, Mosby.

Heuscher DJ, Vembar M: Reduced partial volume artifacts using spiral computed tomography and integrating spiral interpolator, *Medical Physics* 26: 276-287, 1999.

Heuscher DJ, Vembar M: Improved 3D and CT angiography with spiral CT, *Radiology* 197: 222-227, 1995.

Hounsfield GN: Potential uses of more accurate CT absorption values by filtering, *Am J Roentgenol* 131: 103-106, 1978.

Hsieh J: Image artifacts, causes and correction. In Goldman LW, Fowlkes JB, eds: *Medical CT and ultrasound: current technology and applications,* Md, 1995, American Association of Physicists in Medicine.

Hsieh J: Nonstationary noise characteristics of the helical scan and its impact on image quality and artifacts, *Medical Physics* 24:1375-1384, 1997.

Hsieh J: Adaptive artifact reduction in computed tomography resulting from x-ray photon noise, *Medical Physics* 25:2139-2147, 1998.

Hsieh J: Personal communication, 1999.

Hupke R: The advantages of fast and continuously rotating CT systems. In Fuchs WA, ed: *Advances in CT,* New York, 1990, Springer-Verlag.

Joseph PM, Ruth C: Method for simultaneous correction of spectrum hardening artifacts in CT images containing both boe and iodine, *Medical Physics* 24: 1629-1643, 1997.

Kalender WA, Polacin A: Physical performance characteristics of spiral CT scanning, *Medical Physics* 18:910-915, 1991.

Kalender WA et al: Causes of artifacts in spiral CT angiography with MIP displays, *Radiology* 197:221-224, 1995.

Kalender WA: Principles and performance of spiral CT. In Goldman LW, Fowlkes JB, eds: *Medical CT and ultrasound: current technology and applications,* College Park, Md, 1995, American Association of Physicists in Medicine.

Mayo JR: High-resolution computed tomography: technical aspects, *Radiol Clin North Am* 29:1043-1048, 1991.

McCullough ED: Factors affecting the use of quantitative information from a CT scanner, *Radiology* 124: 99-107, 1977.

Meziane MA: High-resolution computer tomography scanning in the assessment of interstitial lung diseases, *J Thorac Imaging* 7:13-25, 1992.

Morgan CL: *Basic principles of computed tomography,* Baltimore, 1983, University Park Press.

Pfeiler M et al: Some guiding ideas on image recording in computerized axial tomography, *Electromedica* 1:19-25, 1976

Riederer SJ et al: The noise power spectrum in computer x-ray tomography, *Phys Med Biol* 23:446-454, 1978.

Robb RA, Morin RL: Principles and instrumentation for dynamic x-ray computed tomography. In Marcus JL et al, eds: *Cardiac imaging: a comparison to Braunwald's heart disease*, Philadelphia, 1991, WB Saunders.

Shen Y et al: Improvement of image quality of CT angiography by using deblurring techniques, *Radiology* 197:221-223, 1995.

Siemens Aktiengesellschaft: *The technology and performance of the Somatom Plus*, Henkestrasse, Germany, 1989, Siemens AG.

Sprawls P: *Physical principles of medical imaging*, Rockville, Md, 1995, Aspen.

Swensen SJ et al: High-resolution CT of the lungs: findings in various pulmonary diseases, *Am J Roentgenol* 158:971-979, 1992.

Villafana T: Physics and instrumentation of CT and MRI. In Lee SH, Rao K, eds: *Cranial computed tomography and MRI*, ed 2, New York, 1987, McGraw-Hill.

Measuring Patient Dose from Computed Tomography Scanners

ROBERT CACAK

Two questions often asked regarding CT scanners are "How much radiation dose is my CT scanner delivering to the patient?" and "How does the radiation dose from my CT scanner compare with the dose from other CT scanners?" The radiation dose must be known to estimate the patient's potential risk from the radiation and to weigh this risk against the benefits of CT scanning. In addition, most radiation regulatory agencies require the measurement or estimation of radiation dose to patients from medical x-ray units.

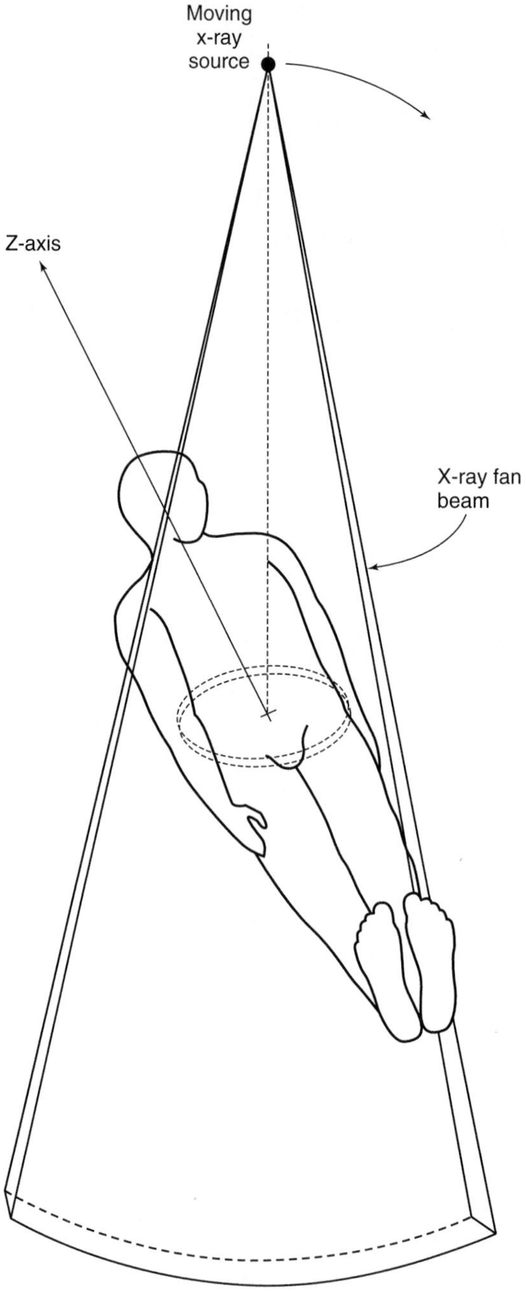

CT SCANNER X-RAY BEAM GEOMETRY

Most modern CT scanners emit a fan-shaped x-ray beam that usually has a quite narrow cross-section. Along the longitudinal axis of the patient, the beam is quite thin, typically only a few millimeters thick. A diagram of a typical x-ray beam striking a patient is shown in Fig. 12-1.

Fig. 12-2, A shows the same fan-shaped x-ray beam viewed from the side with the thickness exaggerated for clarity. If the longitudinal (cranial-caudal) axis of the patient is defined as the z axis,

FIG. 12-1. Most modern scanners employ a fan-shaped x-ray beam. The dimensions of the radiation beam in the fan dimension are large enough to cover the patient. The dimension along the axis of the patient (z axis) is typically only a few millimeters thick.

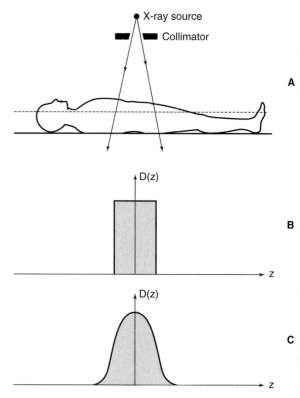

FIG. 12-2. The width of the x-ray beam is viewed from the side (**A**). The collimator near the x-ray source (the width is exaggerated for clarity) determines the beam width. An ideal dose distribution along the z axis is shown (**B**). It has a flat top and steep sides and is the same width as the x-ray beam. A more realistic bell-shaped dose distribution curve is typical of most CT scanners (**C**).

then in theory, the intensity of the radiation beam along that axis can be graphed. Ideally the radiation intensity measured along the z axis would have equal intensity everywhere inside the beam and would have no intensity on either side. Fig. 12-2, *B*, shows this ideal rectangular intensity profile of the radiation beam. In reality, the radiation intensity measured along the z axis has smoother edges and appears as a bell-shaped curve. The dose distribution is almost always wider than the nominal slice width (SW). CT scanner manufacturers design the x-ray beam somewhat wider than the nominal SW to allow for slight misalignments of the x-ray beam and the fact that the x-ray beam does not have the ideal rectangular shape.

The dose distribution is given by the function $D(z)$, which describes an arbitrarily shaped dose intensity along the patient axis. In general, the shape of $D(z)$ varies between CT scanners.

METHODS OF MEASURING PATIENT DOSE

Radiation doses from CT scanner examinations are among the highest in diagnostic radiology. Accurate determination of dose from CT scanners is therefore especially important. Although there are many dose measurement methods, only the pencil ionization chamber method, or CT dose index (CTDI) method, is described in this chapter. The ionization chamber method is the easiest and probably the most accurate, and it is used almost exclusively to report dose.

Historical Perspective

Historically, there have been many schemes for measuring the dose profile $D(z)$. Some schemes have involved film dosimetry; other schemes have placed thermoluminescent dosimeter (TLD) crystals end to end across the width of the x-ray beam, exposing them, and measuring the dose absorbed by each crystal (Jucius and Kambic, 1977; Dixon and Eckstrand, 1978; Shope et al, 1982; Cacak and Hendee, 1979). Other techniques have used special ionization chambers that are capable of measuring dose at several points across the width of the x-ray beam (Moore, Cacak, and Hendee, 1981) and reconstructing the shape of the dose curve from these measurements. These measurement schemes may be quite time consuming and require highly specialized equipment. Although profile data provide information on shapes of the dose

curves, profile data are not usually necessary to yield meaningful CT scanner dose measurements.

In 1981, the staff at the Bureau of Radiological Health (now the Center for Devices and Radiological Health) suggested an easy and accurate method to measure patient dose that relied on CT dose index (CTDI) and multiple scan average dose (MSAD) (Shope, Gagne, and Johnson, 1981). This technique uses a single ionization chamber measurement and a subsequent simple calculation to determine the average dose delivered to a patient who has received a series of scans at a given technique with a specified bed indexing (BI, the distance between scans). Since then, other improvements have been suggested (Spokas, 1982; Poletti, 1984). MSAD appears to be sufficiently accurate for the newer types of spiral/helical CT scanners, as well as single-slice scanners.

Ionization Chamber

Recall that an ionization chamber is an instrument used to accurately quantify radiation exposure. An ionization chamber consists of a small air-filled container with thin walls that allow radiation to pass through easily. As the high-energy photons (x-ays) collide with air molecules enclosed within the ionization chamber, some of the molecules are "ionized" (i.e., one or more electrons are knocked from some molecules). These free electrons can be collected on a conducting wire or plate and measured as electric charge. The amount of collected charge is proportional to the amount of ionization, which is proportional to the amount of radiation that passes through the chamber. The charge is removed from the ionization chamber and measured with a very sensitive instrument known as an *electrometer*. The total electric charge generated by an x-ray beam is represented by Q and measured in coulombs (one coulomb = 1.6×10^{19} electrons).

Multiple Scan Average Dose

In the multiple scan average dose (MSAD), a series of CT scans is performed on a patient (Fig. 12-3). Between each scan, the patient is moved a bed index (BI) distance. Each slice delivers the characteristic bell-shaped dose represented by the curves in the top of Fig. 12-3. If the doses from all scans are summed, the resulting total patient dose resembles the oscillating curve in the bottom of Fig. 12-3. In the regions where the bell curves overlap, the resultant dose is higher than that from just one scan. If the total dose distribution curve is known (bot-

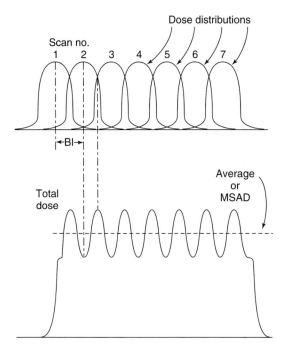

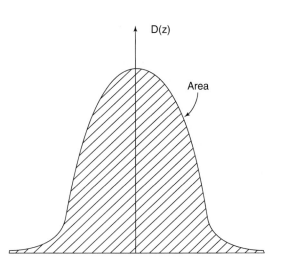

FIG. 12-3. A series of seven scans spaced (bed indexing) apart along the z axis disburses seven bell-shaped dose distribution curves (*top*). When the doses from this series of curves are summed, the resultant total dose appears as the bottom curve. The total dose curve has peaks where the bell-shaped curves overlap. The dotted line through the total dose curve is the multiple scan average dose.

FIG. 12-4. The integral in Equations 1 and 3 is numerically equal to the area (*shaded region*) of the dose distribution curve.

tom curve), the MSAD (dotted straight line) can be calculated by mathematically sampling the peaks and valleys of the multiple scan dose curve.

Dose Index

The CT dose index (CTDI) is defined as:

$$CTDI = \frac{1}{n \cdot SW} \int_{-\infty}^{\infty} D(z)dz \qquad (12\text{-}1)$$

where n is the number of distinct planes of data collected during one revolution, SW is the nominal slice width (in mm), $D(z)$ is the dose distribution, and z is the dimension along the patient's axis. For axial (nonspiral) CT scanners and spiral scanners with a single array of detectors, $n = 1$. For multislice CT scanners, n is the number of active arrays during the scan.

This seemingly formidable equation is not as complicated as it appears. The integral sign merely instructs the user to determine the area under a single curve $D(z)$. Fig. 12-4 demonstrates the value of this integral by shading the area under a typical dose distribution curve. If this area is divided

by the number of slices times the slice width $(n)(SW)$, the result is the CTDI.

This definition is good for essentially all shapes of dose distribution curves $D(z)$ that are emitted by CT scanners. Note that the CTDI can be increased by increasing the area under the curve. The area can be increased by either increasing the intensity of radiation, which raises the height of the curve, or by widening the curve, usually by opening the x-ray collimators near the x-ray tube. Either case increases the CTDI and ultimately icreases the radiation dose to the patient.

The BRH researchers recognized that if the CTDI could be measured, it could easily be related to the MSAD regardless of the shape of the dose distribution curve. They proved that the MSAD may be calculated by multiplying the ratio of SW to BI by the CTDI. Mathematically, this becomes

$$MSAD = CTDI\left(\frac{SW}{BI}\right) = \frac{1}{n \cdot BI} \int_{-\infty}^{\infty} D(z)dz \qquad (12\text{-}2)$$

In this equation, BI is the bed index or slice spacing (in mm), SW is the slice width (in mm), and n is the number of active arrays of detectors.

The part of the equation to the right of the second equal sign (=) is derived from the definition of the CTDI (Equation 12-1). Because the values for n and BI are known, it is only necessary to measure the dose integral to arrive at a value for MSAD; this can be easily done with a single scan and a "pencil" ion chamber.

As the value of BI is increased, the value of MSAD generally decreases. This means that if the slices are spaced farther apart, the radiation is spread over a greater distance within the patient and the average dose becomes smaller. Of course, as the slice spacing increases, there is a greater likelihood that relevant tissue will be "missed" (it falls between the slices) in the scan sequence, thus limiting the amount that the BI can be increased. Conversely, when the bed index is made smaller, the slices become closer together, more overlap of adjacent dose distributions occurs, and the average dose increases. When the slice width equals the BI, the MSAD is numerically equal to the CTDI.

Strictly speaking, the MSAD is only valid in the center of the scan series. Upon examination of the dose near either end of the scan series, it may be seen that the MSAD slightly overestimates the true average dose. Nevertheless, the MSAD is sufficiently accurate for the center portion of the CT scan series and is valuable despite this rather minor shortcoming.

Measuring the CTDI

After the measurement of CTDI, the calculation of the MSAD is straightforward using Equation 12-2. The only term of any concern is the integral in Equation 12-1. Fortunately, it is very easy to measure the integral term in the CTDI equation with a long cylindric ionization chamber and the radiation dose from a single slice. One benefit of the MSAD is that the average dose for a series of slices, which is usually the clinical case, can be determined by measuring the CTDI from a single slice.

The ionization chamber receives radiation from all parts of the dose distribution $D(z)$ because its length is several times the width of the x-ray beam. The total charge from the ionization chamber is proportional to the integral in the CTDI definition. Mathematically, this is expressed as:

$$Q = \frac{1}{C_f} \int_{-\infty}^{\infty} D(z)dz \qquad (12\text{-}3)$$

where Q is the total charge collected during a single scan and C_f is the calibration factor of the ionization chamber. Because the ionization chamber measures exposure and not the dose, a conversion factor (the f-factor) must be included in C_f, which

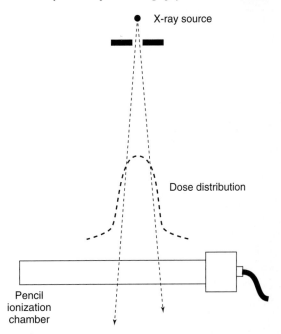

FIG. 12-5. An ionization chamber effectively performs the integral in Equation 12-3 by intercepting the radiation beam and sensing the dose from all parts of the dose distribution curve. The charge emitted from the chamber is proportional to the area under the dose distribution curve.

converts exposure (Roentgen) to dose (cGy; recall that 1 cGy = 1 rad). The value of the f-factor at CT scanner x-ray energies is approximately 0.94 cGy/Roentgen.

The long ionization chamber is often called a *pencil chamber* because of its shape and size. The entire narrow width of the x-ray beam is intercepted by the chamber placed perpendicular to the fan of the radiation beam (i.e., the chamber is placed parallel to the longitudinal axis of the patient) (Fig. 12-5). The x-ray beam must merely be positioned in the center of the chamber, and the radiation beam is turned on while a single scan is made.

To standardize the measurement of the dose and provide a clinically realistic geometry, the BRH researchers suggested that the ionization chamber be placed in one of two cylindric phantoms during the radiation measurement. The smaller phantom simulates a patient's head and the larger phantom simulates a "body" or torso (Fig. 12-6). Both phantoms are 15 cm in length. The diameter of the "head" phantom is 16 cm, and the diameter of the "body" phantom is 32 cm. Both phantoms are solid acrylic with holes drilled through the phantom at specified locations to accommodate the pencil

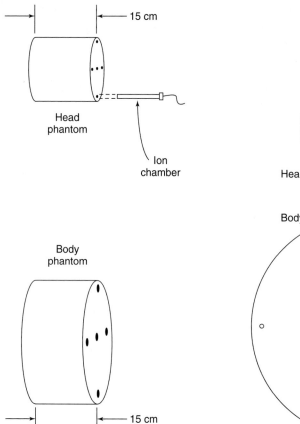

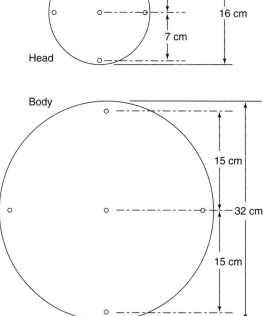

FIG. 12-6. The "head" and "body" CT scanner dosimetry phantoms are solid acrylic with holes placed strategically to receive a pencil ionization chamber. Although the phantoms differ in diameter, they are both 15 cm long.

FIG. 12-7. A view of the face of a "head" phantom (*top*) and a "body" phantom (*bottom*). Dimensions and location of the ionization chamber holes are shown. Diameters of the holes are typically 1 cm and should be drilled to match the outer diameter of the ionization chamber.

ionization chamber (Fig. 12-7). Acrylic plugs are placed in the holes unoccupied by the ionization chamber. Fig. 12-8 shows a pencil ionization chamber about to be inserted into a CT scanner dosimetry phantom. The holes that are not being used for the ionization chamber are filled with acrylic plugs. Careful examination of the plug reveals a small hole that can be seen through its diameter. This hole is centered end-to-end in the plug and is visible in the CT image of the dosimetry phantom if the x-ray beam is centered on the phantom and passes through the hole. The appearance of the hole in the image verifies that the x-ray beam is striking the center of the phantom.

The procedure for measurement is to place the ionization chamber in one of the phantom holes, take a scan, and record the amount of charge emitted from the chamber. Then the chamber is moved to the next hole, the plug is placed in the original chamber hole, and the procedure is repeated. Mov-

ing the chamber to another hole (e.g., from the anterior to the posterior) allows the dose to be determined at a variety of locations within the phantom. Generally, the dose varies between locations, even when the same technique is used. For example, the dose at the anterior location of the phantom differs from the dose at the posterior location, which differs from the dose on the patient's right side, and so on. It is usually prudent to measure the dose at several locations for a given technique.

MEASUREMENT PROCEDURE
Basic Steps

The measurement of MSAD may be performed as follows:

1. Select the technique needed to measure dose. In general, the technique will require the operator to select the kVp, mAs, SW,

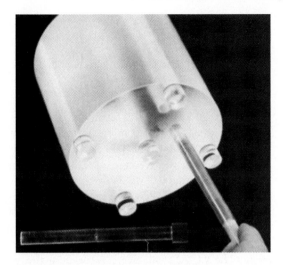

FIG. 12-8. A pencil ionization chamber about to be inserted in a "head" CT scanner dosimetry phantom. The holes that are not being used for the ionization chamber are filled with acrylic plugs (*bottom*). The appearance of the hole in the image verifies that the x-ray beam is striking the center of the phantom.

NOTE: If the CT scanner starts its scan at the same location for all scans, this single measurement is sufficient. However, some CT scanners are bidirectional (i.e., they make even-numbered scans in a clockwise motion and make odd-numbered scans in a counter-clockwise direction). These bidirectional CT scanners will usually have different doses for the clockwise and counter-clockwise scans, depending on the location of the ionization chamber in the phantom relative to where the scans start and stop. If the CT scanner operates in a bidirectional scan mode, two successive scans (one clockwise and one counter-clockwise) should be performed and the average of the two readings should be used for the value of Q.

7. Calculate the MSAD using the following expression derived from Equations 12-2 and 12-3:

$$MSAD = \frac{(C_f)(Q)}{(n)(BI)} \qquad (12\text{-}4)$$

where C_f is the ionization chamber calibration factor (in cGy-mm coulomb) provided by an accredited dosimetry calibration laboratory or by a physicist equipped to calibrate pencil ionization chambers.

8. Move the ionization chamber to a different location in the phantom and repeat the measurement. Perform the measurement at each location in the phantom. Be careful not to move the phantom as the ionization chamber's location is changed.

9. Repeat the measurements at each technique requiring dosimetry data. Change the phantom size from "head" to "body" when appropriate.

x-ray filters (if any), BI, scan time, and perhaps other parameters (e.g., x-ray pulse length).

2. Choose the appropriate phantom for the technique being measured. For example, if a head technique is to be measured, then the smaller "head" size phantom should be used. For a spine or body technique, the larger "body" phantom is appropriate.

3. Place the phantom where the patient would be located for a scan. Orient the phantom so the phantom axis will be parallel to the axis of the patient. Usually, the phantom is placed on the bed; perhaps a head holder is used for a head phantom. The bed is raised or lowered until the phantom is approximately centered vertically in the CT scanner.

4. Move the bed and the phantom in or out until it is positioned so that the center of the x-ray beam will intersect the center of the phantom as measured from end to end.

5. Place the pencil ionization chamber in the desired hole in the phantom where the dose is to be measured. Fill the remaining holes with acrylic plugs. Connect the ion chamber to a charge-measuring instrument such as an electrometer that operates in the "charge" or "integrate" mode.

6. Make a single scan and record the charge from the ion chamber. Call this charge Q.

Spiral/Helical CT Scanner Dosimetry

The above CTDI procedure may also be used with reasonable accuracy to estimate patient dose delivered when the CT scanner is operated in the spiral mode. In this case, the slice width must be set equal to that for the spiral scan, and a single scan measurement is performed. The CTDI is measured with the bed stationary, and the value of the BI in Equation 12-2 is set equal to the distance the bed travels during one revolution of the scanner. If measurements are performed on a CT scanner with more than one set of detector arrays, then the appropriate value of *n* in the equations must be selected.

The CTDI slightly overestimates the true spiral scan dose for rather subtle reasons. The CTDI procedure requires a measurement of a single scan only. However, when a single scan is performed, the x-ray tube usually begins to emit radiation a few degrees in its travel before the actual start of the data accumulation. At the end of the scan, the tube is often left on for a few degrees after data accumulation. The net result is that the radiation is emitted for a few degrees more than the 360 degrees usually required for a complete spiral scan. The measured radiation is slightly higher than a single scan because during spiral scans, the tube is on continuously and the data are accumulated for exactly 360 degrees before the next data cycle is begun. In general, this overestimation of dose is small, and the CTDI procedure is a reasonably accurate method for determining patient dose, even for spiral scans.

The sample data in the box below are an example of a measurement of patient dosimetry.

Calculate using Equation 12-4:

$$MSAD = \frac{(C_f)(Q)}{(n)(BI)}$$

First scan: $Q = 2.52 \times 10^{-10}$ coulomb; however, because the CT scanner does not rewind between scans, there is probably a radiation output difference between the clockwise and counterclockwise scan directions. Therefore measure the radiation output for the second scan and average. The second scan measures $Q = 3.46 \times 10^{-10}$ coulomb. The average of two scans is $Q = 2.99 \times$

10^{-10} coulomb. Insert the numbers in the equation for MSAD:

$$MSAD = \frac{(102.0 \times 10^9 \text{ cGy}^{-mm})(2.99 \times 10^{-10} \text{ coul})}{(1)(7 \text{ mm})}$$
$$= 4.36 \text{ cGy}$$

Therefore the MSAD for this technique is 4.36 cGy. The average dose to the patient on the anterior portion of the head will be 4.36 cGy (rad). At another location in the phantom, the MSAD using the same technique will probably be different.

If the BI is increased (i.e., greater distance between scans) the MSAD will decrease even though the measured charge from the ionization chamber Q will be the same for the single scan measurement. The MSAD will decrease because the BI term is in the denominator of Equation 12-4.

REDUCTION OF PATIENT DOSE

The operator of a CT scanner should know the approximate radiation dose that is delivered to a patient during a CT examination. It is even more important to know what can be done to keep the dose to a minimum and the way the CT scanner image will be affected by reduced MSAD. From an examination of Equation 12-2, it can be determined that to reduce the MSAD, either the value of the integral can be reduced:

$$\int_{-\infty}^{\infty} D(z)dz$$

or the BI can be increased. The BI is easy to change on most CT scanners. Unfortunately, there are practical limits to the amount that BI can be increased. If the BI is increased too much and the SW is kept constant, a gap will appear between the slices. Tissue that falls in these gaps may not appear in the image and relevant anatomic features may be missed. If the SW is increased to match the increased BI, the beam dose profile curve widens and causes the area under the curve in Fig. 12-4 to increase. Because the integral in Equation 12-2 equals the area under the dose profile curve, the MSAD will increase as the beam is widened. In addition, increased beam width reduces the ability to resolve objects that have small dimensions in the z-direction.

The other way to reduce MSAD is to reduce the area under the dose profile curve. This can be done by reducing either the width or the height of the curve. The width of the curve can be reduced by bringing the collimators near the x-ray tube

DATA

Date	December 13, 1999
Institution	Any hospital
CT scanner	Brand X Super-1000
Technique name	Routine head
KVp	120
MA	300
Duration of scan	5 sec
Slice width	10 mm
Bed index	7 mm
X-ray filter	Standard
Phantom size	Head
Location in phantom	Anterior
Ion chamber calibration factor	102.0×10^9 cGy-mm/ coulomb
Q = Charge collected	2.99×10^{-10} coulomb
n = number of active detector arrays	1

closer together, thus narrowing the slice width. This effectively squeezes the x-ray beam into a narrower profile. However, this method has its limitations because arbitrary beam narrowing can cause other problems. First, as the beam width is reduced, it becomes narrower than the detectors and the full width of the detector is not used. In this case, the detector's geometric efficiency decreases and fewer x-rays are counted. This causes the statistical noise to increase, which in turn causes the image noise to increase and reduces the low-contrast perceptibility.

Second, if the beam is too narrow, small imperfections in the mechanical alignment of the x-ray source, collimators, and detectors can become a problem. Slight misalignments may produce a wobbling of the x-ray beam across the face of the detectors as the x-ray tube is rotated around the patient. The wobbling x-ray beam may cause fluctuations in the output that manifest themselves as circular artifacts in the image. Ideally, the width of the x-ray beam would be exactly the same as the width of the detectors. In practice, the x-ray beam is usually slightly larger than the detectors to allow for inevitable mechanical misalignments.

Third, as the beam is narrowed, more scans are required to cover the relevant patient anatomy. This increases the time necessary to complete a series of scans.

The height of the dose profile curve can also be reduced to reduce patient dose. This is most easily accomplished by reducing the mAs. Reducing mAs is an effective means to reduce patient dose, but like most other dose reduction schemes, image quality will usually be compromised. As previously mentioned, when the dose is reduced, the noise in the reconstructed image increases. Acceptable image quality usually dictates the amount of dose reduction that can be tolerated.

The relationship between image noise and dose is as follows (Brooks and Di Chiro, 1976):

$$\sigma = \frac{k\sqrt{\mu E}}{\sqrt{D(SW)P^3}} \qquad (12\text{-}5)$$

where σ is the standard deviation of pixel values, a measure of statistical noise present in the image (this should be as small as possible); k is a constant; μ is the mass energy attenuation coefficient of tissue for x-rays with effective energy E; D is the dose; SW is the slice width; and P is the size of the pixels in the image.

The noise increases with the inverse square root of the dose, D. This implies a moderate to slow dependence of σ on D, which means that patient dose can usually be reduced before the noise in the image becomes objectionable.

From a cursory examination of this equation, it is tempting to try to reduce the x-ray energy E by turning down the kVp to decrease the image noise. However, as the energy is reduced, the tissue attenuation coefficient μ increases rather rapidly, causing σ to increase. There appears to be an optimum energy (kVp) at which noise is minimized, and this energy is usually recommended or set by the manufacturer.

An increase in the pixel size P will also reduce the image noise; however, larger pixels obscure visualization of small objects and spatial resolution suffers. SW can also be increased in an attempt to reduce σ, but the problems of selecting too large a slice width have already been discussed.

In summary, it is very difficult to find a satisfactory means to reduce dose without compromising some other aspect of the image. Manufacturers of CT scanners can help to reduce patient dose by carefully aligning the x-ray beam and making sure that the beam is no wider than necessary. Increasing the detection efficiency of the radiation detectors makes better use of the radiation that passes through the patient and is also helpful to reduce image noise.

DOSIMETRY SURVEY

In 1990, the Center for Devices and Radiological Health (CDRH) surveyed the MSAD from about 250 randomly chosen CT scanners throughout the United States (Conway et al, 1992). The survey included many models from several manufacturers (Table 12-1). The data presented in Table 12-1 are averages from CT scanners most frequently encountered in 1990. The data are old but represent the most recent nationwide survey. They are presented as representative doses only. The dose values in Table 12-1 may have no correlation with the CT scanner used in the clinic or hospital; therefore it is important to measure the MSAD of a particular CT scanner. Do not rely on these values to accurately represent the patient dose delivered by a scanner, even if it is listed in the table.

When considered in the context of other radiographic exams, patient dose from a CT scanner exam is moderately high. For comparison, the patient entrance surface dose from most routine radiographs falls in the range from 0.03 cGy (chest radiograph) to about 1.4 cGy (lateral pelvis radio-

TABLE 12-1

Dosimetry Survey of CT Scanners

MULTIPLE SCAN AVERAGE DOSE (CENTRAL AXIS OF PATIENT)*		
MANUFACTURER & MODEL	GEOMETRY	MSAD (MUSCLE)†
General Electric 8800	Rotate-rotate	5.1 cGy
General Electric 9000	Rotate-rotate	4.2 cGy
General Electric 9800	Rotate-rotate	6.3 cGy
General Electric CT-M/P	Rotate-rotate	6.3 cGy
Philips 60	Rotate-rotate	4.2 cGy
Picker 1200	Rotate-stationary	5.9 cGy
Siemens DR	Rotate-rotate	4.1 cGy
Technicare 1440	Rotate-stationary	8.2 cGy
Technicare 2060	Rotate-stationary	8.2 cGy

*These scans are only *representative* of head techniques. No body scan data are provided. Note that the average central axis dose lies in the range of 4 to 8 cGy. If the same region of the patient is scanned twice (e.g., with and without contrast media), then these doses must be doubled. All listed CT systems used between 120 and 130 kVp. A very large majority of these CT systems used SW = BI = 10 mm. All scans used head techniques and the "head" phantom described in the text. Recall that 1 cGy = 1 rad.
†The MSAD values here are not numerically equal to the values listed in the original article. The original article listed "dose to PMM" values. PMM is polymethyl methacrylate, the acrylic plastic in which the measurements were made. To convert the values in the original table to "dose to muscle" values, the original values were multiplied by the ratio of mass energy absorption coefficients of muscle to PMM at 70 keV (=1.21). The "dose to muscle" values are listed here. "Dose to muscle" values are consistent with the factors used to calculate MSAD earlier in the chapter and are probably more representative of the true dose delivered to patients. To calculate dose to PMM, use f-factor = 0.78 cGy/R to determine C_f in Equation 12-4.
Modified from Conway et al: Average radiation dose in standard CT examination of the head: results of the 1990 NEXT survey, *Radiology* 184:135-140, 1992.

graph). However, fluoroscopic procedures can easily deliver doses higher than CT scanner exams, especially if the procedure requires lengthy fluoroscopic visualization as with some cardiac and interventional procedures.

REFERENCES

Brooks RA, Di Chiro G: Statistical limitations in x-ray reconstructive tomography, *Med Phys* 3:237-240, 1976.

Cacak RK, Hendee WR: Performance evaluation of a fourth-generation computed tomography (CT) scanner, *Proc Soc Photoopt Instr Eng* 173:194-207, 1979.

Conway BJ et al: Average radiation dose in standard CT examinations of the head: results of the 1990 NEXT survey, *Radiology* 184:135-140, 1992.

Dixon RL, Eckstrand KE: A film dosimetry system for use in computed tomography, *Radiology* 127:255-258, 1978.

Jucius RA, Kambic GX: Radiation dosimetry in computed tomography (CT), *Proc Soc Photoopt Instr Eng* 127:286-295, 1977.

Moore MM, Cacak RK, Hendee WR: Multisegmented ion chamber for CT scanner dosimetry, *Med Phys* 8:640-645, 1981.

Poletti JL: An ionization chamber-based CT dosimetry system, *Phys Med Biol* 29:725-731, 1984.

Shope TB et al: Radiation dosimetry survey of computed tomography systems from 10 manufacturers, *Brit J Radiol* 55:60-69, 1982.

Shope TB, Gagne RM, Johnson GC: A method for describing the doses delivered by transmission x-ray computed tomography, *Med Phys* 8:488-495, 1981.

Spokas JJ: Dose descriptors for computed tomography, *Med Phys* 9:288-292, 1982.

13

Single-Slice Spiral/Helical Computed Tomography: Physical Principles and Instrumentation

I n 1990 the first CT scanner to perform volume data acquisition was introduced (Kalender, 1995). This scanner was invented to overcome the problems imposed by conventional (slice-by-slice scanning) CT. Additionally, the need for shorter scan times to subsecond levels and improvement in 3D imaging has been met by volume scanners. These scanners are referred to *spiral/ helical CT scanners* based on the beam geometry of data acquisition.

HISTORICAL BACKGROUND
In the Beginning

An early pioneer in the development of the technique of volume scanning in CT was Dr. Willi A. Kalender (see Fig. 1-16) of the Institute of Medical Physics at the University of Erlangen, Germany. Kalender started work on spiral CT in 1988 with Peter Vock from Switzerland, and in 1989, he described the technical details and clinical applications of spiral CT to the Radiological Society of North America (RSNA) meeting in Chicago. Other early investigators included Mori (1987), various Japanese researchers, and Bresler and Skrabecz (1993).

Terminology Controversy

Kalender and Vock's presentation at the RSNA in 1989 resulted in a flurry of activities related to volume scanning. An interesting debate that surfaced in the early literature was related to the terminology to best describe the method of volume data ac-

quisition. Should volume scanning be called spiral CT or helical CT? In a letter to the editors of the *American Journal of Roentgenology* (AJR), Towers (1993) used an illustration (Fig. 13-1) to describe the fundamental differences between spiral CT and helical CT. Towers noted that the term *helical* describes a cylindric configuration, whereas *spiral* refers to both cylindric and conic configurations. He therefore recommended the use of the term *spiral CT*.

In another letter to the editors of *AJR,* Silverman, Corboy, and Zeeman (1994) argued that the term *helical CT* "best describes this new CT technology." Dr. Mark Bahn of the Mallinckrodt Institute of Radiology offered mathematical definitions to support this view. He pointed out that mathematical dictionaries (Baker, 1961, James and James, 1976) provide more technical definitions of these two terms: a spiral describes a curve on a plane surface; a helix describes a curve in 3D space.

In response, Kalender (1994) submitted a letter (Appendix A) to the editors of *Radiology* to support use of the term *spiral CT,* which convinced the editors to accept either term for CT papers published in *Radiology.* This book uses both terms as synonyms, as suggested by Kalender (1994).

CONVENTIONAL SLICE-BY-SLICE DATA ACQUISITION
Scanning Sequence

In conventional CT scanning, the x-ray tube rotates around the patient to collect data from a single slice of tissue, followed by table indexing so that the next contiguous slice can be scanned. This process is repeated until data from several contiguous slices have been collected. The scanning sequence for this type of data acquisition consists of four distinct steps (Fig. 13-2).

In the first step, the x-ray tube must be accelerated to a constant speed of rotation. This means that the cables that supply power to the x-ray tube must be long enough to allow for the full 360-degree rotation. During this rotation (step 2), the x-ray tube produces x-rays that are transmitted through the patient to fall on the detectors, which measure the relative transmission values (data). At this particular point, the patient holds a breath, and data are collected from a specific axial slice. In step 3, the patient resumes breathing while the x-ray tube slows to a stop. In step 4, it is necessary to unwind the cable because of the 360-degree ro-

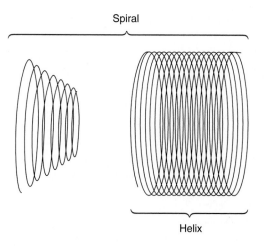

Spiral

Helix

FIG. 13-1.   Spiral geometries. The helix is one type of spiral. (From Towers MJ: Spiral or helical CT? (letter), *Am J Roentgenol* 161:901, 1993.)

tation and to move the patient and table so that the next contiguous slice can be scanned.

This four-step process is repeated until all the required contiguous axial slices have been scanned. The time it takes to accomplish steps 1, 3, and 4 is referred to as the *interscan delay time* (ISD) (Crawford and King, 1990).

Slices are usually collected in groups while the patient holds a breath, with the ISD after each pair of slices. Between two groups of slices is an inter-group delay (IGD), and it is at this point that the patient breathes. Crawford and King (1990) have defined the scan rate as the following ratio:

$$\text{Scan rate} = \frac{\text{No. of scans per group}}{\text{sum of time to collect slices} + \text{IGD}}$$

If the study requires more slices, its duration would have to be increased. This requirement places an additional burden on the patient to remain still to ensure images obtained are free of motion artifacts.

Limitations

The limitations imposed by slice-by-slice sequential CT scanning include the following:

1. Longer examination times because of the stop-start action necessary for patient breathing, table indexing, and cable unwinding. This gives rise to the ISD. The cable wrap-around and unwinding is shown in Fig. 13-3, A. This wraparound results from the fixed length of the high-voltage cable,

which follows the x-ray tube as it rotates through 360 degrees around the patient. The cable is unwound during the imaging of the next slice. In Fig. 13-3, B, the cable wraparound process is eliminated through the use of slip-ring technology, which allows the x-ray tube to rotate continuously as the patient moves continuously through the gantry. This is spiral/helical CT scanning.

2. Certain portions of the anatomy are omitted because the patient respiration phase may not always be consistent between scans (Fig. 13-4). For example, it has been reported that lesions in the liver smaller than 1 cm may be missed because of inconsistent levels of inspiration (Regauts et al, 1990). This omission of anatomy is often referred to as *slice-to-slice misregistration.*

3. Inaccurate generation of 3D images and multiplanar reformatted images, attributed to the inconsistent levels of inspiration from scan to scan. The result is the appearance of "step-like" contours in 3D images (Kalender et al, 1990a). Fig. 13-5 illustrates production of the stair-step artifact and its elimination with spiral/helical CT.

4. Only a few slices are scanned during maximum contrast enhancement when the contrast enhancement technique is used (D'Agincourt, 1991). These problems may be overcome if the scan rate is increased and the ISD is eliminated, both of which are technologically feasible. The scan time can be increased by decreasing the time

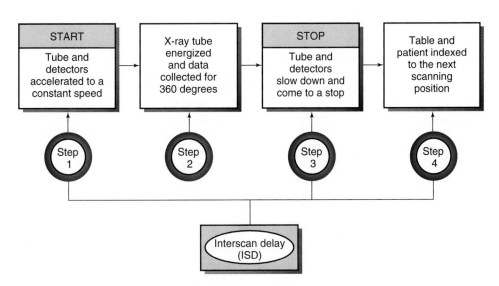

FIG. 13-2. Characteristic four-step process of slice-by-slice sequential CT scanning.

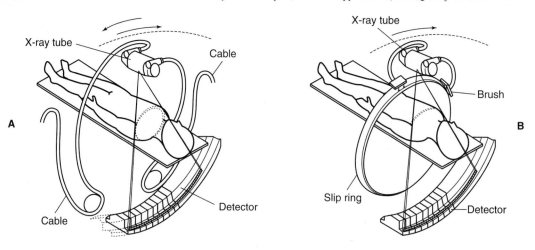

FIG. 13-3.   One advance in CT technology that facilitates CT fluoroscopy is continuous scanning using slip ring technology. The cable wrap-around typical of conventional slice-by-slice CT results in a delay that prevents real-time image reconstruction and display. **A,** Reciprocating rotation; **B,** fast continuous rotation. (From Ozaki M: Development of a real-time reconstruction system for CT fluorography, *Toshiba Med Rev,* 1995.)

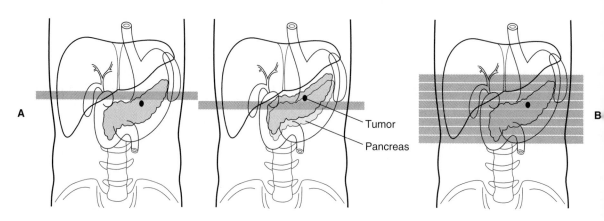

FIG. 13-4.   Removal of the effects of different levels of respiration. **A,** Conventional scanning. In spiral/helical CT scanning (**B**) there is no shifting of lesions because of different levels of respiration. (Courtesy Toshiba America Medical Systems; Tustin, Calif.)

to accomplish the four steps shown in Fig. 13-2. The ISD can be eliminated by having the tube (and detector) rotate continuously around the patient (instead of the start-stop action characteristic of slice-by-slice sequential CT scanning) while simultaneously translating the patient through the gantry aperture at a faster speed. Data are acquired during the patient translation.

This chapter concentrates on methods to remove the ISD with the goal of acquiring the data continuously rather in slices. This technique is only possible with continuous rotation scanners based on slip-ring technology.

SLICE-BY-SLICE VOLUME SCANNING

The introduction of continuous rotation CT scanners that can scan rapidly with scan times shorter than 1 second has led to the development of new scanning techniques. One such technique, spiral/helical CT, has become commonly used and has gained widespread attention.

According to the particular manufacturer, various terms are used to describe the action of continuous data collection during continuous patient translation. As the x-ray tube rotates continuously around the patient, it traces a path with respect to the patient (Fig. 13-6). The path geometry describes a spiral or helical winding and there-

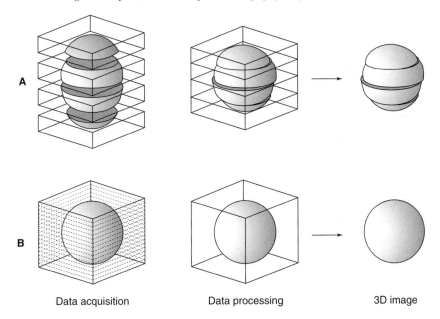

FIG. 13-5. Comparison of the accuracy of 3D reconstruction for conventional (**A**) and spiral/helical (**B**) CT scanning. (Courtesy Toshiba America Medical Systems; Tustin, Calif.)

fore has been referred to as *spiral/helical* CT, or volume scanning. Other terms considered synonymous are *spiral volume* CT (Kalender et al, 1990b) and *helical volumetric* CT (Jirjian et al, 1991).

Requirements for Volume Data Acquisition

Because the data in spiral/helical CT are collected in volumes rather than slices, the following requirements must be met:

1. Continuously rotating scanner based on slip-ring technology
2. Continuous couch movement
3. Increase in loadability of the x-ray tube, capable of delivering at least 200 mA per revolution continuously throughout the time it takes to scan the volume of tissue
4. Increased cooling capacity
5. Spiral/helical weighting algorithm
6. Mass memory buffer to store the vast amount of data collected

Physical Principles

Kalendar et al (1990a) described the need to reduce scanning times and improve 3D and reformatted images. In addition to other factors such as increased x-ray tube loadability, these needs provided the motivation to develop new scanning se-

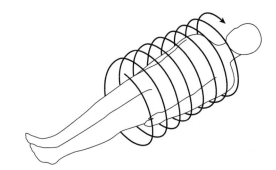

FIG. 13-6. The spiral/helical geometry created when the x-ray tube rotates continuously around the patient with simultaneous patient translation.

quences and gave rise to a renewed interest in slip-ring technology and the subsequent birth of continuous rotation scanners. The fundamental principles of spiral/helical CT include two major steps that are significantly different from those of non-spiral/helical CT systems.

Data Acquisition

The first step in volume scanning is data acquisition (Fig. 13-7). The x-ray tube traces a spiral/helical path with a radius equal to the distance from the focal spot to the center of rotation. This results in an entire volume of tissue being scanned during a single breath hold compared with slice-by-slice imaging (Fig. 13-8).

Transporting the patient too quickly leads to image degradation caused by motion artifacts, or may cause the patient to experience motion sickness. It is therefore important that the patient move at a constant speed. In general, patients are moved at a table speed of about 10 mm/sec during a continuous 1-second scanning. If a 24-second scan is taken, then the anatomic volume scanned is 240 mm (24 cm). Scanning times differ by manufacturer but average about 32 seconds. In addition the slice thickness may range from 1 to 10 cm. The technical data for the acquisition process are listed in Table 13-1.

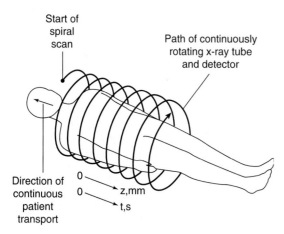

FIG. 13-7. First step in spiral/helical CT: data acquisition. As the patient is transported through the gantry aperture, the x-ray tube traces a spiral path around the patient, collecting data as it rotates.

Several problems can result from data acquisition using spiral geometry:

1. There is no defined slice and thus localization of a particular slice is difficult.
2. The geometry of the slice volume is different for spiral/helical scans compared with conventional CT scans (Fig. 13-9). Fig. 13-10 explains the origin of the slice volume shown in Fig. 13-9, *B*. In conventional slice-by-slice CT the tube rotates around the patient for 360 degrees to collect a complete set of data in planar geometry for each individual slice shown in Fig. 13-9, *A*. This data set is said to be consistent; that is, it is collected from one slice or plane. In spiral/helical volume CT scanning, the x-ray tube rotates continuously as the patient moves through the gantry continuously as well. In this situation, data are now collected in nonplanar geometry, resulting in the diagram shown in Fig. 13-9, *B*. The data are collected from different regions of the volume and not through a particular plane.
3. The effective slice thickness increases because it is influenced by the width of the fan beam and the speed of the table.
4. Because of the absence of a defined slice, the projection data are inconsistent (consistent projection data are needed to satisfy the standard reconstruction process).
5. When inconsistent projection data are used with the standard reconstruction process, streak artifacts akin to motion artifacts are clearly apparent on the image.

TABLE 13-1

Technical Data Typical of the Acquisition Process in Spiral/Helical CT

PARAMETER	SPECIFICATION
Rotational velocity of measurement system	360 degrees/sec
Scan time	Maximum 24 sec
Table feed (selectable in 1-mm steps)	1 to 10 mm/sec
Slice thickness (selectable, standard 1, 2, 3, 5, and 10 mm)	1 to 10 mm
Effective slice thickness for spiral scanning (at nominal value of 10 mm)	12.8 mm at 10 mm/sec, 10.2 mm at 5 mm/sec, and 10.0 mm at 0 mm/sec (corresponding to Dynamic Multiscan mode)
Tube current	75 to 250 mA
Tube voltage	12 kV / 137 kV
Start delay after scan start	minimum 3 sec, maximum 60 sec (selectable)

Courtesy Siemens Medical Systems; Iselin, NJ.

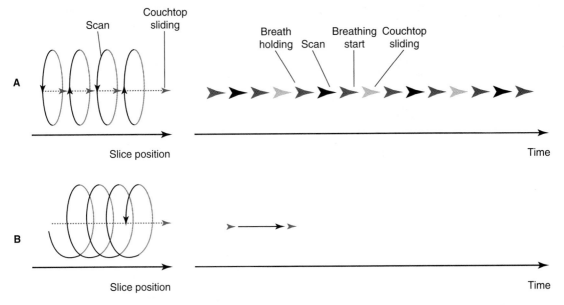

FIG. 13-8. Comparison of conventional (**A**) and spiral/helical (**B**) CT scanning sequences. (From Tohki Y: The helical scanning technique, *Toshiba Med Rev* 38:1-5, 1991.)

These problems can be solved through the use of special postprocessing techniques. One such method involves a "dedicated reconstruction algorithm that synthesizes raw data representing a perfectly planar slice from the original spiral data by interpolation" (Kalender et al, 1990b). Interpolation is a mathematical technique whereby an unknown value can be estimated given two known values on either side (see Chapter 6). Interpolation and extrapolation are illustrated in Fig. 13-11.

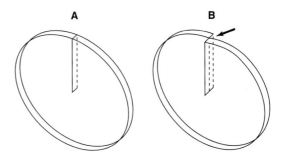

FIG. 13-9. Geometry of the slice volume characteristic of conventional CT scanning (**A**) and spiral/helical (**B**) CT scanning.

Image Reconstruction

Inconsistent data that are obtained from 360-degree spiral/helical scan rotation are used directly in the image reconstruction process. Motion artifacts are apparent as shown in Fig. 13-12, A for phantom images and in Fig. 13-13, A for patient images.

To eliminate these motion artifacts arising the continuous movement of the patient during scanning, two steps are needed:

1. Calculation (using interpolation) of a planar data set from the tissue volume data set for every image (Fig. 13-14). The planar data set (the image plane in Fig. 13-14) approximates the transverse axial section as with conventional CT. Within the volume scanned, a slice can be selected anywhere between the start and end positions in addition to the spacing and the number of slices (Fig. 13-15).

2. Reconstruction of images similar to conventional CT, using the filtered back-projection algorithm. The results of these two processes are free of blurring as shown in Fig. 13-13, B.

A number of interpolation algorithms are used to produce the planar data set, and linear interpolation (LI) represents the "simplest approach" (Kalender, 1995). Two interpolation algorithms for single-slice spiral/helical CT are the 360-degree LI algorithm and the 180-degree LI algorithm.

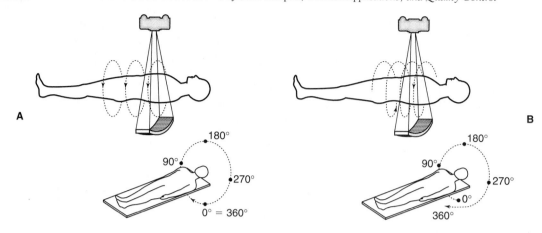

FIG. 13-10. Data acquisition geometries for conventional slice-by-slice CT (**A**) and spiral/helical CT (**B**).

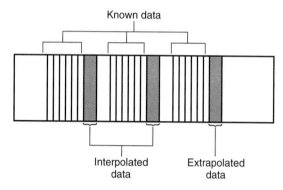

FIG. 13-11. A comparison of interpolated and extrapolated data

360-degree Linear Interpolation Algorithm

The 360-degree LI algorithm was the interpolation algorithm used during the initial development of spiral/helical CT scanners (Fig. 13-16). The basis for this algorithm is illustrated in Fig. 13-16. The planar slice is interpolated using data points measured 360 degrees apart. The fundamental problem with the 360-degree LI algorithm is related to the image quality of the planar slice. This algorithm broadens the slice sensitivity profile (SSP) and hence degrades image quality. To overcome this problem, the 180-degree LI algorithm was introduced.

180-degree Linear Interpolation Algorithm

The 180-degree LI algorithm improves the image quality of the 360-degree LI algorithm by using points that are closer to the planar slice to be interpolated (Fig. 3-17). The basic difference between the 360-degree and the 180-degree LI algorithms is that a second spiral (the dotted line in Fig. 13-17) is calculated from the measured spiral/helical data set and is offset by 180 degrees. In this situation the planar slice can then be interpolated using data points that are closer to it, compared with the 360-degree LI algorithm. This process improves on the SSP and therefore enhances image quality.

Additionally, as noted by Kalender (1995), "higher-order nonlinear interpolation algorithms can be implemented. While they preserve the shape of the sensitivity profiles even better, their influence on noise and image quality is not easy to predict and control. On a given scanner, the exact algorithm and above all its implementation, which may have significant influence on image quality and artifact behavior are not documented as they are considered confidential by the manufacturers in most cases."

INSTRUMENTATION

Spiral/helical CT scanners (Fig. 3-18) are not different in external appearance from conventional CT scanners. However, there are significant differences in several major equipment components.

Equipment Components

A block diagram of the major equipment components of a spiral/helical CT scanner is shown in Fig. 13-19. The most noteworthy feature is the use of slip rings to connect the stationary and rotating parts of the scanner.

The rotating part of the system consists of the x-ray tube, high voltage generator, detectors and detector electronics (DAS). The stationary part

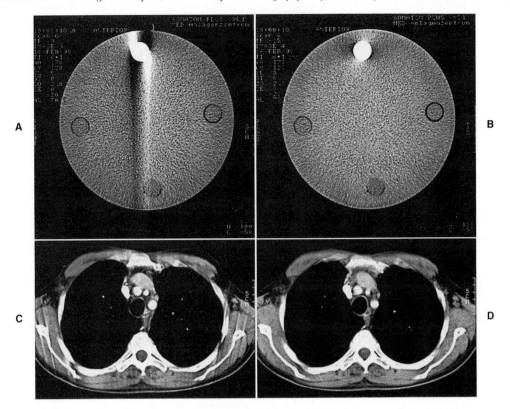

FIG. 13-12. Comparison of image quality using direct reconstruction of the spiral data (**A, C**) as opposed to reconstruction using the interpolation algorithm (**B, D**) for phantom (**A, B**) and mediastinal (**C, D**) studies. Note that the streak artifacts are removed when the interpolation algorithm is used. (From Kalender WA, Vock P, Seissler W: Spiral CT scanning for fast and continuous volume data acquisition. In Fuchs WA, ed: *Advances in CT*, New York, 1990, Springer-Verlag.)

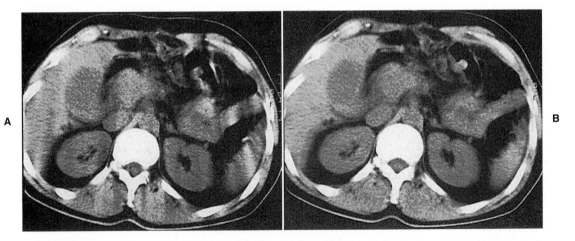

FIG. 13-13. Image reconstruction principles in spiral/helical CT. **A,** Direct reconstruction of an image from a 360-degree spiral segment results in motion artifacts. **B,** Image reconstruction from a planar data set calculated by slice interpolation from the spiral data set results in images free of artifacts. (From Kalender W: Principles and performance of spiral CT. In Goldman LW, Fowlkes JB, eds: *Medical CT and ultrasound: current technology and applications,* Maryland, 1995, American Association of Physics in Medicine.)

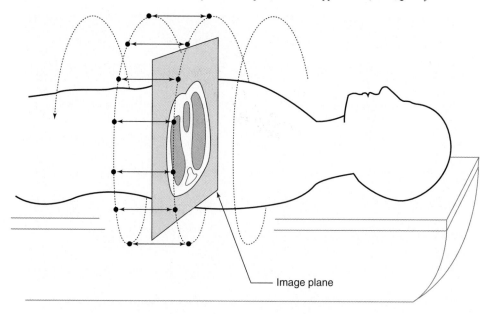

FIG. 13-14. The first step to produce an image in spiral/helical CT scanning is to calculate a planar data set (image plane) from the volume data set (measured data). This is accomplished using linear interpolation.

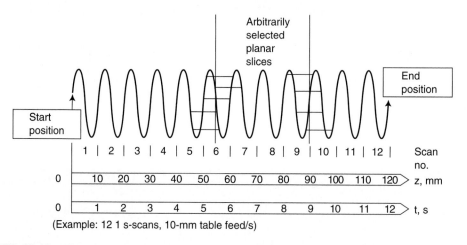

FIG. 13-15. The second major step in spiral/helical CT is interpolation. Images of arbitrarily selected slices can be reconstructed using an interpolation algorithm. (Courtesy Siemens Medical Systems, Iselin, NJ.)

consists of the front-end memory and computer and the first stage high-voltage component.

The x-ray tube and detectors rotate continuously during data collection because the cable wraparound problem has been eliminated by slip-ring technology. Because large amounts of projection data are collected very quickly, increased storage is needed. This is accommodated by the front-end memory, fast solid state, and magnetic disk storage.

In spiral/helical CT scanners, the x-ray tube is energized for longer periods of time compared with conventional CT tubes. This characteristic requires x-ray tubes that are physically larger than conventional x-ray tubes and have heat storage capacities greater than 3 million heat units (MHU) and anode cooling rates of 1 MHU per minute (Bushong, 1997).

X-ray detectors for single-slice spiral/helical CT scanning are one dimensional (1D) array and

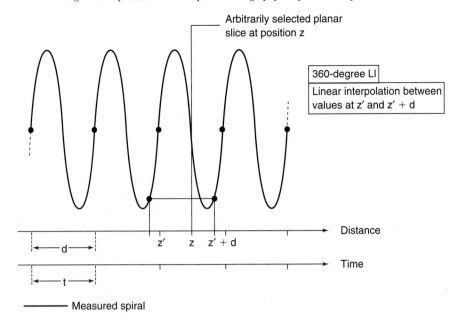

FIG. 13-16. The 360-degree linear interpolation (LI) algorithm. LI between points Z' and $Z' + d$ was most commonly used in the early days of spiral/helical scanning to estimate data that would have been obtained in planar geometry for an arbitrarily selected image position Z.

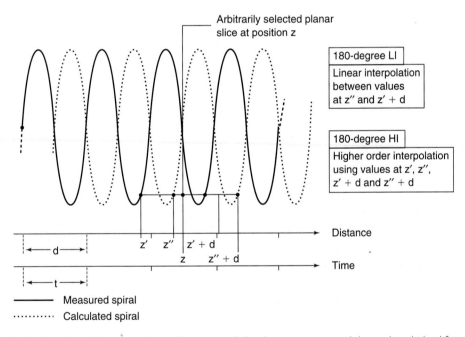

FIG. 13-17. The 180-degree LI algorithm. Interpolation between measured data points derived from 180-degree opposite views allows to limit the scan range used per image. Higher order interpolation schemes can also be implemented.

should be solid-state because their overall efficiency is greater than gas ionization detectors.

The high-voltage generator for spiral/helical CT scanners is a high-frequency generator with high power output. The high-voltage generator is mounted on the rotating frame of the CT gantry and positioned close to the x-ray tube (Fig. 13-19). X-ray tubes operate at high voltages (about 80 to 140 kVp) to produce x-rays with the intensity needed for CT scanning. At such high voltages,

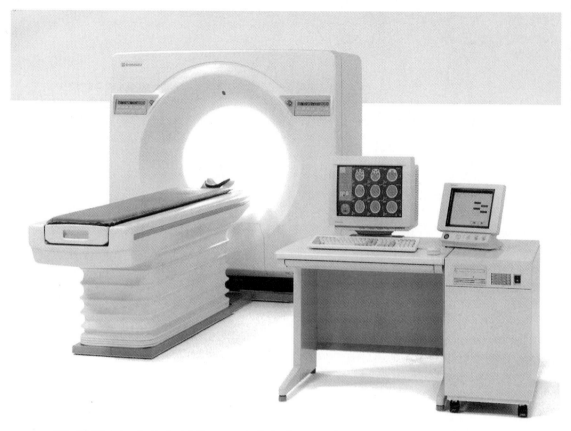

FIG. 13-18. A spiral/helical CT scanner is similar in external appearance to conventional CT scanners. (Courtesy Shimadzu Medical Systems, Seattle, Wash.)

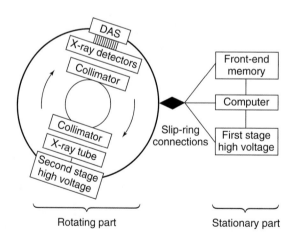

FIG. 13-19. The major equipment components of a spiral/helical CT scanner. Connection between the stationary and rotating parts of the scanner is made possible by slip-ring technology.

arcing between the brushes and rings of the gantry may occur during scanning. To solve this problem, one approach (high-voltage SR) is to divide the power supply into a first stage on the stationary part of the scanner, where the voltage is increased to an intermediate level, and a second stage on the rotating part of the scanner, where the voltage is increased to the required high voltages needed for x-ray production and finally rectified to direct current potential (Fig. 13-19) (Napel, 1995). Another approach passes a low voltage across the brushes to the slip rings, the high-voltage genera-

PARAMETERS FOR SPIRAL/HELICAL CT

SCAN PARAMETERS IN CONVENTIONAL CT

Voltage: 80 to 140 kVp
Tube current: 100 to 400 mA
Power: 10 to 60 kW
Slice collimation (S): 1 to 10 mm
Scan time per 360-degree rotation (T): 0.75 to 2.0 sec
Scan increment (SI): arbitrary, mostly equal to S
Number of scans (n): 20 to 60
Scan volume (V): $(n - 1) \cdot SI + S$ mm

SCAN AND RECONSTRUCTION PARAMETERS UNIQUE TO SPIRAL CT

Spiral scan time (T): 24 to 100 sec
Table feed per 360-degree rotation (d): 1.0 to 20.0 mm
Table speed (d'): 1.0 to 20.0 mm/sec
Number of revolutions (n): 20 to 60
Scan range (R): 30 to 1500 mm

$$R = T \cdot d' = n \cdot d$$

Z-interpolation algorithm: various, mostly 360-degree or 180-degree linear interpolation
Reconstruction increment (RI): 0.1 to 5 mm

SOME TERMINOLOGY COMMONLY USED IN SPIRAL/HELICAL CT

Pitch (P): 1.0 to 2.0; $P = d/S$ (dimensionless); the table feed per 360° rotation divided by the slice thickness
$S/d/RI$: a triple of numbers specifying the scan and reconstruction parameters (e.g., 3/5/1 means a scan with
$\quad S = 3$ mm, $d = 5$ mm, $RI = 1$ mm
Z-axis: the scanner's axis of rotation and, for all practical purposes, the body's longitudinal axis
Z-interpolation: calculation of planar attenuation data for desired table position interpolation between data
$\quad$ points measured for the same projection angle at neighboring z-axis positions (synonyms: slice
$\quad$ interpolation, section interpolation, z-axis interpolation)

(From Kalender WA: Principles and performance of spiral CT. In Goldman LW, Fowlkes JB, eds: *Medical CT and ultrasound: current technology and applications,* Maryland, 1995, American Association of Physics in Medicine.)

tor, and then the x-ray tube. In both designs, only a low to intermediate voltage is applied to the brush/slip-ring interface, thus decreasing the chances of arcing.

Slip-Ring Technology

One of the major technical factors that contributes to the success of spiral/helical CT scanning is slip-ring technology (Fig. 13-19). The purpose of the slip ring is to allow the x-ray tube and detectors (in third-generation CT systems; see Fig. 13-19) to rotate continuously so that a volume of the patient, rather than one slice, can be scanned very quickly in a single breath hold. The slip rings also eliminate the long, high-tension cables to the x-ray tube used in conventional start-stop CT scanners. As the x-ray tube rotates continuously, the patient also moves continuously through the gantry aperture so that data can be acquired from a volume of tissue.

The technical aspects of using slip rings for data acquisition were described in Chapter 5. These include the design and power supply to the rings and a comparison of low-voltage and high-voltage slip-ring CT scanners in terms of the high voltage supplied to the x-ray tube.

BASIC SCAN PARAMETERS

Several scan parameters for spiral/helical CT are the same as for conventional CT; however, there are a few parameters as well as a set of terms associated only with spiral/helical CT. Typical values for these parameters are given in the accompanying box. It is not within the scope of this chapter to describe all these parameters; however, pitch is of particular significance because it affects image quality and patient dose and also plays a role in the overall outcome of the clinical examination.

Other parameters that affect the performance of spiral/helical CT and demand effective communication between the radiologist and technologist are collimation, table speed, duration of the scan, and the reconstruction increment (Brink et al, 1994; Kalender 1995; Cinnamon, 1998).

Pitch

The *pitch* is a term associated with a fastener, and it is actually the distance between the turns on the fastener. In spiral/helical CT, the pitch is defined as the distance (in mm) that the CT table moves during one revolution of the x-ray tube (Fig. 13-20). The pitch is used to calculate the pitch ratio, which is a ratio of the pitch to the slice thickness or beam collimation. The pitch ratio is as follows:

$$\text{Pitch} = \frac{\text{distance the table travels during 360-degree revolution}}{\text{Slice thickness or beam collimation}}$$

When the distance the table travels during one complete revolution of the x-ray tube equals the slice thickness or beam collimation, the pitch ratio (pitch) is 1:1, or simply 1. A pitch of 1 results in the best image quality in spiral/helical CT scanning. The pitch can be increased to increase volume coverage and speed up the scanning process (Fig. 13-21).

Volume Coverage

The volume coverage is given by the following relationship:

Volume coverage = pitch × slice thickness, or beam collimation × scan time

for fixed scan time and fixed slice thickness (Bushong 1997).

Another factor that influences the volume coverage is gantry rotation time. The volume coverage in this case becomes:

$$\text{Volume coverage} = \frac{\text{pitch} \times \text{collimation} \times \text{scan time}}{\text{gantry rotation time}}$$

Collimation and Table Speed

Collimation determines the slice thickness and in most cases is equal to the table increment (a pitch of 1). Collimation selection also depends on the type of tissue to be examined. Smaller structures usually require narrow collimation, whereas larger structures are imaged with wider collimation.

Another parameter of importance is the table increment (mm/sec), also referred to as the *table feed* or *table speed*. As the table increment increases with respect to the collimation, pitch increases, resulting in a loss of image quality. To cover a certain

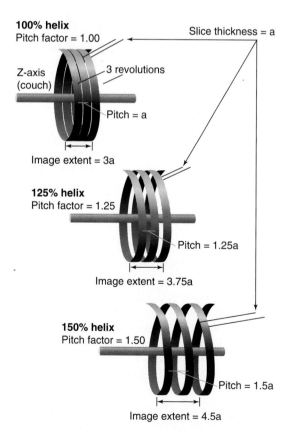

FIG. 13-21. The pitch can be increased to increase volume coverage quickly, although image quality degrades.

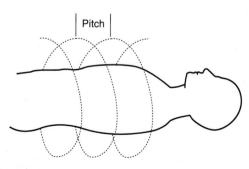

FIG. 13-20. The pitch is the distance the CT table moves during one complete revolution of the x-ray tube.

volume, it is important to keep in mind two parameters that influence image quality: collimation and table incrementation. In this regard, Brink et al (1994) suggest the use of the chart presented in Table 13-2, which summarizes the reconstruction lengths performed with various collimation widths and table speed values. The goal is to use the smallest possible collimation at a pitch of 2 (with 180-degree interpolation algorithm). Hence, for a volume length of 30 cm, either a 5-mm or 8-mm collimation can be used with a table speed of 10 mm.

Scan Time

Another operator-defined parameter in spiral/helical CT that affects the outcome of the examination is scan time, which refers to the duration of the scan. The choice of scan time depends on the patient's respiratory condition. Most current scanners feature various spiral/helical scan modes (Fig. 13-22) for patients who have difficulty holding their breath. For example, in a multistep spiral/helical scan mode, multiple scans are obtained with a pause between scans to enable patients to breathe, so that the required length of tissue can be imaged successfully.

Reconstruction Increment

Another parameter unique to spiral/helical CT is the reconstruction increment (RI), also referred to as the *reconstruction interval* or *reconstruction spacing*. The RI determines the degree of sectional overlap to improve image quality. As RI decreases, image quality increases "but with trade-offs of in-creased image processing time, data storage requirements, and physician time for image review" (Brink et al, 1994). Urban et al (1993) found that for the detection of small lesions in the liver, a 50% overlap (Fig. 13-23) resulted in better visualization of these lesions by 10%. In a set of simulations conducted by Brink et al (1994) to find whether an increased degree of overlap would provide better results, the researchers recommended "reconstructing one or two sections per table increment for routine diagnosis and at least three sections per table increment for multidimensional imaging."

IMAGE QUALITY CONSIDERATIONS

A number of workers have investigated the physical performance characteristics of spiral/helical CT (Rigauts et al, 1990; Kalender et al, 1994; Jerjian et al, 1990; Kalender and Polacin, 1995; Polacin et al, 1992). These characteristics include image quality parameters such as spatial resolution, image uniformity, and contrast; image noise and slice sensitivity profiles; radiation dose; and artifacts.

In general, most characteristics appear to be affected only slightly. As noted by Kalender (1995) image quality in spiral/helical CT is equivalent to that of conventional CT "in every respect" because the basic imaging parameters are the same.

Spatial and Contrast Resolution

For the same image reconstruction parameters, contrast and spatial resolution should be about the same for both spiral/helical CT and conventional CT. For example, measurements of the scan plane

---

TABLE 13-2

Reconstruction Lengths for 32-sec Spiral/Helical Scans Performed with Different Collimation Settings and Table Increment Values

| | TABLE INCREMENT (mm) | | | | | | | | | | | | | | |
COLLIMATION (mm)	2	3	4	5	6	7	8	9	10	11	12	13	14	15	16
2	6	9	12												
3		9	12	15	18										
5				15	18	21	24	27	30						
8							24	27	30	33	36	39	42	45	48
10									30	33	36	39	42	45	48

From Brink JA et al: Helical CT: principles and technical considerations, *Radiographics* 14:887-893, 1994.

(image plane) spatial resolution conducted by Kalender (1995) using a standard perspex hole pattern phantom demonstrate this similarity between spatial resolution for conventional CT and spiral/helical CT. The visual evidence is shown in Fig. 13-24. However, as noted by Kalender (1995), the contrast for small objects and the spatial resolution along the z-axis (longitudinal direction) may be somewhat different. For example, in simulations, phantom experiments, and specimen studies that compared contrast and spatial resolution along the z-axis for both conventional and spiral/helical CT, Kalender et al (1994) found that spiral/helical CT provides "significantly better" contrast and spatial separation of 5-mm spheres imaged with a 5-mm slice thickness.

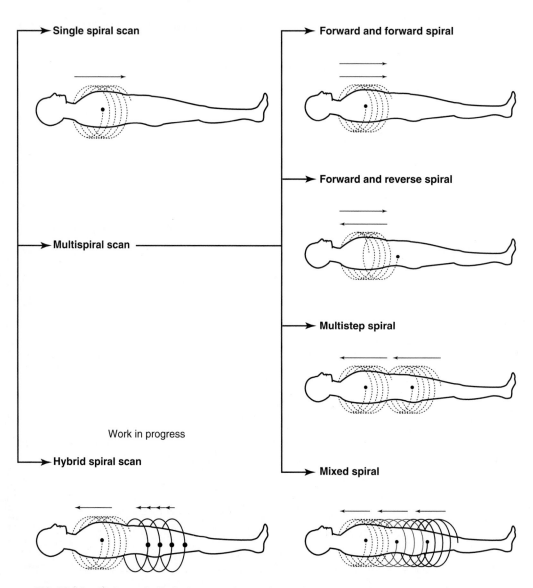

FIG. 13-22. Various spiral/helical scan modes can be used to accommodate the needs of the examination. For example, the multistep spiral scan mode can accommodate patients who have difficulty holding their breath for prolonged scan times.

Noise

Noise in spiral/helical CT is affected by a range of parameters including beam intensity, beam quality (energy), slice thickness, and matrix size (pixel size). Additionally, noise in spiral/helical CT is also affected by the interpolation algorithm. When compared with conventional CT (all other factors held constant), the 360-degree LI algorithm produces less noise; however, when the 360-degree LI and the 180-degree LI algorithms were compared, it was found that the 180-degree LI algorithm produced more noise and thus degraded image quality (Kalender, 1994). However, Cinnamon (1998) reports that this problem has little effect on the image quality of bony structures because the subject contrast of bone is greater than its surrounding soft tissues (Fig. 13-25).

Slice Sensitivity Profile

The SSP "describes how thick a section is imaged and to what extent details within the section contribute to the signal" (Kalender, 1994). For conventional CT, the shape of the SSP is rectangular

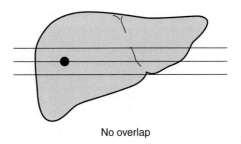

No overlap

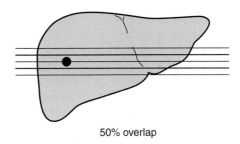

50% overlap

FIG. 13-23. Overlapping sections may result in better visualization of lesions.

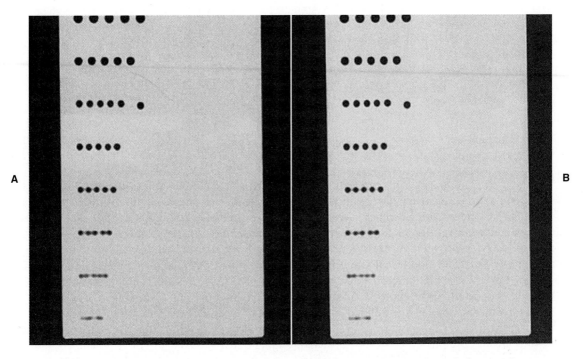

FIG. 13-24. The spatial resolution as measured by a perspex hole pattern phantom is the same for conventional CT (**A**) and spiral/helical CT (**B**) for the same reconstruction parameters. (From Kalender WA: Technical foundations of spiral CT, *Semin Ultrasound CT MRI,* 15:81-89, 1994.)

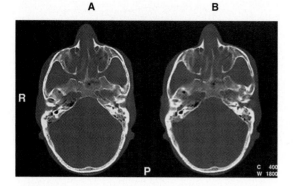

A **B**

FIG. 13-25. The difference in image quality and noise in studies carried out using a pitch of 1 (360-degree interpolation algorithm) and a pitch of 2 (180-degree interpolation algorithm) may be inconsequential in bone studies because of the high inherent subject contrast, especially when other imaging parameters are optimized, as evidenced by these phantom studies. **A,** Pitch 1, 360 degrees. **B,** Pitch 2, 180 degrees. (From Cinnamon J: *Multislice volumetric spiral CT: principles and applications,* 1998, Massoz.)

(Fig. 13-26, A). The section thickness is measured in the middle of the rectangle. This point is referred to as the full width at half maximum (FWHM). For spiral/helical CT, the SSP also depends on the pitch and the interpolation algorithm. Fig. 13-26, B shows the SSPs for a pitch of 1 and 2. Fig. 13-26, C shows SSPs for a 180-degree LI algorithm and a 360-degree algorithm. The SSP degrades with a pitch of 2 and a 360-degree LI algorithm. (The FWHM does not approximate closely the actual slice thickness selected.) As the SSP widens, image quality degrades.

RADIATION DOSE CONSIDERATIONS

Radiation dose in CT was described in detail in Chapter 12, including the factors affecting the dose in CT and two dose descriptors: the computed tomography dose index (CTDI) and the multiple scan average dose (MSAD). This section explores the nature of radiation dose in spiral/helical CT.

Dose Factors

The same factors that affect dose in conventional CT affect dose in spiral/helical CT because most of the scan parameters are identical. As the mAs and kVp increase, dose increases proportionally. As noise, pixel size, and slice thickness decrease, pa-

tient dose increases (Seeram, 1999). Additionally, the dose in spiral/helical CT decreases with increasing pitch.

Dose Descriptors

McGhee and Humphreys (1994) showed that the dose descriptors, CTDI and MSAD, are both valid for use in spiral/helical CT and can be used directly to estimate the dose.

Dose Comparison and Effective Doses

During the early development and use of spiral/helical CT, it was thought that the dose would be higher simply from volume data acquisition. Comparison studies show that the dose in conventional CT is about equal to that of spiral/helical CT.

There are several reasons why patient dose is less in spiral/helical CT than in conventional CT, as follows:

1. Tube currents in spiral/helical CT are set to lower values than in conventional CT.
2. Spiral/helical CT largely eliminates the need to retake single scans.
3. Spiral/helical CT arbitrarily calculates overlapping images from one spiral scan without renewed exposure, whereas conventional CT must take many overlapping images to obtain high display quality.
4. Unlike contiguous scanning, spiral/helical CT can reduce patient dose by using pitch values >1. (Kalender, 1994)

The effective doses from spiral/helical CT for the head, chest, abdomen and pelvis are 1.1, 6.7, 4.3, and 2.7 mSv, respectively (Kalendar, 1994). The effective dose allows the quantification of the risk from partial body exposure based on that received from an equal whole-body dose.

More recently, Huda et al (1997) reported effective dose range from 1.5 to 5.3 mSv for abdominal examinations in pediatric and adult patients. To place all this in perspective, the effective dose from natural background radiation is about 2.4 mSv per year (Kalender, 1994).

MULTIDIMENSIONAL IMAGING

In addition to the routine imaging modes that generate transverse axial images, the volume scanning capability of spiral/helical CT opens new dimensions in CT imaging. The vast amount of data collected from the patient volumes, when subjected to appropriate computer processing, have created

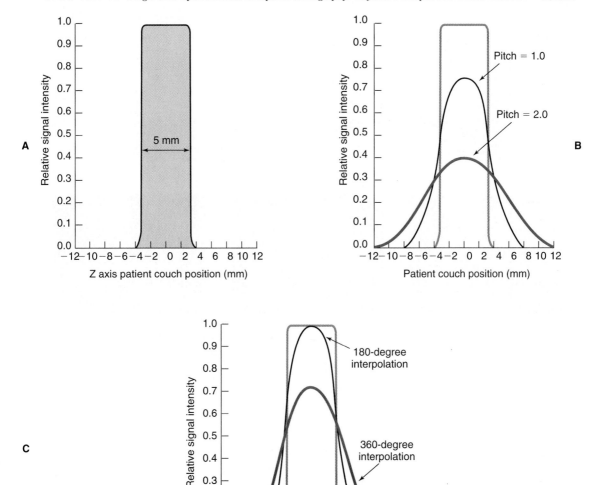

FIG. 13-26. The slice sensitivity profile (SSP) for conventional CT and spiral/helical CT. **A,** The SSP is almost a rectangle and closely approximates the slice thickness. **B,** The SSPs for spiral/helical CT are shown for a pitch of 1 and a pitch of 2. **C,** The influence of two linear interpolation algorithms on SSP. SSP is wider for the 360-degree LI, resulting in a loss of image quality.

techniques such as real-time CT fluoroscopy (continuous imaging), 3D imaging, CT angiography, and virtual reality imaging or CT endoscopy.

ADVANTAGES AND LIMITATIONS
Advantages

In a recent article, Gay and Matthews (1998) discuss 10 advantages of CT scanning in spiral/helical geometry, as follows:

1. Complete organs or volumes can be scanned in short times because of continu-

ous data acquisition synchronized with continuous patient transport through the gantry aperture.
2. The examination time is reduced because of the elimination of the ISD.
3. Gapless scanning is possible because a volume of tissue is scanned rather than a slice as in conventional, nonspiral CT systems.
4. Artifacts caused by patient motion are reduced.
5. Slices can be obtained for any arbitrary position with the volume.

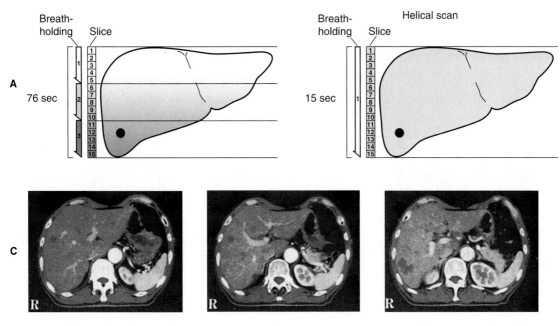

FIG. 13-27. Lesion detection comparison between conventional rapid sequence scanning (**A**) and spiral/helical CT scanning (**B**). Lesion detection is optimized with spiral/helical CT (**C**). (Courtesy Toshiba America Medical Systems; Tustin, Calif.)

6. The effects of different levels of respiration are removed. There is no shifting of anatomic structures between the slices, and lesions can be localized accurately.

7. New perspectives in contrast medium studies are possible because contrast medium administration times are shorter and smaller amounts are required.

8. In spiral/helical CT, contrast enhancement is more uniform throughout the scanning sequence and lesion detection is optimized. This is not the case with conventional, rapid sequential CT (Fig. 13-27).

9. There is greater accuracy in multiplanar reconstruction and 3D processing (see Fig. 13-5).

10. Multidimensional imaging including CT fluoroscopy, 3D imaging, CT angiography, and CT endoscopy. These techniques expand the scope of clinical applications.

Limitations

Although CT scanning in spiral geometry offers significant advantages over the use of conven-

tional slice-by-slice CT scanning, it also has the following drawbacks:

1. Spiral/helical CT places additional demands on the x-ray tube. The tube must be able to sustain higher power levels for longer periods of time compared with the tube used in nonspiral CT systems. Therefore tubes with improved cooling rates and higher capacity are needed. This area is receiving much attention from manufacturers of continuous rotation scanners.

2. Although the interpolation algorithm removes streak artifacts (see Fig. 13-12), unsharp images may appear as a result of partial volume averaging.

Additional limitations of single-slice spiral/helical CT will be outlined in Chapter 15, which deals with multislice spiral/helical CT.

REFERENCES

Baker CCT: *Dictionary of mathematics*, New York, 1961, Hart.

Brink JA et al: Helical CT: principles and technical considerations, *Radiographics* 14:887-893, 1994.

Gay SB, Matthews AB: Ten reasons why spiral CT is worth a million bucks, *Diag Imag* Nov:111-113, 1998.

James G, James R, eds: *Mathematics dictionary*, ed 4, New York, 1976, Van Nostrand Reinhold.

Kalender WA: Technical foundations of spiral CT, *Semin Ultrasound* CT MRI 15:81-89, 1994.

Kalender WA, Polacin A, Suess C: A comparison of conventional and spiral CT: an experimental study on the detection of spherical lesions, *CAT* 18:167-176, 1994.

Kalender WA: Spiral or helical CT: right or wrong? *Radiology* 193:583, 1994.

McGhee PI, Humphreys S: Radiation dose associated with spiral computed tomography, *J Can Assoc Radiol* 45:124-129, 1944.

Mori I: *Computerized tomographic apparatus utilizing a radiation source*, U.S. Patent 4630202, 1987.

Napel SA: Basic principles of spiral CT. In Fishman ED, Jeffrey RB Jr, eds: Spiral CT: principles, techniques, and clinical applications, New York, 1995, Raven Press.

Seeram E: Radiation dose in computed tomography, *Radiol Tech* 70:534-556, 1999.

Urban BA et al: Detection of focal hepatic lesions with spiral CT: comparison of 4-mm and 8-mm interscan spacing, *Am J Roentgenol* 160:783-787, 1993.

BIBLIOGRAPHY

Bresler Y, Skrabacz C: Optimal interpolation in helical scan 3D computerized tomography, *National Science Foundation* (MIP88-10412):1472-1475, 1993.

Huda W et al: An approach for the estimation of effective radiation dose in CT for pediatric patients, *Radiology* 203: 417-422, 1997.

Kalender WA: Principles and performance of spiral CT. In Goldman LW, Fowlkes JB, eds: *Medical CT and ultrasound: current technology and applications*, Maryland, 1995, American Association of Physics in Medicine.

14

Advances in Volume Scanning

BRYAN R. WESTERMAN

CHAPTER *Outline*

The performance of computed tomography scanners has improved greatly since their introduction in 1972 in areas such as scan time, data processing speed, and x-ray tube heat capacity. Some major events have moved CT scanning into another gear and thereby have had considerable impact on clinical applications. The introduction of spiral/helical scanning, near real-time reconstruction, and multislice detectors will significantly affect the future use of CT.

CONTINUOUS IMAGING

Continuous imaging, or near real-time CT, was introduced at the 1993 Radiological Society of North America meeting in Chicago (Katada et al, 1994). Its first clinical application was the guidance of a free-hand puncture of an intracerebral hemorrhage. Key technologies leading to this advance were the slip-ring gantries necessary for spiral/helical scanning, rapid parallel processing of the CT data to hasten image reconstruction, and the introduction of a new processing algorithm (Ozaki, 1995). Instead of reconstructing each image from a unique 360-degree raw data set as the gantry advances each 60 degrees, new data are added to the image file while the oldest 60-degree data are discarded. Using this reconstruction technique, a 1-second scanner can display six CT images each second, each of which represents a full 360 degrees of data (Fig. 14-1), thus efficiently using the continuous data stream generated by the slip-ring gantry.

The first image appears 1.17 seconds after the x-ray beam is activated, and a new image appears every 0.17 seconds thereafter. Images are reconstructed in a 256 × 256 matrix to reduce processing time, but image quality is generally more than adequate for the intended purpose. Continuous images may be displayed while the table and gantry are moved.

Although continuous imaging (CI) was proposed to aid in CT guidance of interventional procedures, the technology has found additional applications in both routine spiral/helical scanning and contrast tracking.

The use of CI during routine spiral/helical scanning provides considerably more control over an examination than was previously available. Because the operator can see the images as they are obtained, studies can be immediately aborted if improperly set up or terminated when the volume of interest has been covered. Physicians can get a rapid indication of how to proceed in the handling of trauma cases before the examination is complete and the final images are reconstructed and filmed. Used as a routine tool, CI can save time and minimize radiation dose to the patient (Katada, 1995).

The ability to observe anatomy at six frames/sec also greatly simplifies the task of timing the beginning of scans in contrast studies. With continuous observation of the target vessel, the arrival of contrast medium can easily be seen and the spiral/helical data acquisition can be initiated (Fig. 14-2). This visual cueing of contrasted studies has been

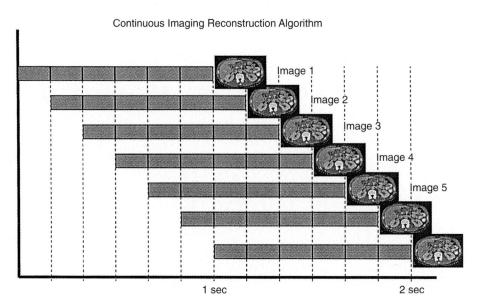

Continuous Imaging Reconstruction Algorithm

Image 1
Image 2
Image 3
Image 4
Image 5

1 sec   2 sec

FIG. 14-1. A new image is displayed each one sixth of a second by adding the latest 60 degrees of data and discarding the first 60 degrees. In this way, each image represents a full 360 degrees.

shown to be more reliable than setting a target threshold in a region of interest (ROI) and can significantly reduce the volume of contrast required without loss of image quality (Schweiger et al, 1998). An ROI is often unreliable to initiate scanning because of patient motion as the contrast material approaches the target vessel. When the contrast arrives, the ROI may no longer be over the selected vessel, particularly if it is small. The use of CI for contrast tracking complements spiral/helical scanning by providing accurate timing for optimal opacification, whether in routine contrasted abdominal studies or in CT angiography. The time between the observation of the arrival of contrast and the start of the spiral/helical scan is typically 3 to 5 sec. As CT scanning becomes faster, the need for reliable contrast tracking will be even more important.

Perhaps the most dramatic application of CI is in the guidance of interventional procedures. Instead of leaving the room each time an image is needed, technologists now may work within the room while continuously observing the progress of the procedure in near real-time. The addition of x-ray and table controls at the couchside has enormously reduced the time for CT-guided intervention and increased patient safety and comfort (Fig. 14-3). Careful evaluations have estimated between 40% and 80% reduction in the time required for CT guided interventional procedures. CT fluoroscopy has proven valuable in neuro-

logic, chest, and abdominal procedures involving biopsy and drainage (Meyer et al, 1998; Daly and Templeton, 1999). One advantage is the ability to observe critical structures near the path of a biopsy needle so that technologists can avoid them by changing the angle of approach (Fig. 14-4). Targets in the chest that move during respiration can be more reliably sampled. As the lesion moves into view on the monitor, the patient suspends respiration so that the lesion is immobile until the completion of the biopsy. Such control provides access to smaller targets, including those near the heart, than is practical with conventional CT guidance.

An exciting development that has accompanied CT fluoroscopy is the expansion of CT-guided intervention into new areas. Spinal interventional procedures have been reported to be faster and safer under CT fluoroscopy guidance. Brachytherapy catheter placement for implant radiation therapy can also benefit from this technique. CT fluoroscopy has been used to guide sacroiliac joint injection, vertebral repair, and gastrostomy tube placement. This application of CT technology may have considerable impact on the operation of a radiology department. CT guidance of interventional procedures no longer has to burden a scanner for hours.

Both operator and patient dose are kept within acceptable limits by using tube currents of 30 to 50 mA and, in the case of at least one manufacturer, introducing a dedicated x-ray filter into the

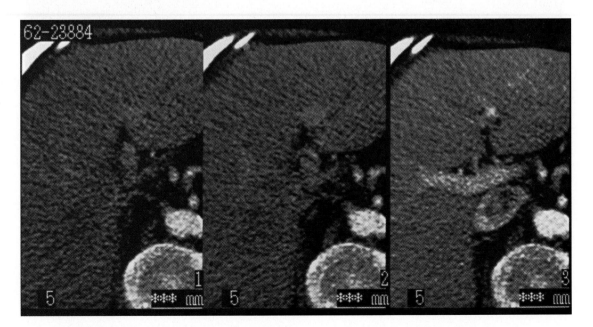

FIG. 14-2. A continuous imaging sequence that shows the arrival of contrast at the portal vein. Spiral/helical scanning is initiated when the presence of contrast is visually confirmed. (Courtesy University of Iowa; Iowa City.)

beam to reduce dose by 50% (Kato et al, 1996). Tools that allow the interventionalist to manipulate a needle in the image plane while keeping the hands out of the primary beam are also essential.

SUBSECOND SCANNING

Scanning time continues to decrease from the 5 minutes needed by the original EMI scanner to as low as one half second at present. The engineering barriers to be overcome in reaching this gantry speed are formidable. The acceleration on gantry components such as the tube and generator can reach 13 Gs, considerably more than experienced by the space shuttle at lift off. Some interesting technologic developments have accompanied the design of these high-speed CT systems.

To prevent anode movement under the stress of subsecond acceleration, new x-ray tubes have the anode mounted on a shaft that extends along the tube, providing support on both sides of the anode. This design has distinct advantages over the traditional method of supporting a massive anode from the rear only. Other innovative developments in tube design for CT include grounded anodes and a technique to reduce off-focal x-rays. Virtually all medical x-ray tubes have applied the potential difference equally between cathode and anode so that the cathode can be at -75 kV while the anode is at $+75$ kV. This requires a substantial gap between the anode and the tube housing to reduce the possibility of arcs. With all the voltage placed on the cathode and the anode at ground potential, the tube housing can be brought into close proximity to the anode, which facilitates heat transfer and markedly improves anode cooling rate (Fig. 14-5). Recoil electrons, which normally are re-attracted to the anode and generate off-focal x-rays, can now be collected on a special collimator located near the anode. This eliminates off-focal x-rays that can reduce image quality and reduces the anode heat loading by about 30%, thereby reducing tube cooling delays during routine scanning.

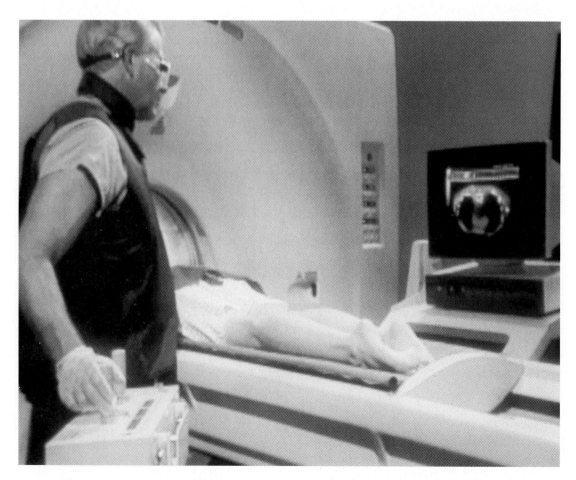

FIG. 14-3. CT fluoroscopy allows the physician to continuously observe the progress of the needle while controlling x-rays and table and gantry movement.

The clinical benefits of subsecond scanning include reduced motion artifact and greater scan coverage. Patient movement during CT scanning, whether by cardiac motion, breathing, or peristalsis, may cause artifacts because filtered back-projection reconstruction combines all the views acquired during the scan rotation to cancel artifacts. Movement of any object in the field of view (FOV) during gantry rotation prevents accurate elimination of artifacts with consequent loss of im-

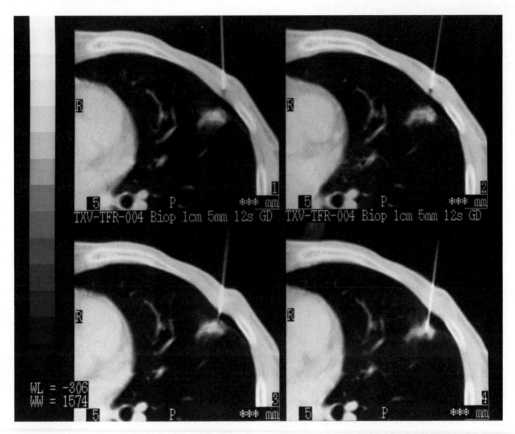

FIG. 14-4. A lung biopsy that illustrates how the needle approach can be changed in real time to reach the target and avoid critical structures. (Courtesy University of Maryland; Annapolis, Md.)

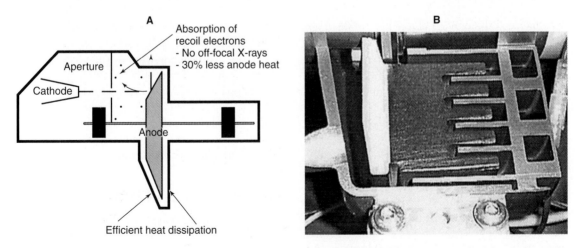

FIG. 14-5. Innovative developments in tube technology include (**A**) extended anode support, absorption of recoil electrons to prevent off-focal x-rays, and operations with the anode at ground potential. With no potential difference between anode and tube housing, these two structures can be very close together (**B**) for rapid heat transfer and tube cooling.

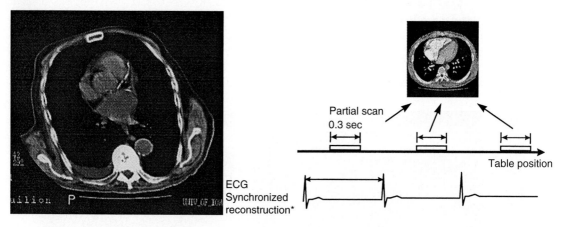

FIG. 14-6. Partial (320-ms) images can be reconstructed during diastole using ECG triggering. Images of thoracic anatomy are sharper than those using longer scan times. Calcium can be seen in the coronary artery of the patient image.

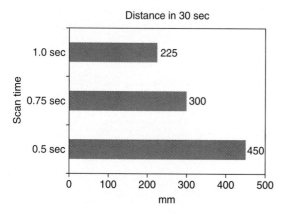

FIG. 14-7. Distance traveled in 30 sec with a 5-mm slice and pitch 1.5 at different scan times.

age quality. If the moving object has notably high or low contrast, such as bone, calculi, or air, the artifacts are particularly noticeable. Unfortunately, the left ventricle and pulmonary vessels near the heart move so quickly that scans would have to be completed in less than 20 to 25 ms to completely eliminate all blurring (Ritchie, 1992). This is a far shorter time than is possible with conventional CT scanners and is even difficult for electron-beam CTs, which are extremely fast. Even so, the new half-second scanners, which can acquire "partial" (i.e., less than 360-degree rotation) images in 250 to 320 ms have made it feasible to obtain considerably better images of the heart and chest than is possible with a 1-second system. An example is the ability of these scanners to employ gated reconstruction, in which the raw scan data for image reconstruction can be selected based on the patient's electrocardiogram (ECG). Reconstruction of a gated "partial" image during cardiac diastole when the heart is relatively quiescent can show fairly sharp ventricular borders and calcium in the coronary arteries (Fig. 14-6).

Prospective gating can also be employed, in which the patient's ECG triggers the actual scan acquisition. This is a relatively simple technique, although it is not applicable to spiral/helical scanning.

A less dramatic but very practical benefit of subsecond scan times is the increased spiral/helical coverage that can become available. For the same pitch and scan duration, a half-second scanner will cover twice the anatomy that can be acquired with a 1-second scanner (Fig. 14-7).

Alternatively, the half-second scanner could cover the same area using 50% of the slice thickness, which improves z axis resolution and leads to better image quality in 3D and multiplanar reconstructions. Clinical applications such as CTA can benefit from increased patient coverage without increasing pitch. This assumes that the system generator is able to produce enough power to accommodate the faster scans. For example, a 250-mA image of the abdomen requires a tube current of 500 mA in a half-second scanner.

MULTISLICE DETECTORS

The first clinical scanner, the EMI Mark 1, and several of its successors recorded two image slices simultaneously in an effort to offset their agonizingly slow scan speeds. In 1992, Elscint introduced the first modern multislice scanner, which employed dual detector banks. A major difference be-

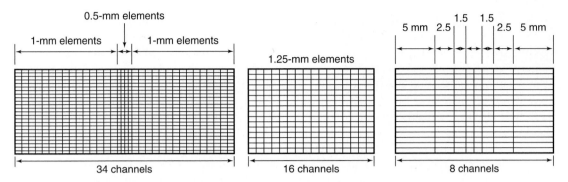

FIG. 14-8. Multirow CT detector designs. Detector elements may be uniform or nonuniform.

tween the EMI Mark 1 and Elscint scanners was that a particular image from the Elscint system could take advantage of data acquired by both detector banks, whereas the old EMI scanner, which predated spiral/helical acquisition, simply generated two independent images.

Detectors capable of providing more than two slices for CT scanners were introduced in 1998. At present, they allow acquisition of up to four slices simultaneously, and their design suggests that this number may increase in the future. This dramatic technical advance promises to have a major impact on the way CT is used in clinical practice. The tremendous increase in the rate of data collection will influence routine CT applications and create new areas for CT imaging.

Several different approaches to the construction of these detectors are available (Fig. 14-8). As can be seen from Fig. 14-8, detector arrays in the z-axis can be uniform, with all elements of the same dimensions or nonuniform to reduce the number of elements needed for thicker slices. An advantage of the nonuniform elements is the reduction of dead space (the gap between detector elements to ensure optical isolation). On the other hand, this arrangement offers less flexibility for the future, when slice numbers greater than four will be practical. Element dimensions shown are "effective" detector sizes, calculated at the center of gantry rotation where slice thickness is measured. The size and distribution of detector elements in the x-y plane are similar to those in current single-slice systems. Consequently, spatial or high-contrast resolution is unlikely to change significantly. Such arrays can involve more than 30,000 individual detector elements.

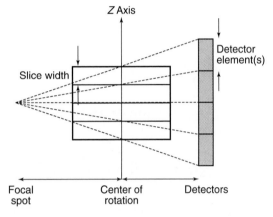

FIG. 14-9. Slice geometry in multislice scanners. The number of detector elements grouped together determines the size of the slice. Slice width is defined at the center of gantry rotation.

Slice Thickness

Individual slice widths (Fig. 14-9) are generally defined by the number of detector elements grouped into each data channel. The smallest slice width available is determined by the smallest single detector element. An exception to this generalization occurs in the nonuniform array shown in Fig. 14-9, in which two 0.5-mm slices can be acquired by moving the collimator leaves inward so that only the inner half of the two central 1-mm elements are exposed to the x-ray beam. Similarly, four 1-mm slices are acquired by irradiating the two central elements and two thirds of the adjacent 1.5-mm elements. Slice width is defined at the center of rotation (center of the gantry aperture) so the actual detector dimensions for that slice will be greater because of the magnification produced by beam divergence. The x-ray beam width, as defined by the pre-patient collimators, will be approximately four times the slice width.

The slice, as defined by the tissue irradiated during the rotation of a multislice detector, is significantly different from that of a single detector scanner (Fig. 14-10). This is an extension of the problem with the earlier dual-detector scanners. In this case, however, the outer two slices are considerably more affected by beam divergence than the inner two slices.

The significance of this geometric nonuniformity may be most severe in the case of conventional scanning. Reconstruction of the CT image involves all views acquired throughout the 360 degrees of data collection. When views from different angles are actually measuring quite different tissue pathways, there will be varying degrees of volume averaging with an increased likelihood of artifact and inaccurate reconstruction. If detector size is increased in future scanners to add more slices, this geometric situation will be further exaggerated. With the x-ray beam fan extended in the z axis, as well as the x-y plane, a reconstruction algorithm that is different from those used for single-slice scanners is needed to process the raw data (Taguchi and Aradate, 1998; Hu, 1999.)

The signals from the individual detector elements are fed to four data acquisition systems (DAS) through a bank of switches that combines the signals from the appropriate number of elements into the slice width selected by the operator (Fig. 14-11).

Detector elements outside the selected slices are switched off and do not contribute any signal to the DAS. Patient dose is controlled by prepatient collimators that restrict the x-ray beam to only those detector elements needed for the four data slices. At present, the slice thickness must be selected before scanning, and it is not possible to narrow the slice width after data collection. Summing slices after scanning to create fewer, thicker images is certainly feasible and can have clinical value. In this case, it would be possible to return to the thinner slices if clinically indicated and if the raw data were still available.

So far, all multislice detectors that have been introduced employ solid-state materials (either scintillation crystals or ceramics). Although it is feasible to construct a multislice xenon detector,

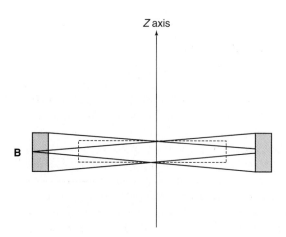

FIG. 14-10. Comparison of slice geometry between multislice (**A**) and single-slice (**B**) scanners. The x-ray beams are shown at opposite sides of gantry rotation. Although the diagram is exaggerated, there is more beam divergence with the multislice system.

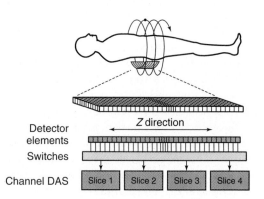

FIG. 14-11. Switches group the signal from individual detector elements. The signals are then transferred to one of four data acquisition systems that generate the four simultaneous slices. Additional DAS channels can be added in the future.

the reduction in sensitivity would increase image noise. This would be particularly troublesome because of the move towards scanning with thinner slices.

Another consideration is the way in which multislice detectors will affect scanner geometry. Only a few commercial scanners are designed as rotate-stationary (fourth-generation scanners). It seems that the cost and complexity of developing multislice detectors for fourth-generation geometry cannot be justified by any perceived advantages. The future of CT appears firmly tied to rotate-rotate systems.

SPIRAL/HELICAL SCANNING WITH MULTISLICE DETECTORS

Pitch is an important and familiar parameter in spiral/helical scanning that combines the table distance traveled per 360-degree rotation with the slice thickness. Pitch relates to the volume covered and also to patient dose. A spiral/helical pitch of less than 1 is effectively the same as overlapping slices and imparts a high dose. Conversely, spiral/helical pitches of greater than 1 result in reduced patient dose. The introduction of multislice detectors requires a reevaluation of the definition of pitch.

$$\text{Beam pitch} = \frac{\text{Table distance traveled per gantry rotation}}{\text{Beam width}}$$

Beam pitch is comparable to the familiar parameter used with single-slice scanning in terms of its effect on patient dose.

$$\text{Slice pitch} = \frac{\text{Table distance traveled per gantry rotation}}{\text{Slice width}}$$

Slice pitch is defined in terms of individual slice width, as is the case with single-slice scanners.

Slice pitch = N × Beam pitch,
where N = the number of slices

Therefore a slice pitch of 3 would correspond to a pitch of 0.75 for a single-slice scanner, whereas a slice pitch of 6 would be equivalent to a single-slice pitch of 1.5.

For a patient dose comparable to current single-slice scanners at a pitch of 1, a four-slice scanner would require a beam pitch of 1 or a slice pitch of 4. As an example, selection of 4 × 5-mm slices with a table speed of 20 mm/rotation should result in approximately the same patient dose as from a single-slice scanner operated with a 5-mm slice at 5 mm per rotation table speed. Whether this is true in practice depends on the collimator design of the specific scanner.

Spiral/Helical Data Reconstruction

Reconstructing images from spiral/helical data is more complicated than conventional CT reconstruction. For a single slice, all views accumulated from the 360-degree gantry rotation are processed to create the image. However, with spiral/helical scans in which the couch moves continuously through the gantry as data are collected, only a few views are actually measured at the table position where the image is to be reconstructed. Interpolation overcomes this limitation. When a view from a particular gantry angle is needed but not directly measured, it is created by averaging the nearest views from the same angle in front of and behind the image position. This form of interpolated reconstruction (360-degree linear interpolation) works well but has the drawback of substantially increasing the effective slice thickness of the image. Because the data used for reconstruction could extended from 360 degrees before to 360 degrees after the image plane, slices reconstructed with this interpolated data could easily be 30% to 40% thicker than the actual collimator width.

A different algorithm was developed based on the mathematical fact that a CT view from a specific angle contains the same information as a view in the opposite direction (at 180 degrees). The 180-degree view, when flipped and used for interpolated reconstruction, is referred to as *complementary data*, as opposed to the direct, measured data (Fig. 14-12).

To reconstruct a spiral/helical image, it is not necessary to search as far for a view at the desired angle. Simply follow the z axis until the complementary view is located, flip it for interpolation, and carry out the reconstruction. This algorithm, known as 180-degree linear interpolation, results in thinner effective slices and is now used for most routine patient studies. However, because the image involves fewer data points along the z axis, it is noisier than a 360-degree interpolated reconstruction. Thus the choice of a spiral/helical interpolation routine involves a trade-off between thinner slices and gives better z axis resolution and less volume averaging compared with a thicker, less noisy image.

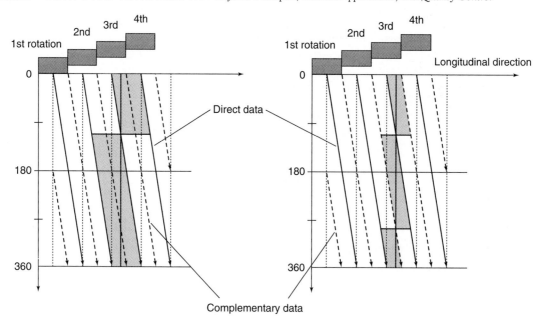

FIG. 14-12. Single-slice spiral/helical data are generated from many gantry rotations. Reconstruction of an image in a single plane on the patient axis involves the interpolation of views in front of and behind the image plane. The use of complementary data reduces effective slice thickness but increases noise.

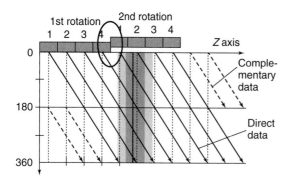

FIG. 14-13. Rotation of a multislice detector with an even integer pitch causes the overlap of direct and complementary data from different slices. This duplication reduces the amount of information available for image reconstruction and affects image quality.

Multislice Reconstruction

The reconstruction of spiral/helical images from multislice data adds another level of complexity to an already confusing situation. Because the patient now moves past four rows of contiguous detectors, if the scan pitch is poorly chosen, direct data from one detector will overlap the complementary data from an adjacent detector (Fig. 14-13). If this type of duplication occurs, less data are available for reconstruction and image quality is reduced. Conse-

quently, in the selection of a spiral/helical slice pitch for a multislice scanner, it is better to avoid even integers such as 4.0 or 6.0 (Fig. 14-14). To simplify setting up scan techniques, manufacturers may limit the number of available pitches.

Any spiral/helical beam pitch of less than 1 or any slice pitch less than 4 represents overlapping acquisition and will increase patient dose.

Another unique aspect of multislice data reconstruction involves averaging data in the z axis direction. Interpolation of spiral/helical data is still needed, but the fact that the density of data points in this dimension is greater than with single-slice scanners is advantageous. One approach to image reconstruction employs a filter in the z axis to select and weight the data points to be used in the averaging (Taguchi and Aradate, 1998) (Fig. 14-15). A practical advantage of this technique is that the size and shape of the filter can be selected by the operator for more control over the effective slice thickness versus noise tradeoff. As can be seen from Fig. 14-15, the selection of different filter widths provides considerably more control over effective slice thickness than has generally been available with single-slice spiral/helical reconstruction. Filter width can also substantially affect image noise compared with conventional 180- or 360-degree linear interpolation.

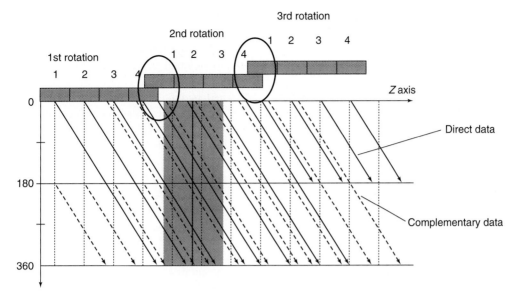

FIG. 14-14. Careful choice of multislice pitch avoids the duplication of direct and complementary data so that image quality is not compromised.

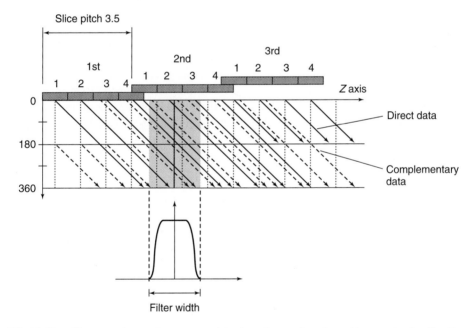

FIG. 14-15. Filters may be used to average data along the z axis and provide more trade-off options between effective slice thickness and image noise to the operator.

CLINICAL APPLICATIONS

The immediate advantages of multislice CT are the speed of volume acquisition and the reduced loading on the x-ray tube. The same anatomic coverage may be obtained in one fourth the time and at one fourth the anode heating with all other parameters remaining the same. The implications for the x-ray tube are enormous. Not only is it possible to perform many more acquisitions before the necessary pause for tube cooling, but the wear and tear on the tube is also greatly reduced for the same scan volume.

For example, a full body scan from head through the pelvis, which would require more than

95 seconds of data collection in a 1-second, single-slice scanner (excluding interscan delays), could be performed in less than 12 seconds of data collection for a half-second, multislice system. (See Table 14-1.)

Such amazing speed should have immediate value in examinations of trauma and pediatric patients. Better phase differentiation in contrasted studies is now possible, which hopefully will lead improved diagnostic information. However, just as the introduction of spiral/helical CT emphasized the need for accurate contrast timing, the speed of multislice scanning will make this accuracy even more critical. Accurate contrast tracking techniques such as those available from continuous imaging technology will play an even greater role in the optimization of contrast opacity in both routine and special examinations.

As with spiral/helical scanning, speed may be exchanged for improved image quality. With the single-slice scanner, technique selection must balance the volume to be covered against slice thickness and pitch. Multislice systems offer the possibility of extended coverage with thin slices, which improves z axis resolution and reduces partial volume averaging (Fig. 14-16). These effects should be particularly noticeable in 3D and multiplanar reconstructions of scan data in CT angiography, for example.

As can be seen in Table 14-2, 0.5-mm slices can be achieved in reasonable scan times, which brings isotropic resolution in 3D reconstructions within reach. This is particularly valuable in cerebral CT angiography for the more accurate visualization of small vessels (Fig. 14-17). Aneurysms and stenoses may be characterized quantitatively to yield better diagnostic information and allow the presurgical preparation of customized stents and other devices for more effective therapy. Similar improvements in CTA of the neck, aorta, and renal vessels are available with these scanners because of the combination of speed and thin slices for high axial resolution. Indeed, examples of peripheral runoff studies are appearing in which superb CT angiograms of the aorta and lower extremities can be completed in 75 seconds with substantially less contrast volume. In addition to more accurate CT angiography, the ability to cover large volumes with excellent spatial resolution should also provide more accurate data sets for the performance of CT endoscopy and the diagnosis of pulmonary embolism. Although experience with these scanners is very limited at present, the early indications are that in all situations, the multislice CT is preferred over a single-slice system.

Another exciting prospect with multislice detectors is the development of functional CT imaging. Examples of the usefulness of CT in the evaluation of perfusion and other functions in various parts of the body have occasionally been reported, but the limitation of single-slice acquisition has

TABLE 14-1

Speed of Volume Acquisition

REGION	DISTANCE	SLICE THICKNESS	SINGLE-SLICE, 1-SEC SCAN, PITCH 1.5	MULTISLICE, 0.5-SEC SCAN, SLICE PITCH 6.0
Head	20 cm	8 mm	16.7 sec	2.1 sec
Neck	15 cm	5 mm	20.0 sec	2.5 sec
Chest	30 cm	8 mm	25.0 sec	3.1 sec
Abdomen	20 cm	8 mm	16.7 sec	2.1 sec
Pelvis	20 cm	8 mm	16.7 sec	2.1 sec
		Total	95.1 sec	11.9 sec

TABLE 14-2

Coverage and Slice Thickness with Multislice Systems

COVERAGE AT SLICE PITCH OF 3.5	2-mm SLICE THICKNESS	1-mm SLICE THICKNESS	0.5-mm SLICE THICKNESS
40 mm	2.9 sec	5.7 sec	11.4 sec
60 mm	4.3 sec	8.6 sec	17.1 sec

prevented routine applications. Now that a larger volume of data can be continuously acquired, the potential of CT in functional studies may be realized. An early application of this technique will likely be the evaluation of brain perfusion through the observation of first-pass contrast flow in patients suspected of acute infarction.

THE CATCH

Although multislice scanners have dramatic advantages, they also have some potential problems. Cases that are currently scanned with thin slices, overlapped reconstruction, and possibly two or more reconstruction algorithms can generate huge numbers of images. Routine studies consisting of 300 to 400 images are common, and special examinations might involve nearly 1000 images. Obviously, such large data sets present problems for in-

terpretation, recording, distribution, and archiving. Radiologists will be forced to move away from film diagnosis to "soft" reading of images on workstations. There will also be pressure to read MPR and 3D reconstructions instead of individual axial images because of the need for fast and efficient workstations. Reliance on remote locations for diagnosis may strain existing transmission capabilities and necessitate considerably faster systems for the future.

It will no longer be practical to record all CT images on film, and even archiving to digital media may require new strategies such as "stacking" slices or selective archival. Some departmental PACS systems have already been stretched beyond their capabilities by the flood of new data, and great care is needed in future facility design. The handling of image data may be the next big problem area for CT.

WHERE NOW?

Hardware development in CT will continue, of course. Scan times may be further reduced with partial scan times perhaps approaching 150 ms, but the demands on the gantry components will be severe. In particular, generators will need to supply much larger tube currents to maintain image noise at current levels.

Area detectors for CT are currently under investigation. The most likely prospects appear to be the flat plate detectors that are currently being introduced into general radiography. These devices could extend z axis coverage substantially and result in the scanning of most organs in one or two gantry revolutions. Potential drawbacks are the acquisition speed of these devices, which leads to image lag at fast scan speeds, and the inevitable increase in scattered radiation with larger field sizes. Cone beam reconstruction algorithms would be needed to accommodate the extended x-ray fan beam. Such a development may be associated with volumetric image reconstruction instead of axial slices, as is the case with MRI.

Image reconstruction times will continue to decrease, partly from the pressure of the vast number of images that will be generated by CT examinations. Added flexibility during reconstruction will become available as software permits the operator more latitude in the trade-off between spatial and temporal resolution.

It is also highly likely that new options for image handling, display, and processing will develop for both PACS systems and 2D or 3D workstations.

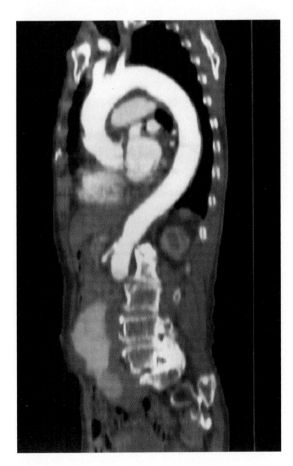

FIG. 14-16. Sagittal reconstruction of an aortic aneurysm study. Scanned with 4 × 5-mm slices, 0.5-second rotation, and a slice pitch of 4.5. The data was acquired in 11.5 seconds. (Courtesy Fujita Health University; Japan.)

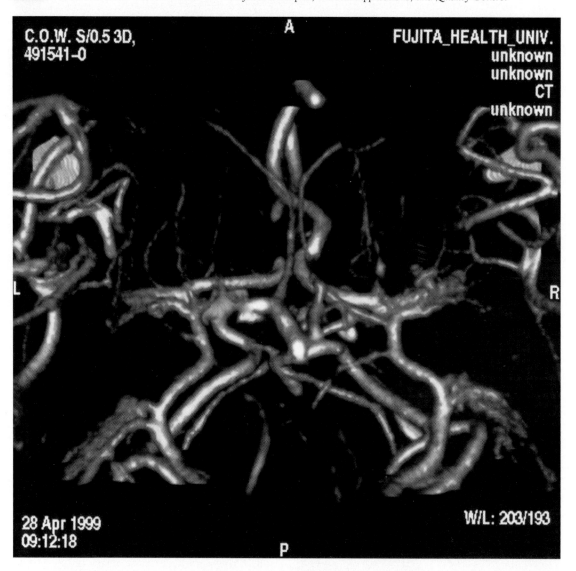

FIG. 14-17. CT angiogram of the circle of Willis reconstructed on a Vital Images workstation with a half-second scan time, 4 × 0.5-mm slices, 120 kV, and 300 mA. Data acquired in 18 seconds. (Courtesy Fujita Health University; Japan.)

REFERENCES

Daly B, Templeton PA: Real-time CT fluoroscopy: evolution of a clinical tool, *Radiology* 211:309, 1999.

Hu H: Multislice helical CT: scan and reconstruction, *Medical Physics* 26:5, 1999.

Katada K et al: Early clinical experience with real-time CT fluoroscopy (abstract), *Radiology* 193:339, 1994.

Katada K: Further innovations in CT technology: CT fluoroscopy and real-time helical scan CT, *Toshiba Medical Review* 53:1, 1995.

Kato R et al: Radiation dosimetry at CT fluoroscopy: physician's hand doses and development of needle holders, *Radiology* 201:576, 1996.

Meyer CA et al: Real-time CT fluoroscopy: utility in thoracic drainage procedures, *Am J Roentgenol* 171:1097, 1998.

Ozaki M: Development of a real-time reconstruction system for CT fluorography, *Toshiba Medical Review* 53:12, 1995.

Ritchie CJ et al: Minimum scan speeds for suppression of motion artifacts in CT, *Radiology* 185:37, 1992.

Schweiger G D, Chang PJ, Brown BP: Optimizing contrast enhancement during helical CT of the liver, *Am J Roentgenol* 171:1551, 1998.

Taguchi K, Aradate H: Algorithm for image reconstruction in multislice helical CT, *Medical Physics* 25:550, 1998.

15

Multislice Spiral/Helical Computed Tomography: Physical Principles and Instrumentation

LIMITATIONS OF SINGLE-SLICE VOLUME CT SCANNERS

Ever since its introduction in 1990, single-slice volume CT has been used successfully in many body CT imaging applications, in which speed and volume coverage are important. Volume coverage and speed can be increased by using higher pitch ratios; however, higher pitch ratios in single-slice volume CT scanning degrade image quality (z axis resolution) and produce image artifacts. In describing the volume coverage and speed, Hu (1999a) introduces the term *volume coverage speed performance* to refer to "the capability of rapidly scanning a large longitudinal (z) volume with high longitudinal (z axis) resolution and low image artifacts."

In single-slice volume CT, the volume coverage speed performance is limited, especially in clinical applications that demand large volume scanning with critical timing requirements and optimum image quality (z axis resolution and low image artifacts), such as CT angiography with 3D,

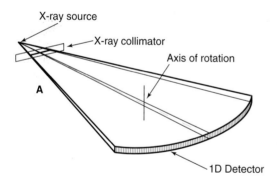

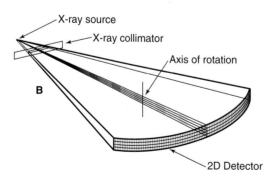

FIG. 15-1. One of the most conspicuous differences between a single-slice volume CT scanner and a multislice CT scanner is the detector design. **A,** A 1D detector is used in single-slice systems. **B,** A 2D detector array is characteristic of multislice CT systems.

MPR, and MIP techniques (Hu, 1999a). Single-slice volume CT is based on the use of a single row of detectors (1D detector array). Because the x-ray beam is highly collimated to the size of the detector array, only a small percentage of x-rays emitted by the tube is used in the imaging process. This situation is described as poor geometric efficiency. Also, single-slice volume CT uses the 360-degree linear interpolation algorithm (LIA) and the 180-degree LIA to improve the problems imposed by the 360-degree LIA, such as poor image quality and artifact production. However, the 180-degree LIA produces more noise while preserving the detail (slice sensitivity and spatial resolution).

Additionally, the time duration for covering defined volumes in single-slice volume CT (several seconds) is limited by several factors, such as the ability of some patients, particularly those who are critically ill, to maintain a single breathhold during volume scanning, and the heat loading of the x-ray tube.

Single-slice volume CT is also limited in its ability to meet the needs of time-critical clinical examinations such as multiphase organ dynamic studies and CT angiography, in which both arterial and venous phases are extremely important, using smaller amounts of contrast media. The use of higher pitch ratios to solve these problems degrades the slice sensitivity profile (detail). Therefore other methods are needed to overcome these limitations, to improve the performance of single-slice volume CT in terms of better use of the x-ray output (improved geometric efficiency), and scan parameters affecting image quality and volume coverage.

Multislice CT offers "substantial improvement of the volume coverage speed performance" (Hu, 1999a). This means that multislice CT provides faster scanning and higher resolution for a number of clinical applications (Taguchi and Aradate, 1998). One of the most conspicuous differences between multislice CT and single-slice volume CT is that the former uses a multiple-row of detectors (2D detector array), whereas the latter uses a single-row of detectors (1D detector array) (Fig. 15-1).

EVOLUTION OF MULTISLICE CT SCANNERS

The evolution of multislice CT technology is outlined in Fig. 15-2. Its overall goal is to improve volume coverage speed performance; therefore scanning is at higher speeds with higher pitch ratios to cover large volumes with equivalent image quality, compared with single-slice volume CT scanners introduced in the 1990s. The last set of boxes in Fig. 15-2 indicates some room for improvement of multislice CT. For example, the Toshiba Corporation Medical Systems Division plans to introduce a high-speed 3D CT scanner (Fig. 15-3) as part of their development continuum for CT technology. The high-speed 3D scanner will use larger area detectors to scan larger volumes at high speeds and subsequently display all images in 3D.

Dual-Slice CT Scanners

The history of scanning more than one slice at a time dates 20 years to one of the early EMI CT scanners (second-generation scanner). This scanner used two detectors and is based on the rotate/translate method of data collection over 180 degrees. The next major step to multislice CT scanning appeared in the 1990s, with the introduction of the first dual-slice volume CT scanner, the Elscint CT-Twin (Elscint, Hackensack, NJ). The most significant difference between the dual-slice volume CT scanner and its single-slice counterpart is shown in Fig. 15-4. As can be seen, the dual scanner slice geometry is based on a fan-beam of x-rays falling on two rows of detectors (Fig. 15-4, A) instead of one row of detector characteristic of the single-slice CT scanner beam geometry (Fig. 15-4, B). The Elscint CT-Twin has been ac-

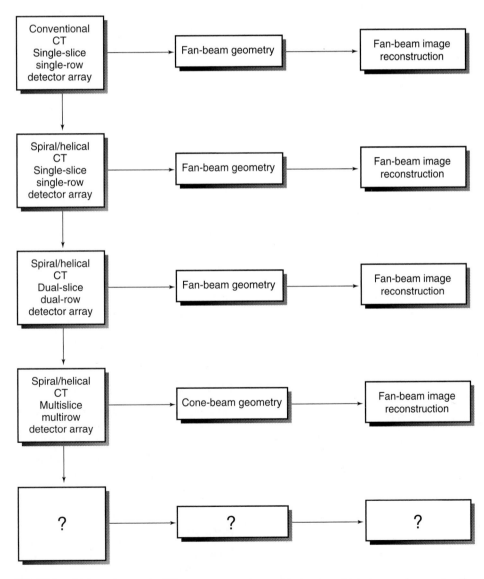

FIG. 15-2. Major advances in CT scanner geometry and technology (detectors and reconstruction algorithms) since the introduction of CT scanners in the 1970s.

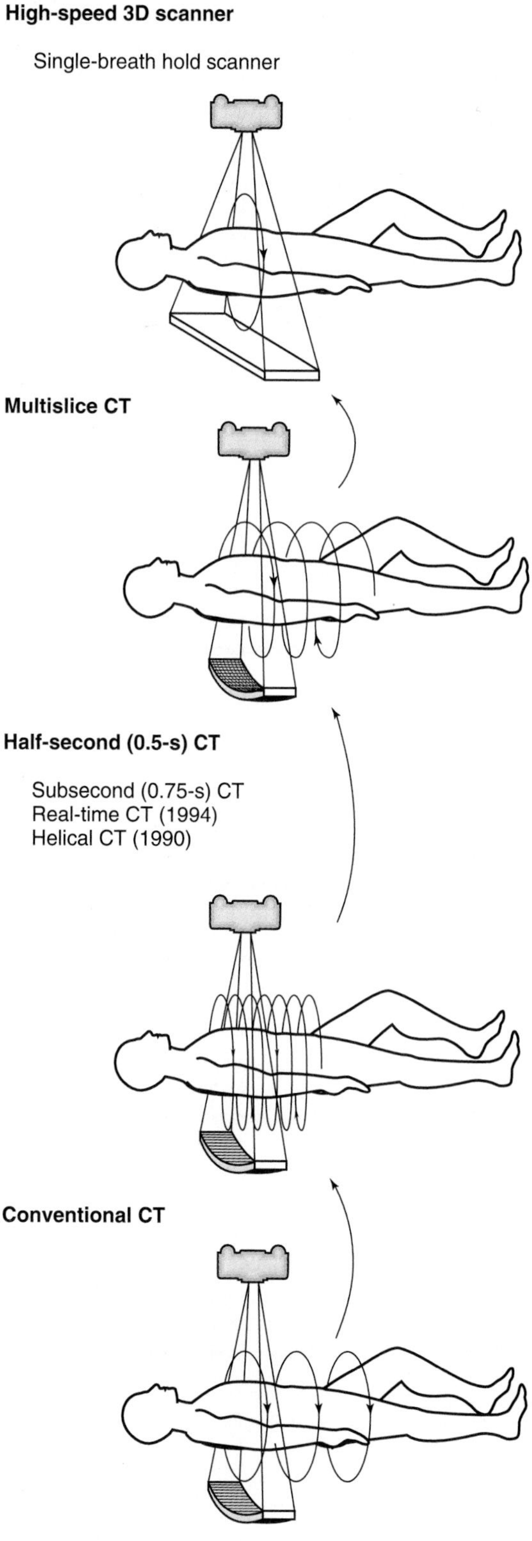

High-speed 3D scanner

Single-breath hold scanner

Multislice CT

Half-second (0.5-s) CT

Subsecond (0.75-s) CT
Real-time CT (1994)
Helical CT (1990)

Conventional CT

FIG. 15-3. The development continuum and milestones for Toshiba's CT scanners.

quired by Picker International and is now marketed as the Mx-Twin.

The dual-slice CT scanner offers improved volume coverage speed performance compared with single-slice volume CT scanner, reducing the scan time by 50% while maintaining image quality for the same scanned volume. Liang and Kruger (1996) compared the performance characteristics of the dual-slice CT scanner with a single-slice CT scanner and found that "the image quality is equivalent in most respects for the two scanners. Based on noise and low-contrast resolution measurements, no increase was found in the x-ray noise in the dual-slice mode. The trade-off between the double speed and the longitudinal resolution for the dual-slice scanner is very small when 180-degree linear interpolation (LI) is employed. This work indicates multiring detector technology does offset faster scans with minimized degradation of image quality."

Multislice CT Scanners

The dual-slice CT technology paved the way for the development of multislice CT scanners. These scanners were introduced at the 1998 meeting of the Radiological Society of North America in Chicago. They are based on spiral/helical scanning using multiple detector rows ranging between 8, 16, 24, and 34 depending on the manufacturer.

The overall goal of the multislice CT scanner is to improve the volume coverage speed performance of both single-slice and dual-slice CT scanners. For example, a multislice CT scanner with N-row detector array will be N times faster than its single-row counterpart. Thus multislice CT with its new technology opens new avenues and opportunities to improve the quality of care afforded to patients (Berland and Smith, 1998).

PHYSICAL PRINCIPLES

Although the fundamental physics and flow of data are the same as conventional nonspiral/nonhelical and spiral/helical CT scanners, multislice CT scanners introduce several new concepts relating to detector technology, the geometry of data acquisition, and multislice image reconstruction algorithms.

Data Acquisition

Data acquisition is one of two mechanisms that affect image quality in CT (the other is image reconstruction). This section examines data acqui-

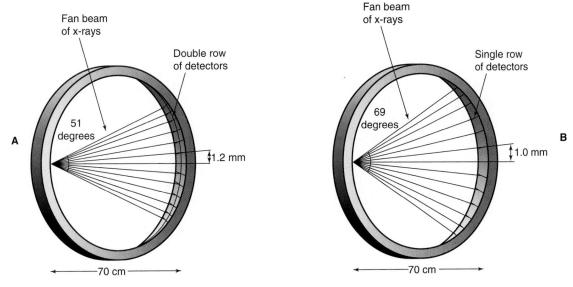

FIG. 15-4. **A,** Dual scanner slice geometry based on far beam of x-rays falling on two rows of detectors. **B,** Single-slice CT scanner based on far beam of x-rays falling on one row of detectors.

sition in multislice CT with respect to beam geometry and basic parameters such as collimation, slice thickness, and pitch, but first, a brief review of data acquisition in single-slice CT is in order.

Single-Slice CT

The basic data acquisition geometry for single-slice volume CT is shown in Fig. 15-5. This is a third-generation scheme in which the x-ray tube is coupled to a single-row detector array positioned in the z axis.

Collimation. The x-ray beam collimation system is designed to ensure a constant beam width because the pre- and postcollimator widths are equal. The beam may or may not be collimated at the detector array. The width of the precollimator defines the slice thickness (z axis resolution or spatial resolution) and affects the volume coverage speed performance. Although thin collimation results in better resolution and takes longer to scan a specified volume, wide collimation results in less resolution but provides better volume coverage speed. The beam width (BW) is measured in the z axis at the center of rotation for single-row detector array, and it is defined by the precollimator width, which determines the thickness for a single slice. A collimator width of 8 mm falling upon a 1D detector array will provide a slice thickness of 8 mm.

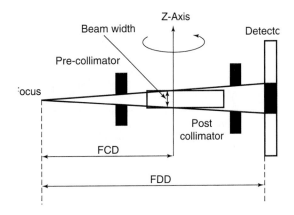

FIG. 15-5. A side view of the basic data acquisition geometry for single-slice volume CT scanners.

Beam Geometry. The x-ray beam geometry for single-slice CT describes a small fan (see Fig. 15-5) and is referred to as a *parallel fan-beam geometry.*

Pitch. The pitch for single-slice volume CT is defined as the ratio of the distance the table translates per gantry rotation to the beam width or precollimator width. As noted by Hu (1999a), "the table advancement per rotation of twice the x-ray beam collimation appears to be the limit of the volume coverage speed performance of a single-slice CT, and further increase in the table translation would result in clinically unusable images."

Slice Thickness. In single-slice volume CT, the thickness of the slice is determined by the pitch and the width of the precollimator (which also defines the beam width, [BW]) at the center of rotation (see Fig. 15-5).

Multislice CT

The data acquisition geometry for multislice CT is shown in Fig. 15-6 (see also Fig. 15-1, B). Perhaps the most conspicuous difference between the data acquisition geometry in Fig. 15-1 and Fig. 15-6 is the multirow detector array (specifically 4) cou-

pled to the x-ray tube to describe a third generation geometry (see Fig. 15-6, A). This 2D detector array is what Hu (1999a) refers to as the "enabling component" of a multislice CT scanner. Other important and unique features of multislice data acquisition relate to collimation, beam geometry, and pitch.

Collimation. The fundamental collimation scheme is shown in Fig. 15-1, B. The beam is collimated by a precollimator to fall on the entire multirow detector array. The beam width (BW) is still defined in the z axis at the center of rotation but now is for a four-row multislice detector array as shown in Fig. 15-6, B. This width will be for four slices and is prescribed by the precollimator. A precollimator width of 8 mm that falls on a four-row multislice detector array will produce four slices, each with a thickness of 2 mm (i.e., 8 mm—the total beam width in the z-axis at the center of rotation divided by 4). This is unlike the single-slice counterpart, which provides a slice thickness of 8 mm with its 8 mm wide precollimator. In addition, the four slices are a result of the division of the total x-ray beam into multiple beams, depending on the number of arrays in the 2D detector system. These multiple beams are the result of the detector row collimation or the detector row aperture (Hu, 1999a).

Fig. 15-7 is a cross-section view of a multislice CT scanner beam from the x-ray tube to the detectors. D is the width of the x-ray beam collimator and is measured at the axis of rotation; N is the number of detector rows; and d represents the detector row collimation. Hu (1999a) explains that if the gaps between the adjacent detector rows are small and can be ignored, the detector row spacing is equal to the detector row collimation (d). The detector row collimation d and the x-ray beam collimation D, has the following relationship:

$$d \text{ (mm)} = D \text{ (mm)} / N$$

where N is the number of detector rows. In single-slice CT, the detector row collimation equals and is interchangeable with the x-ray beam collimation. "In multislice CT, the detector row collimation is only $1/N$ of the x-ray beam collimation." This makes it possible "to simultaneously achieve high volume coverage speed and high z axis resolution. In general, the larger the number *of* detector rows N, the better the volume coverage speed performance."

For example, if the x-ray prepatient collimation width (x-ray beam collimation) is 20 mm and

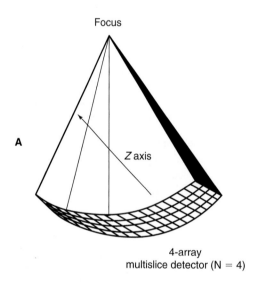

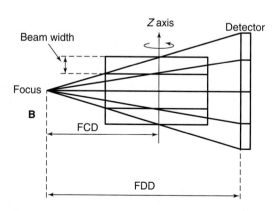

FIG. 15-6. Data acquisition geometry for multislice CT. **A,** The coordinate system. **B,** A cross-section *(side view).*

the scanner has a four-row detector array, the detector row collimation is as follows:

d (mm) = D (mm) / N

in which d is the detector row collimation, N is the number of detector rows, and D is the x-ray beam collimator width (20 / 4 = 5mm).

Alternatively,

d = 1 /N × x-ray beam collimator width
d = 1 /4 × 20
= 5 mm

As the beam width increases in the z direction to cover the number of rows in the 2D detector system, the amount of scattered radiation increases because a wide area of the patient is scanned. To minimize scattered radiation, antiscatter collimation may be used at the detector array (post collimation). One such scheme is shown in Fig. 15-8.

Beam Geometry. As the number of detector rows in a multirow detector array increases, the beam becomes wider to cover the 2D detector array (see Figs. 15-7 and 15-9). The beam must cover the length of the detector array. This coverage is influenced by the fan angle of the beam, in which a wider fan angle will cover a longer detector array. The beam must also cover the width of the detector array, which is defined by the number of rows in the detector array. A larger number of rows will result in a wider beam (large cone beam) in the z-axis direction.

A cone beam geometry produces more beam divergence along the z axis compared with fan-beam geometry. For this reason, increasing the number of detector rows in multislice CT creates a need for a different approach to the interpolation process (compared with single-slice spiral/helical interpolation) because the rays that contribute to the imaging process are more oblique. In addition,

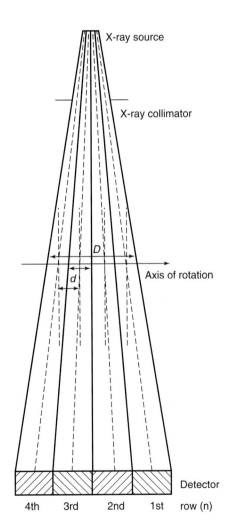

FIG. 15-7. A side view or cross-section of a multislice CT beam geometry from the x-ray tube to a four-row multislice detector array system.

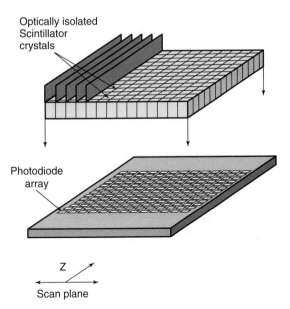

FIG. 15-8. A proposed scheme for the use of post collimation in multislice CT to reduce scattered radiation falling on a 2D detector array. The collimators are positioned between detector columns similar to conventional CT single-row detector arrays.

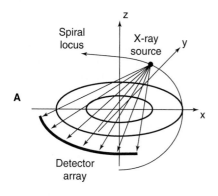

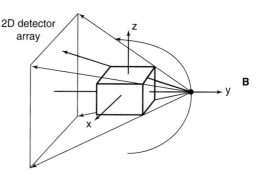

FIG. 15-9. **A,** The fan-beam geometry of single-row 1D detectors, in which the rays at the detector array are almost parallel and close together. **B,** The concept of cone-beam geometry typical of multi-row 2D detectors. The cone beam results in a wider divergence of rays at the detector array than the fan-beam geometry of single-row 1D detector.

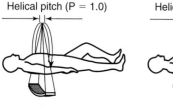

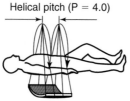

FIG. 15-10. A comparison of the pitch between single-slice and multislice CT data acquisition. In the multislice case, the pitch is increased by a factor of 4, which allows for increased volume coverage in less time without a loss of image quality.

the number of detector rows plays an important role in slice thickness selection and volume coverage.

Pitch. The pitch, P, for single-slice CT is defined as the ratio of the distance, L, the tabletop travels for one complete rotation of the x-ray tube to the x-ray beam collimation. This collimation defines the BW for a single-row detector array at the center of rotation (see Fig. 15-5). The thickness of the slice is determined by the BW at the center of rotation.

The definition of pitch is somewhat varied and controversial. For example, Hu (1999a) extends the single-slice pitch definition (Equation 15-1).

> multislice CT pitch = table movement per rotation/detector row collimation (or spacing)
>
> (15-1)

As noted by He (1999), "the key difference here is that multislice CT beam collimation is much wider than the smallest detector row used for data acquisition. In the 4-slice scanner case, for example, one scan mode is 4×2.5 mm, table speed is 7.5 mm/rotation, beam width is 10 mm. So if we used our definition, the pitch value would be 7.5 mm/2.5 mm = 3. However, one could also argue that the pitch should be 7.5 mm/10 mm = 0.75. There are good arguments for either definition here."

Taguchi and Aradate (1998) define the pitch, P, in a 4-slice scanner (four-row detector array) as:

$$P = L / BW \qquad (15\text{-}2)$$

where L is table speed per rotation and BW is the beam width in the z axis for a 1-row detector array, at the center of rotation (see Fig. 15-5). For a four-slice scanner, each slice is defined by BW (see Fig. 15-6). In this case, four slices are acquired at the same time, and the helical pitch is increased by a factor of four, compared with single-slice volume CT (Fig. 15-10).

In addition, Kalender (1997) defines pitch for a multislice CT scanner with a four-row detector array as "the table feed, d, per full rotation relative to the slice width, S, of a single detector row (rather than relative to the total detector width)." Mathematically, this can be expressed as shown in Equation 15-3:

$$Pitch = d/S \qquad (15\text{-}3)$$

Finally, Cinnamon (1998) explains the multislice pitch concept using the dual-slice volume CT scanner as a reference point. This scanner has a dual-detector system (two detectors used to collect data from the slice). In this case, a pitch of Dual-1 means that the table travels the same distance per rotation as the beam collimation. Therefore if the table travels 10 mm per rotation and the beam is 10 mm thick, the dual pitch is 1 (10/10), even though two 5 mm slices are obtained. He extends this notion to the multislice CT scanner by pointing out that "to arrive at the same 5 mm slices using the multislice scanner, one would use a beam collimation of 20 mm and a table speed of 20 mm per scan rotation, and the pitch in this case is quad-1." The term *quad* is used to refer to four-row detector array. Cinnamon also points out that for multislice CT, the beam collimation does not equal the slice thickness.

Although pitch for single-slice volume CT is defined in terms of the table speed per rotation, the definition of pitch for multislice CT is varied and is based on the table speed per rotation and either the slice thickness, the detector row collimation, or the beam width at the center of rotation, depending on the manufacturer. In time, perhaps there will be a stable definition of pitch in multislice CT.

Slice Thickness. In multislice CT, the slice thickness is determined by the BW (see Fig. 15-6), the pitch, and other factors such as the shape and width of the reconstruction filter in the z axis.

Image Reconstruction

In conventional step-and-shoot CT (conventional CT), a fan-beam geometry and a single-row detector array are used in the data acquisition process, and all rays pass through the image plane (planar section), the slice of interest. With this condition, a fan-bean reconstruction algorithm, specifically, the filtered back projection algorithm is used for image reconstruction.

Single-Slice CT. In single-slice spiral/helical CT (single-slice CT), the fan-beam geometry is maintained and a single-row detector array is used in the data acquisition process. In conventional CT the patient is stationary during scanning, whereas in single-slice CT, the patient is moving continuously through the gantry aperture during a 360-degree rotation of the x-ray tube and detectors. In this case, all rays do not pass through the image plane. A fan-beam geometry is used, so the fan-beam reconstruction algorithm used in conventional CT is used for image reconstruction. During data acquisition, the fan-beam traces a spiral/helical path around the patient as shown in Fig. 15-11. Because

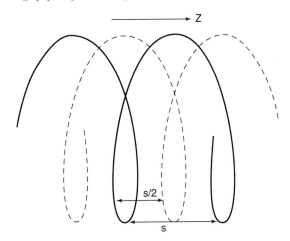

FIG. 15-11. The spiral/helical trace of a single-row detector array in single-slice volume CT. The distance of the data points used for 360-degree LI and 180-degree LI are *s* and *s/2*, respectively.

all rays do not pass through the image plane (planar section), single-slice spiral/helical CT requires an additional step of first calculating a planar section. This is done by interpolation, using data points on either side of the section.

The first interpolation algorithm used was 360-degree linear interpolation (360 degrees LI), in which the distance between the two data points used in the interpolation was represented by *s* in Fig. 15-11. In an effort to improve the image quality resulting from the 360-degree LI, a 180-degree LI was developed, using data points that are now closer to the image plane. The distance between the two points used for interpolation is now *s/2*. This equation involves calculation of a complimentary data set (*dashed lines*) using the direct fan-beam data set or measurements (*solid lines*). The distance between the two points used for interpolation is referred to as the *z-gap* (Hu, 1999a). The z-gap affects image quality such that, the smaller the z-gap, the better the image quality. In single-slice spiral/helical CT, increased volume coverage can be achieved with increased pitch; however, as the pitch increases image quality decreases because the z-gap becomes larger. This is one motivating factor for the development of multislice CT.

Multislice CT. One of the most conspicuous differences between single-slice CT and multislice CT is that the latter uses a new detector technology, in which the number of detector rows can vary from 4 to 34 (at the time of publication). These multiple detector rows result in a large 2D detector array. Because of this, a cone-beam geometry results instead of the fan-beam geometry characteristic of single-slice CT systems. Cone-beam geometry produces an increase in the beam divergence, which now poses a fundamental problem because all the rays do not pass through the image plane. Rays at the periphery of the beam lie outside the image plane. Approximate cone-beam reconstruction algorithms have been developed for solving this problem (Wang et al, 1997; Kudo and Saito, 1991); however, these particular algorithms demand extensive calculations (compared with fan-beam algorithms) and are not suitable for use in medical imaging.

Special fan-beam reconstructions (Hu, 1999a; Taguchi and Aradate, 1998) have been developed for multislice CT in its present state. In deriving an algorithm for image reconstruction in multislice CT, a logical first step is to extend the principles of 360-degree LI and 180-degree LI used in single-slice CT to multislice CT. To examine this extension, consider Fig. 15-12, which shows the spiral/helical path of a four-row detector array used in multislice CT. For a 360-degree LI, the distance between the two points used for interpolation of a planar section is *s*, the same distance as in

Fig. 15-11 for single-slice CT. With a 180-degree LI, the distance of the data points is *s/2* (distance between the solid and dashed lines of the same detector row). The *z*-gap is the same as in single-slice CT.

In multislice CT, the *z*-gap is determined by the pitch (as in single-slice CT) and by the detector row spacing, *d*. "As the helical pitch varies, distinctively different *z* sampling patterns and therefore interlacing helix patterns may result in multislice helical CT" (Hu, 1999a). This is illustrated in Fig. 15-13 for a four-row detector array with for two different pitches. At a pitch of 2:1 (Fig. 15-13, A), the distance between the points used for interpolation, the *z*-gap, is *d*, "which is the same as the displacement from one solid helix to the next. This causes a high degree of overlap between different helices, generating highly redundant projection measurements at certain *z*-positions. Because of this high degree of redundancy (or inefficiency) in *z*-sampling, the overall *z*-sampling spacing (i.e., the *z*-gap of the interlacing helix pattern) is still d, not any better than its single-slice counterpart" (Hu, 1999a).

Increased pitch in multislice CT from 2:1 to 3:1 (Fig.15-13, B) results in a *z*-gap of *d/2*, a much

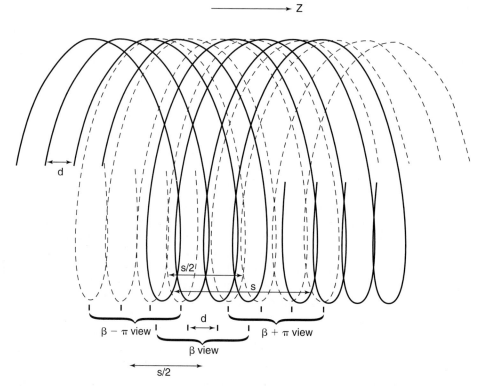

FIG. 15-12.   The spiral/helical trace of a four-row detector array in multislice CT. See text for further explanation.

shorter distance. In this case the volume coverage speed can be increased. In addition because the z-gap is less as the pitch increases, better image quality results. Hu (1999a) points out that "the volume coverage speed performance of the multi-slice scanner is substantially better than its single-slice counterpart, and so the selection of helical pitches is very critical to its performance. The pitch selection is determined by the consideration of the z-sampling efficiency and conventional factors such as volume coverage speed, (which disfavors very low helical pitch); slice profile; and image artifacts, which disfavor very high helical pitch." The preferred helical pitches are those that represent the preferred tradeoffs for various applications.

Alternatively, Figs. 14-12, 14-13, and 14-14 can be used to explain the problem and solution described above. The unwound helical path for single-slice CT is shown in Fig. 14-12 for both direct and complimentary data. The image plane is interpolated using two points from the direct data and the complimentary data on either side of it (image plane). Extending the single-slice concept to the multislice case as shown in Fig. 14-13 results in a superimposition of the complimentary and direct data for each of the detector rows in the four-row array. Note also that the z-gap is larger and this results in image degradation. Additionally, the superimposition does not allow for efficient z-sampling. A pitch of 4 is not preferable as a pitch of 2 because of the redundancy in the data sampling.

Fig. 14-14 provides a solution to the problem imposed by Fig. 14-13. By separating the direct and complimentary data trails, efficient z-sampling can be achieved (Saito, 1998). Taguchi and Aradate (1998) referred to this as *optimized sampling scan.* Fig. 14-14 is with a pitch of 3.5 less than that of Fig. 14-13 (pitch of 4). These figures indicate that a slight compromise in helical pitch (just 0.5) produces amazing improvement in the data sampling pattern.

The detector design for multislice CT allows the operator to select variable slice thicknesses based on the requirements of the examination. The new algorithms for multislice CT also allow for the reconstruction of these variable slice thicknesses. These new algorithms address problems (image quality degradation) arising from the increase in speed (hence volume coverage) of the patient moving through the gantry aperture when the pitch is increased. Additionally, these algorithms provide for the selection of the slice thicknesses that meet the needs of the examination.

Two such algorithms were developed by Taguchi and Aradate (1998) and by Hu (1999a). These algorithms are almost identical (including the algorithm developed by Siemens Medical Systems) and are based on the same philosophy (Hu, 1999b; Taguchi, 1999).

In general, these algorithms are based on the following steps:

1. *Spiral/helical scanning by interlaced sampling.* In this step, smaller z-gaps are obtained by adjusting or selecting the pitch to separate out the complementary data from the direct data.

2. *Longitudinal interpolation by z-filtering.* This is a method of a filtering process in the longitudinal (z) direction. Assuming some range with a width called the *filter width* (FW) in the longitudinal (z) direction (see Fig. 14-15), all data sampled within that range are processed by weighted summation. The filter parameters (e.g., filter width and shape) can control the spatial resolution in the longitudinal direction, the image noise, and the image quality. Because (2) can be applied to single-slice CT, the unique feature in multislice CT is (1). Again, pitch selection is flexible and should be carefully selected.

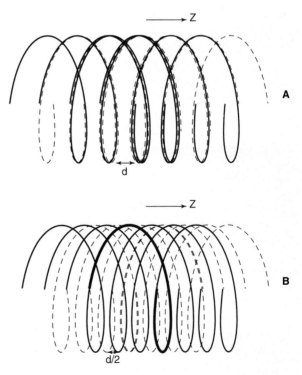

FIG. 15-13. Spiral/helical traces for a four-row detector array in multislice CT at a pitch of 2:1 (**A**) and a pitch of 3:1 (**B**).

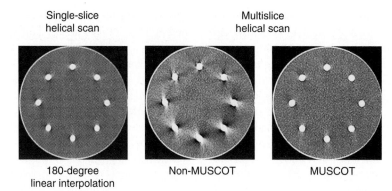

Single-slice helical scan   Multislice helical scan

180-degree linear interpolation   Non-MUSCOT   MUSCOT

FIG. 15-14. The difference in image quality of a ball phantom obtained with a 180-degree LI algorithm (single-slice CT) and with and without the MUSCOT algorithm used for multislice CT imaging. (From Saito Y: Multislice x-ray CT scanner, *Med Rev,* 66:1-8, 1998.)

3. *Fan-beam reconstruction.* This algorithm can be used if the number of detector rows is small. Hu (1999) uses multiple parallel fan-beams to approximate the cone-beam geometry characteristic of multislice CT. The algorithm used by Taguchi and Aradate (1998) is also based on a fan-beam method. Additionally, Saito (1998) labels the algorithm multislice cone-beam tomography reconstruction method (MUSCOT). The effect of MUSCOT on image quality is shown in Fig. 15-14. Compared with single-slice CT (180-degree LI), MUSCOT provides good image quality "at a scanning speed that is about three times faster than that for single-slice CT" (Taguchi and Aradate, 1998).

INSTRUMENTATION

In describing the instrumentation for multislice CT systems, it is essential to focus on the major components responsible for data acquisition, image reconstruction, image display and manipulation, image processing, image storage, and recording.

The flow of data in multislice CT parallels that of conventional step-and-shoot CT and includes x-ray production and transmission through the patient and conversion of x-rays into electrical signals, which are subsequently converted into digital data for processing by a digital computer. Digital data in the computer are then converted into image data through image reconstruction, to be displayed on a monitor for viewing by an observer. However, the detector technology in multislice

CT is one of the most significant developments in the evolution of CT. Other components of significance are the data acquisition system (DAS) and the image reconstruction system for multislice CT scanning.

The major equipment components for multislice CT are the data acquisition components, patient couch or table, the computer system, and the operator console as shown in Fig. 15-15. Detailed specifications for three multislice CT scanners (Toshiba's Acquilion CT Scanner, Picker's Mx 8000 CT Scanner, and Picker's MxTwin, dual-slice CT Scanner) are provided in Appendix B.

Data Acquisition Components

The multislice CT gantry houses the x-ray generator, the x-ray tube, and detectors, as well as the detector electronics (DAS). Almost all multislice CT scanners are based on the third-generation system design, in which the x-ray tube and detectors are coupled and rotate continuously during continuous patient translation through the gantry aperture. Such data collection strategy is possible by the use of slip-ring technology (Fig. 15-16).

X-Ray Generator. The x-ray generator is a compact, lightweight, high-frequency generator that provides a stable high voltage to the x-ray tube to ensure efficient production of x-rays. The power output of these generators is around 60 kW.

X-Ray Tube. The x-ray tube is a rotating-anode tube capable of high heat storage capacity with high anode and tube housing cooling rates.

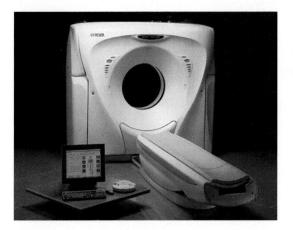

FIG. 15-15. The major equipment components (gantry, patient couch, and computer and operator's console) of a multislice CT scanner. (Courtesy Picker International; Cleveland, Ohio.)

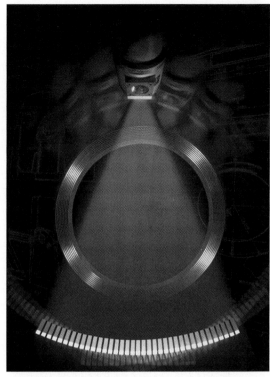

FIG. 15-16. Multislice CT is based on slip-ring technology that facilitates high speed continuous rotation of the x-ray tube and detectors during data acquisition. (Courtesy Picker international; Cleveland, Ohio.).

The x-ray beam is usually fan-shaped and emanates from either a small or large focal spot. X-ray tubes for multislice CT provide for a range of selectable kVp and mAs, such as 80, 100, 120, and 135 kVp and 10 mA to 500 mA in increments of 10 mA. For more specific specifications data on the generator and x-ray tube, refer to Appendix B.

Multislice Detectors. As noted earlier in this chapter, the most significant difference between single-slice CT and multislice CT is the detector technology (Fig. 15-17). These detectors are solid-state scintillation detectors (Fig. 15-18). The design of the multirow detector influences the speed of acquisition of the slices and the thickness of the slices. For example, the number of slices for multislice CT scanners from Toshiba, General Electric, Siemens, and Picker is 4, but the number of detector rows varies from 34, 16, 8, and 8, respectively (at the time of publication). Additionally, the range of the slice thicknesses possible with these scanners is presented in Table 15-1.

The selection of various slice thicknesses is shown in Figs. 15-19, 15-20, and 15-21. Fig. 15-19 compares the slice thickness selection of a single-slice detector array with a multislice multirow detector array. Figs. 15-20 and 15-21 illustrate how the slice thickness is selected for variable area detector arrays. These detectors consist of segments of varying sizes (eight in the case of Fig. 15-20),

TABLE 15-1

*Selectable Slice Thickness for Four Multislice CT Scanners**

SCANNER	SLICE THICKNESS AVAILABLE	
Toshiba	4 × 0.8 mm	4 × 3.0 mm
Acquilion	4 × 1.0 mm	4 × 5.0 mm
	4 × 2.0 mm	4 × 7.0 mm
		4 × 10.0 mm
Picker	4 × 0.5 mm	4 × 5.0 mm
Mx8000	4 × 1.0 mm	4 × 8.0 mm
	4 × 2.5 mm	4 × 10.0 mm
General	4 × 1.25 mm	4 × 5.0 mm
Electric	4 × 2.5 mm	
LightSpeed	4 × 3.75 mm	
Siemens	2 × 0.5 mm	
SOMATOM	4 × 1.0 mm	
M Plus 4	4 × 5.0 mm	

*From manufacturers' specifications.

where each segment or portion of a segment can be turned on or off to provide the appropriate slice thickness.

Data Acquisition System. Another major component of the gantry is the data acquisition system (DAS), the detector electronics responsible mainly for digitizing the signals from the detectors before they are sent to the computer for processing. Fig. 15-21 shows an example of the DAS is coupled to the multirow detector array via switches. In this case, four slices are acquired at the same time because of the presence of four DAS systems (four

times the electrical circuits compared with single-slice CT systems) (Saito, 1998). Regardless of which four slices are required for the examination, the switches can be turned on and off to ensure that the appropriate detector segments are exposed to x-rays.

Patient Table

The patient table, or couch, is shown in Fig. 15-22. The table features are essentially similar to those associated with single-slice CT and conventional step-and-shoot CT scanners. The purpose of the

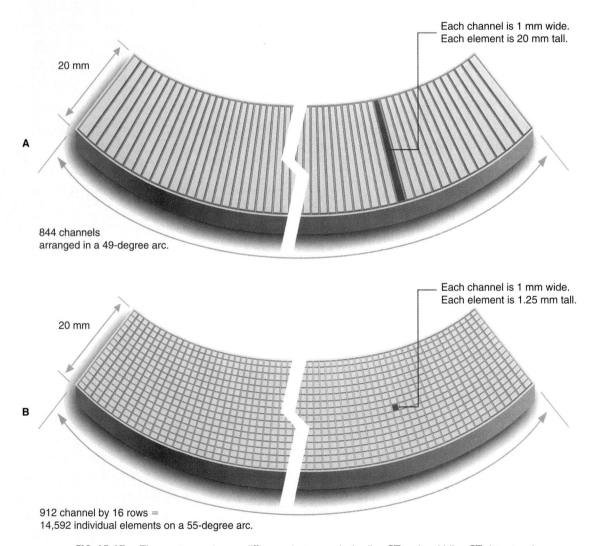

FIG. 15-17. The most conspicuous difference between single-slice CT and multislice CT detectors is the multiple row design approach. Whereas single-slice CT detectors are based on a single-row detector array, multislice CT uses multiple-row detector array, with each row consisting of individual elements. The detectors shown here are from two General Electric CT scanners; the single-slice CT scanner (**A**) and the multislice CT scanner (**B**). (Courtesy General Electric Medical Systems, Milwaukee, Wis.)

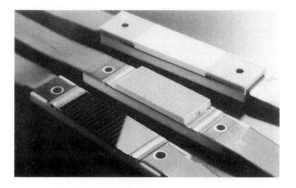

FIG. 15-18. Examples of solid-state multirow matrix detector arrays for multislice CT scanning. These detectors are used in the General Electric LightSpeed QX/I CT scanner, and consist of 16 rows with 912 channels and 14,592 individual elements. (Courtesy General Electric Medical Systems; Milwaukee, Wis.)

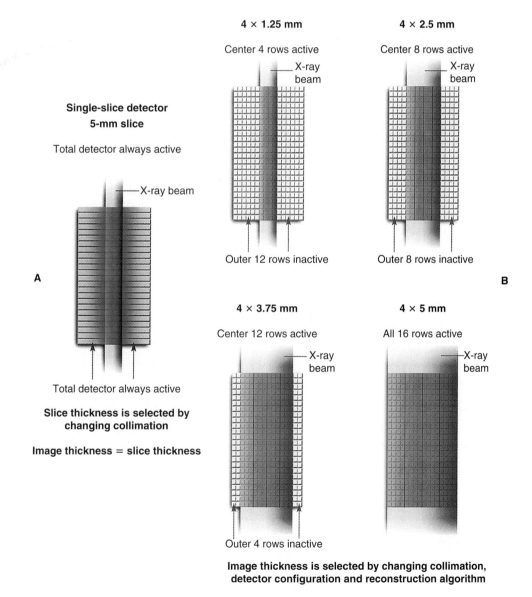

FIG. 15-19. A comparison of slice thickness selection for a single-slice CT detector array (**A**), and a multislice CT matrix detector array (**B**). (Courtesy General Electric Medical Systems; Milwaukee, Wis.)

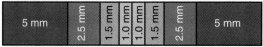

Maximum volume coverage per rotation: 20 mm

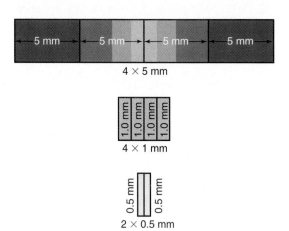

FIG. 15-20. A variable area detector consisting of 8 segments, each of which can be activated to provide the slice thickness appropriate to the needs of the examination. Siemens refers to this detector design as the Adaptive Array Detector. (Courtesy Siemens Medical Systems; Iselin, NJ.)

table is to support the patient and facilitate multislice CT scanning through the variable speed of travel of the tabletop and its wide range of movement. The table can be raised and lowered to accommodate positioning of the patient in the gantry aperture and to facilitate easy transfer of the patient from the scanner to a bed or gurney and vice versa. Movement of the tabletop in the longitudinal direction also facilitates patient position in the gantry aperture, with variable scanable ranges.

Patient tables for CT are equipped with a head holder or headrest (see Fig. 15-22) to ensure patient comfort during the examination. In an emergency during the examination, the movement of the table can be controlled manually to ensure patient safety.

Computer System

The computer system for multislice CT receives data from the data acquisition system and the operator, who inputs patient data and various examination protocols. These systems must be capable of handling vast amounts of data collected by the 2D multirow detector array. These computers have hardware architectures that provide high-speed

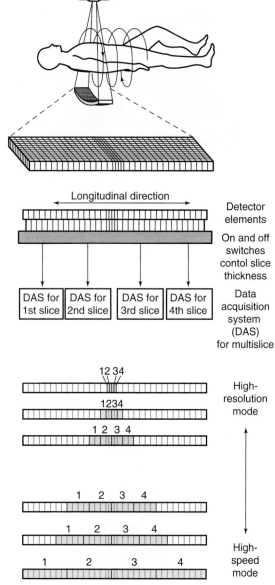

FIG. 15-21. The multirow detector allows for various selections of slice thicknesses to meet the needs of the examination. Thinner slice thicknesses are selected in the high resolution mode, whereas thicker slices are selected in the high speed mode. The slice thickness is varied by turning the switches "on" or "off."

preprocessing, image reconstruction, and post processing operations. Although preprocessing includes various corrections to the raw data, *image reconstruction* refers to the use of multislice reconstruction algorithms for image build-up. On the other hand, postprocessing involves the use of a wide range of image processing and advanced visu-

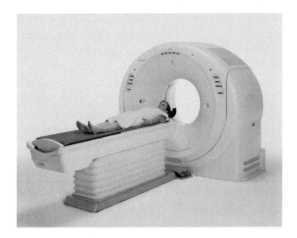

FIG. 15-22. The patient table and gantry for a multislice CT scanner. (Courtesy Toshiba America Medical Systems; Tustin, Calif.)

alization software, such as the generation of 3D and MPR, as well as virtual endoscopic images from the axial data set stored in the computer.

The results of computer processing are displayed for viewing by an observer on a monitor. Several characteristics of the monitor are important to the observer, such as the display matrix, bandwidth, display memory, and the gray level and color resolution.

Data storage devices for holding the raw data and image data include hard disks, usually of the Winchester type with high storage capacities; 3.5-inch microdiskettes, which can typically store 7-512 × 512 images; and erasable optical disks of the magneto-optical type. Typical image storage capacities are provided in Appendix B for two multislice CT scanners.

Operator Console

The operator console allows the operator to interact with the scanner before, during, and after the examination. Two consoles for multislice CT are shown in Fig. 15-23. Essentially the major components include the keyboard, mouse, monitor, and other controls for the execution of specialized functions.

The operator console controls the entire CT scanner system and facilitates the selection of scan parameters and scan control (automatic or manual); image storage, communication, image reconstruction, image processing, windowing, and control of the gantry and x-ray tube rotation.

The console allows for communication of images to other parts of the department and hospital

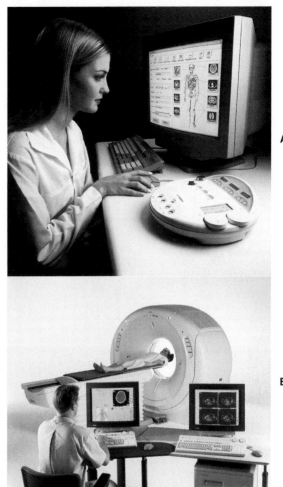

FIG. 15-23. Two operator consoles for multislice CT. (**A,** Courtesy Picker International; Cleveland, Ohio. **B,** Courtesy Toshiba America Medical Systems; Tustin, Calif.)

and other remote sites, through the use of local and wide area networks. The multislice CT console also supports full digital imaging and communication in medicine (DICOM) connectivity to other equipment, such as network printers, for example. Multislice CT consoles also provide for the use of a wide range of software options for image processing, such as 3D imaging, virtual endoscopy, maximum intensity projection, MPR reconstruction, cardiac applications, dental CT and bone mineral analysis.

IMAGE QUALITY CONSIDERATIONS

Spatial resolution is to the ability of the scanner to image fine detail and is measured in line pairs/cm. Contrast resolution or low-contrast resolution or tissue resolution is the ability of the scanner to discriminate small differences in tissue contrast. Noise, on the other hand, is a fluctuation of CT numbers from point to point in the image for a scan of uniform material such as water. Noise degrades image quality and affects the perceptibility of detail. Artifacts can also degrade image quality and cause problems in image interpretation.

In multislice CT, these parameters are the same in terms of definition. Recall that the purpose of multislice CT is to improve on the performance of single-slice CT in terms of speed and coverage. The volume coverage speed performance in multislice CT is better than its counterpart single-slice CT without compromising image quality. The

specifications for spatial resolution, contrast resolution, and noise for three multislice CT scanners are listed in Appendix B.

As these scanners become commonplace, results of acceptance testing and other research studies will provide verification on image quality parameters and more information on the performance of multislice CT scanners in the image quality and radiation dose arenas.

ADVANTAGES OF MULTISLICE CT

The advantages of multislice CT have been outlined by Saito (1998) and Cinnamon (1998), as

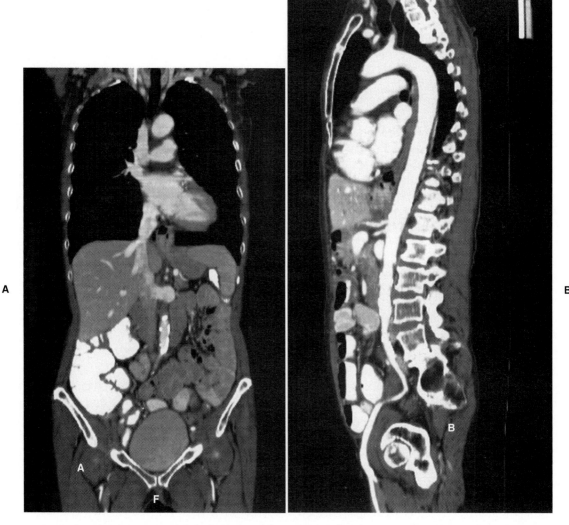

FIG. 15-24. The multislice CT scanner with its increase in pitch and rotation speed capabilities (increased volume coverage speed performance) provides larger volumes of the patient to be scanned in shorter times compared with single-slice CT scanners, with comparable image quality. (Courtesy Picker International; Cleveland, Ohio.)

well as others such as Dr. Westerman, in Chapter 14. Essentially, these advantages include the following:

1. Increase in speed and volume coverage. In multislice CT, the increase in pitch and the increase in rotation speed of the x-ray tube and detectors allow for a larger volume of the patient to be scanned in less time (Fig. 15-24). Hu (1999a), for example, showed that a 4-slice helical/spiral CT scanner is about two times faster than a single-slice CT scanner, for comparable im-

age quality. A comparison of the scanning times for multislice CT and single-slice CT is given in Table 15-2.

2. Improved spatial resolution. Multislice CT images thin slices (Fig. 15-25) with better isotropic resolution. This is sometimes referred to as *isotropic imaging*, in which case, all the sides (axial, vertical, and horizontal) of the voxels in the slice have equal dimensions (Fig. 15-26) compared with single-slice CT. This advantage provides improved MPR (see Fig. 15-24) and 3D images with

TABLE 15-2

Scanning Times for Multislice CT and Single-Slice CT

	SCAN AREA (mm)	RESOLUTION: SLICE THICKNESS (mm)	SCAN TIME (sec) MULTISLICE	SCAN TIME (sec) SINGLE-SLICE
Lung study	300	10	4	30
	300	3	15	100
Trauma case	1300	10	17	130
CTA	40	1	5	40

From Saito Y: Multislice x-ray CT scanner, *Med Rev* 66:1-8, 1998.

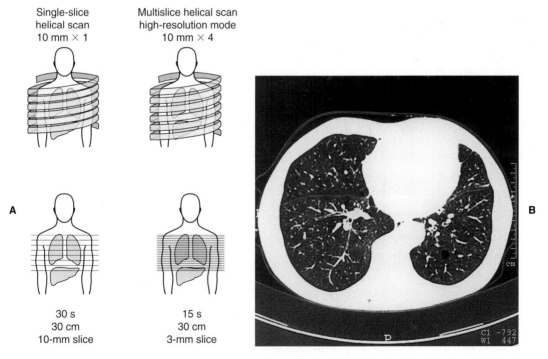

FIG. 15-25. Compared with single-slice CT scanners, multislice CT scanners offer imaging of thinner slices in less time for the same volume scanned (**A**) with excellent resolution (**B**). (*A*, From Saito Y: Multislice X-ray CT scanner, *Med Rev* 66:1-8, 1998. *B*, Courtesy Picker International, Cleveland, Ohio.)

reduced image artifacts. An example of an MIP image is shown in Fig. 15-27.

3. Efficient use of the x-ray beam. In multislice CT, the x-ray beam width has to be opened to fall on the 2D detector array, compared

with a single-row detector array characteristic of single-slice CT scanners. The entire beam is thus used to acquire four slices (images) per 360-degree rotation with-out wasting any portion of the x-ray beam, as opposed to one slice per 360-degree rotation in the single-slice CT case, in which a portion of the x-ray beam is wasted during data acquisition. Such use of the beam increases the life of the x-ray tube. The tube can now be used to produce a large number of thin slices without having to wait for it (x-ray tube) to cool, a problem with single-slice CT systems. Kopecky et al (1999) notes

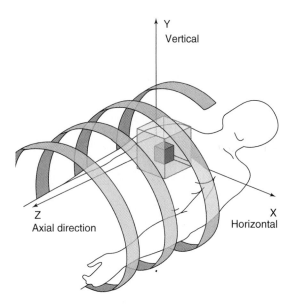

FIG. 15-26. Multislice CT can image thin slices with better isotropic resolution. This means that all sides (axial, vertical, and horizontal) of the voxel have equal dimensions compared with single-slice CT. (Courtesy Toshiba America Medical Systems; Tustin, Calif.)

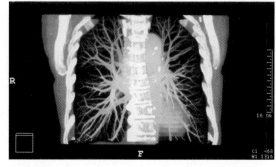

FIG. 15-27. An MIP image from a multislice CT scanner. Multislice CT provides improved 3D images, including MIP images, which enhance visualization of airways and vascular structures, with reduced image artifacts. (Courtesy Picker International; Cleveland, Ohio.)

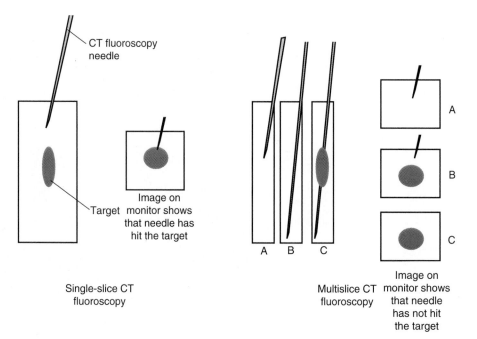

FIG. 15-28. A comparison of the accuracy of needle placement in CT fluoroscopy from single-slice CT and multislice CT systems.

that an x-ray tube with a lifespan of 200,000 secs, a single-slice CT scanner will provide about 200,000 image (one image/sec) compared with 800,000 images for a four-slice multislice CT scanner (same conditions are maintained), "or 1.6 million images if the gantry spins at two revolutions per second, or 3.2 million images if two images are created for each full rotation of 0.5 secs."

4. Reduction of radiation exposure. The development of new reconstruction methods allows for the reduction of patient dose "because more data in the longitudinal direction are utilized for image reconstruction" (Saito, 1998). This results in a decrease in exposure by about 40% for the same image quality as single-slice CT (Saito, 1998).

5. Improved accuracy in needle placement in CT fluoroscopy. One of the problems with needle placement under CT fluoroscopic control using a single-slice CT scanner is illustrated in Fig. 15-28. The image shows that the needle has hit the target, which is simply not the case. This problem is solved with multislice CT fluoroscopy because multiple images are obtained. It is apparent in Fig. 15-28 that the target has been missed.

REFERENCES

Beck T: CT technology overview: state of the art and future directions, *RSNA Categorical Course in Physics* 1996, pp 161-172.

Berland LL, Smith K: Multidetector-array CT: once again technology creates new opportunities, *Radiology* 209: 327, 1998.

Cinnamon J: Multislice volumetric spiral CT: principles and applications, Massoz, 1998, Belgium.

He HD: General Electric medical systems, *Personal Communications* 1999.

Hu H: Multislice helical CT: Scan and reconstruction, *Med Physics* 26:5-18, 1999a.

Hu H: *Personal communications*, 1999b.

Kalender W et al: Spiral CT: Medical uses and potential industrial applications. In Bonse, U, editor: *Developments in x-ray tomography*, Society of Photooptical Instrumentation Engineers, 3149:188-202, 1997.

Kopecky K et al: Multislice CT spirals past single-slice in diagnostic efficacy, *Diagnostic Imaging* April, 36-42, 1999.

Kudo H, Saito T: Helical-scan computed tomography using cone-beam projections, *IEEE Conf. Record 1991 Nuclear Science Symposium and Medical Imaging Conference*, Santa Fe, NM, 1958-1962, 1991.

Liang Y, Kruger RA: Dual-slice spiral versus single-slice spiral scanning: comparison of the physical performance of two computed tomography scanners, *Med Physics* 23:205-217, 1996.

Saito Y: Multislice X-ray CT scanner, *Med Rev* 66:1-8, 1998.

Taguchi K: *Personal communications*, 1999.

Taguchi K, Aradate H: Algorithm for image reconstruction in multislice helical CT, *Medical Physics* 25:550-561, 1998.

Wang G et al: Spiral CT: Current status and future directions. In Bonse U, editor: *Developments in x-ray tomography*, SPIE, 3149:203-21, 1997.

16

Continuous Imaging: Real-Time Computed Tomography Fluoroscopy

The basis for continuous CT imaging or real-time CT fluoroscopy depends on slip-ring technology, high-speed processing of the data collected from the patient and a fast-processing algorithm for image reconstruction. This chapter describes imaging principles, equipment components, and performance considerations, such as image quality and radiation dose and concludes with a brief outline of the application areas of CT fluoroscopy.

CONVENTIONAL CT AS AN INTERVENTIONAL GUIDANCE TOOL
Limitations

Conventional slice-by-slice CT has been used as a clinical tool for guidance in nonvascular interventional radiologic procedures, such as percutaneous interventions as biopsies and drainage, together with other techniques (e.g., ultrasound, conventional fluoroscopy, and magnetic resonance imaging). A problem with conventional CT-guided interventional procedure, compared with ultrasound and fluoroscopy, is the lack of real-time display of images, resulting from a time lag between data collection and image reconstruction. Such image display is especially important during needle puncture of the patient. Conventional CT-guided intervention is also limited in imaging body regions where movement is present, such as the respiratory system and the upper abdominal region. The movement associated with these body regions is responsible for shifting and disappearance of lesions of interest, making localization almost impossible (Froelich et al, 1997; Daly and Templeton, 1999). This results in an unsuccessful examination that must often be repeated (Katada et al, 1996).

This limitation of conventional CT-guided interventional technique has been overcome by the development of new techniques. These allow current CT scanners to reconstruct and display images in real-time with frame rates that can vary from two to eight frames per second, depending on the scanner.

HISTORY

In 1993 Dr. K. Katada of the Fujita Health University, School of Health Sciences, in Japan initiated the idea for real-time imaging using a CT scanner. Dr. Katada subsequently approached Toshiba CT Systems Design Group with a proposal for decreasing the image reconstruction time, the image matrix size, the number of views and the field-of-view (Katada, 1996). This resulted in a modification of one of Toshiba's CT scanners to provide images at a rate of three per second with a time delay of 0.83 second. Having conducted preliminary experiments and clinical trials, Katada and colleagues reported their early clinical experience with real-time CT fluoroscopy at the RSNA in 1994. The first CT scanner capable of real-time imaging was introduced in North America in 1994.

In 1996 the U.S. Food and Drug Administration approved real-time CT fluoroscopy as a useful clinical tool (Daly and Templeton, 1999). Today, several CT scanner manufacturers offer scanners capable of performing real-time CT fluoroscopy, including Toshiba Medical Systems, Picker International, Siemens Medical Systems, and General Electric Medical Systems.

The evolution of CT fluoroscopy has now made it possible to acquire dynamic CT images in real-time (Fig. 16-1), analogous to dynamic images produced in conventional fluoroscopy.

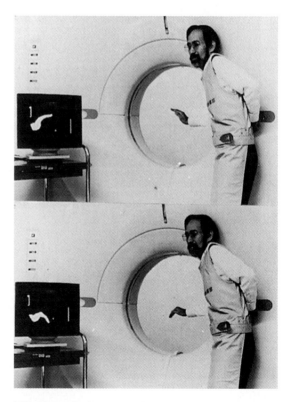

FIG. 16-1. Real-time CT fluoroscopy is capable of producing dynamic CT images. Images of the hand in both flexion and extension are displayed in real-time. (From Katada K: Further innovations in CT technology: CT fluoroscopy and real-time helical scan CT, *Med Rev* 53:1-11, 1995.)

IMAGING PRINCIPLES

The fundamental principles of real-time CT fluoroscopy are based on three advances in CT technology that have also led to other innovations in CT. The imaging principles involved in real-time CT fluoroscopy are illustrated in Fig. 16-2, which shows three steps based on the framework of Ozaki (1995):

1. Fast continuous scanning
2. Fast image reconstruction
3. Continuous image display

Fast Continuous Scanning

Fast continuous scanning was a major technologic development in CT, which resulted in spiral/helical scanning. Spiral/helical scanning is made possible by slip-ring technology (see Fig. 13-3), which allows for continuous rotation of the x-ray tube compared with the stop-and-go scanning characteristic of conventional CT systems, which resulted from cable wraparound. Continuous rotation of the x-ray tube speeds up data collection and allows data to be collected for one rotation (360 degrees) per second.

An important point to note during data acquisition in CT fluoroscopy is that the patient does not move during continuous rotation of the x-ray tube. The patient remains stationary. When data are collected after one rotation (360 degrees), the first image is displayed on the monitor for viewing. Subsequent images are displayed every time a data set has been collected for every 60-degree rotation. The data set for every 60-degree rotation is used to refresh the previous image, which is discarded as new 60-degree data sets are processed. This means that six images per second (360/60) can be displayed as shown in Fig. 16-2.

Fast Image Reconstruction

In real-time CT fluoroscopy, fast image reconstruction is made possible by a set of hardware components dedicated to provide fast computations, together with a new image reconstruction algorithm. An important point to note about CT fluoroscopy is that the interpolation algorithm used in spiral/helical CT scanning is not used. Recall that the purpose of this algorithm is to compute a planar section from which all other sections can be obtained by interpolation. This process removes artifacts resulting from the simultaneous movement of the patient through the gantry while the x-ray tube rotates continuously during data acquisition.

In CT fluoroscopy motion artifacts are therefore present on the image and appear as streaks; however, these artifacts do not restrict visualization of relevant structures. The dedicated hardware components include a fast arithmetic unit,

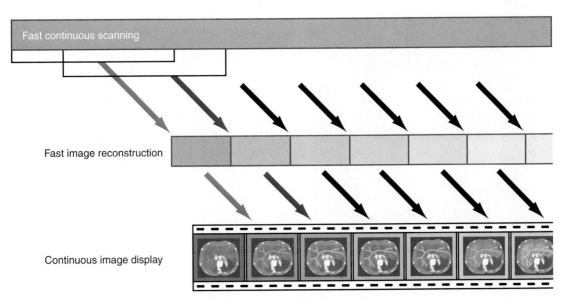

FIG. 16-2. The principles of real-time CT fluoroscopy are based on three steps: fast continuous scanning, fast image reconstruction, and continuous image display.

high-speed memory, and a back projection gate array. All of these components are housed in the image reconstruction unit. Parallel processing of the data is an integral element of real-time CT fluoroscopy.

The other key element of a real-time CT fluoroscopic imaging system is a new image reconstruction algorithm (Ozaki, 1995; Katada et al, 1996). This algorithm is described by Dr. Westerman in Chapter 14 (see Fig. 14-12). In summary, the fast image reconstruction algorithm for CT fluoroscopy processes six images per second (for a 1 second spiral/helical scanner) by first adding the next 60-degree data set acquired and subsequently

subtracting the previously acquired 60-degree data set from the image as the data set is acquired continuously (Fig. 16-3).

Continuous Image Display

As data are collected continuously, it is reconstructed using the fast reconstruction unit, on a matrix size of 256 × 256, and subsequently interpolated to 512 × 512 (Katada et al, 1996) or 1024 × 1024 (Froelich et al, 1997) matrix size to provide better resolution. Images are displayed on a monitor in the cine mode (dynamic display) at frame rates that can vary from two to eight images per second (Daly and Templeton, 1999).

EQUIPMENT COMPONENTS AND DATA FLOW

The basic equipment configuration of a CT fluoroscopic imaging system consists of a number of acquisition, image processing, image display, and recording components (Fig. 16-4).

The acquisition components include the scanner, which utilizes a third-generation spiral/helical data collection geometry with slip-ring technology for continuous data acquisition. The gantry aperture is about 72 cm with a variable field-of-view (18 to 40 cm is not uncommon). The scanner houses the x-ray generator, x-ray tube, detectors, and associated electronics. The x-ray generator is a high-frequency generator, and the x-ray tube is a high-capacity tube capable of producing about 7.0 million heat units (Daly and Templeton, 1999).

Once the raw data are acquired, it is sent to a preprocessor and then to the high-speed memory. The first 360-degree data set is processed using convolution and back projection and the reconstructed image is displayed on a monitor for viewing. Subsequent CT fluoroscopic data are acquired and processed using the real-time reconstruction unit (as described earlier). Using a display interface (I/F) images can be recorded with a video cassette recorder (VCR) and be displayed on a television monitor.

In Fig. 16-5, a scanner for CT fluoroscopy is shown together with an in-suite monitor and a special in-suite control console. This console allows the operator to have full control of the table movement through the gantry, to vary height of the tabletop, and to tilt the gantry during the interventional procedure.

Continuously
updated information

Last ⅙ of data removed

Newest ⅙ of raw data

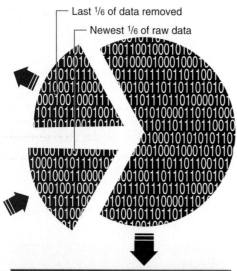

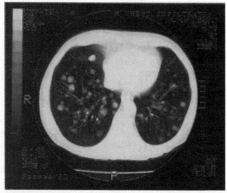

FIG. 16-3. A diagrammatic representation of fast image reconstruction and display of images in CT fluoroscopy. During continuous scanning of the patient, images are reconstructed and displayed every ⅙ second. (Courtesy Toshiba America Medical Systems; Tustin, Calif.)

X-RAY TECHNIQUE PARAMETERS

The x-ray exposure parameters can vary; however, tube currents of 30 to 50 mAs and tube voltages of 80 to 120 kVp are not uncommon (Daly and Templeton, 1999). Additionally, in the CT fluoroscopy mode, a special filter is introduced into the dose to the patient by about 50% (Toshiba's Aspire CT Fluoroscopy data, 1999).

Other technique parameters that must be considered in CT fluoroscopy are slice widths (collimator width), the FOV, and the maximum fluoroscopy time. Although a choice of slice widths ranging from 1, 2, 3, 5, 7, to 10 mm and FOV of 18, 24, 32 or 40 cm is available to the operator, the maximum fluoroscopy time for continuous imaging is 100 seconds (sec). This timer must be reset after 100 sec of fluoroscopy.

IMAGE QUALITY AND RADIATION DOSE CONSIDERATIONS

Measuring the parameters that affect image quality and radiation dose ascertains the performance of a CT scanner.

Image Quality

Image quality parameters in CT fluoroscopy include spatial resolution, density resolution, image noise, and artifacts. These parameters were examined by Ozaki (1995), who compared spatial resolution, density resolution, and image noise of CT fluoroscopy with that of conventional CT. His results are shown in Table 16-1 and demonstrate that the image quality parameters measured for CT fluoroscopy are comparable with that of conventional CT.

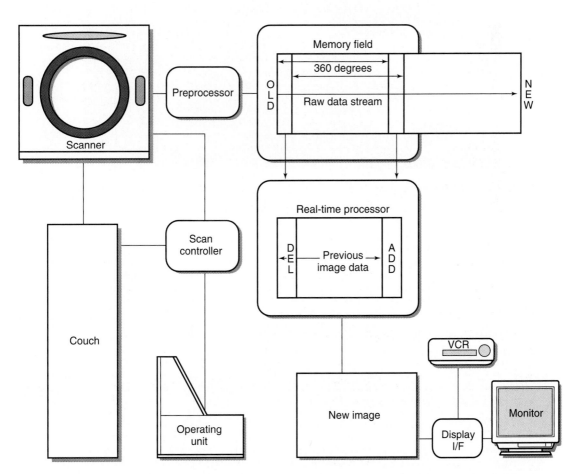

FIG. 16-4. The basic equipment configuration for CT fluoroscopy. See text for further explanation. (From Katada K et al: Guidance with real-time CT fluoroscopy: early clinical experience, *Radiology* 200:851-856, 1996.)

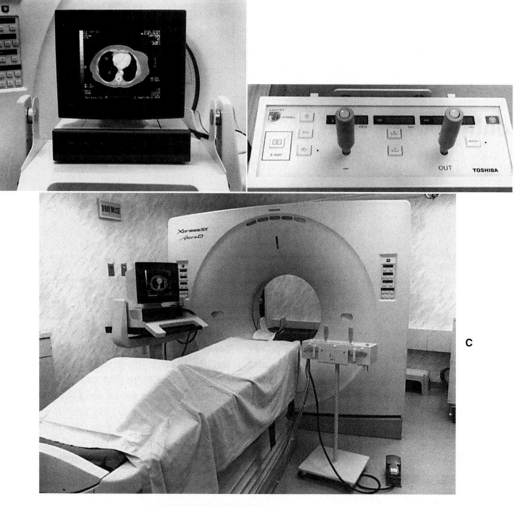

FIG. 16-5. **A,** The in-suite monitor. **B,** The in-suite control console. **C,** A CT scanner capable of CT fluoroscopy. (From Lackner DF, Patrizi JD: Continuous CT imaging, *Med Rev* 60:13-15, 1997.)

TABLE 16-1

A Comparison of Image Quality Parameters Between CT Fluoroscopy and Conventional CT

	CT FLUOROSCOPY	CONVENTIONAL CT
Spatial resolution	6.8 lp/cm	7.5 lp/cm
Density resolution	3 mm 0.45%	3 mm 0.41%
	50 mA	150 mA
Image noise	±3.9 HU	±3.5 HU
10-mm slice	50 mA	150 mA

From Ozaki M: Development of a real-time reconstruction system for CT fluoroscopy, *Med Rev* 53, 1995.
1-s scan, 120 kV, 240-mm FOV, 160-mm phantom

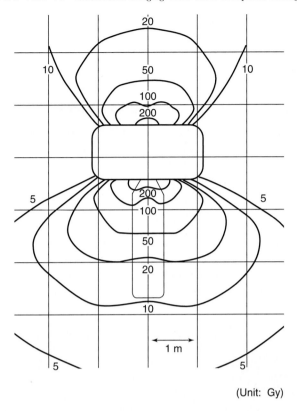

(Unit: Gy)

FIG. 16-6. Scatter radiation dose distribution at CT fluoroscopy.

Artifacts that are commonplace in CT fluoroscopy are those produced by metallic biopsy instruments. In this respect, Ozaki (1995) notes that "both the CT scanner and surgical instruments used in CT-guided procedures should be modified to minimize such artifacts."

Radiation Dose Considerations

The dose in CT fluoroscopy is also important because personnel are present in the room during the procedure. A number of factors influence the dose to the patient and operator in CT. One of the important factors is the length of the time of the exposure because dose is directly proportional to exposure time. Daly and Templeton (1999) report absorbed doses in the range of 3.53 rad (35.3 mGy) for 50 seconds exposure at 80 kVp and 30 mA to 19.81 rad (198.1 mGy) for a similar exposure time at 120 kVp and 50mA. See also Nawfel et al (2000) for more recent information.

During the development and early implementation of CT fluoroscopy, the dose to the hands of the operator was of particular concern because they were directly in the x-ray beam during the procedure. Early studies reported excessively high doses to the operator's hands during the procedure (Katada et al, 1996; Kato et al, 1996). The solution to this problem was the development of needle holders, which are intended to keep the hands of the operator out of the x-ray beam. An early study by Kato et al (1996) showed that the needle holders reduced the absorbed dose rate to the operator's hands. Additionally, the needle holders do not produce image artifacts. A later study by Daly et al (1997) confirmed such dose reduction as a result of using needle holders.

Another concern related to the dose in CT fluoroscopy procedures is that of scatter radiation distribution in the room during the procedure and the dose received by the operator resulting from this scatter. One example of the scattered radiation dose distribution is shown in Fig. 16-6. Using this example, Ozaki (1995) reported the following effective dose equivalent at various measurement positions:

(a) 18.3 mSv/hr at the eye level of the operator (about 93 cm from the scattering object).

(b) 26.4 mSv/hr at the hip level of the operator (about 70 cm from the scattering object)

Ozaki (1995) also reported that when a protective apron is worn during the procedure, the dose equivalent is reduced to 1.9 mSv/hr.

Reducing radiation dose to both patients and personnel is an important goal of radiology. In CT fluoroscopy, one technique that is incorporated in the design of the equipment to reduce the dose to the patient is the use of a special x-ray filter. This filter reduces the patient skin dose by about 50% (Ozaki, 1995; Daly and Templeton, 1999). Lower tube currents and shorter examination times also play a significant role in reducing patient exposures.

Operators standing in the CT room during the procedure must wear protective lead aprons, thyroid shields, and lead glasses or goggles. These protective apparel must be at least 0.5 mm lead equivalent. Additionally, the use of lead drapes in close proximity will result in a marked reduction of exposure to scattered radiation (Wagner, 2000; Nawfel, 2000).

TOOLS FOR USE IN CT-GUIDED INTERVENTIONAL PROCEDURES

A range of tools in addition to needle holders are currently available commercially for use in CT fluoroscopy. These tools are intended to optimize the procedure and assist the operator in improving the efficiency of the examination.

Digital Fluoroscopic CT System: FACTS

Some CT systems utilize conventional C-arm fluoroscopic systems to facilitate interventional CT procedures as shown in Fig. 16-7. Although these

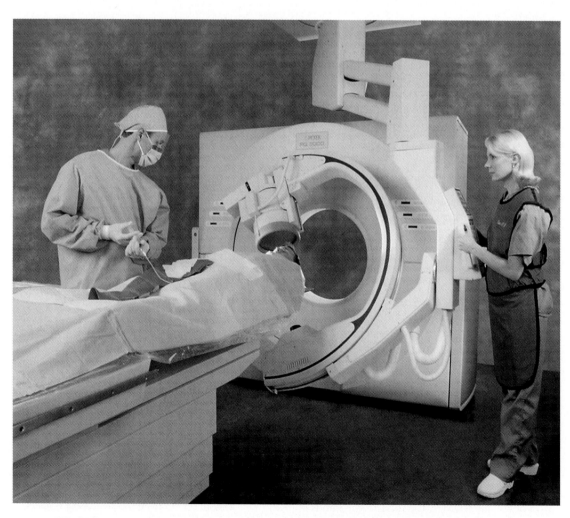

FIG. 16-7. The use of a conventional C-arm image intensifier system for CT interventional procedure. See text for further explanation. (Courtesy Picker International; Cleveland, Ohio.)

systems serve as a useful adjunct to the procedure, they are often difficult to position and use during the procedure because of their physical size. To solve this problem, one manufacturer has developed what they refer to as a fluoro-assisted CT system, FACTS (Picker International. Cleveland, Ohio).

The system shown in Fig. 16-8 consists of a c-arm unto which is mounted an x-ray tube and a flat-panel detector. The flat-panel detector, is a digital detector made of amorphous silicon, which provides uniform image quality across the surface of the detector. In addition the detector unit features an operating panel for controlling the C-arm and the CT scanner during the procedure. The flat panel detector can also be positioned easily to facilitate lateral views of the anatomy. See the box on p. 276.

The performance specifications for FACTS are listed in the box. FACTS can be used in procedures such as tumor biopsies, abscess drainage, bone intervention, and catheter placement for selective organ assessment (CT arterial portography).

Frameless Stereotactic Arm

This frameless stereotactic arm is a tool used in interventional CT under computer control to optimize procedures as follows:

> After the patient has been scanned, the radiologist simply moves the arm's pointer along the patient's skin; the associated computer updates 3D multiplanar reformation (MPR) views in realtime allowing the technologist to visualize the simulated needle path in relation to the target field as well as other critical structures. This allows the radiologist to plot the needle path that best avoids these critical structures and accurately acquires the target.

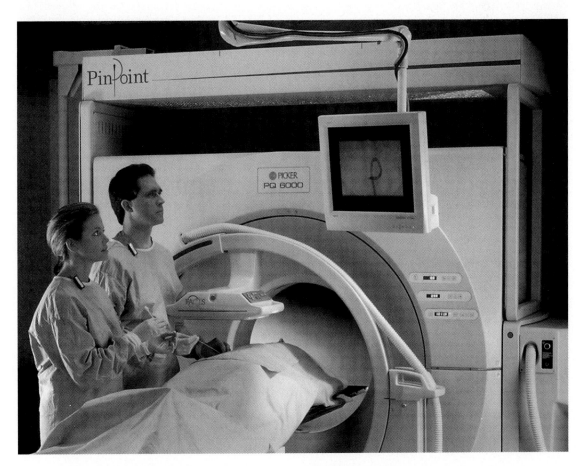

FIG. 16-8. FACTS, a digital fluoro-assisted CT system, with a flat-panel amorphous silicon detector, for use in CT interventional procedures. (Courtesy Picker International; Cleveland, Ohio.)

THE PERFORMANCE SPECIFICATIONS OF FACTS

MECHANICAL

Source-to-image distance: 38 in/96.5cm (fixed)
    C-arm orbit: ±90 degrees
    C-arm vertical travel: 11 in/27.9cm
    C-arm lateral travel: ±5 in/12.7cm
Max. patient clearance with 20 cm cone:
    16.8 in/42.7 cm
Max. patient clearance with 38 cm cone:
    9.8 in/24.9 cm

X-RAY MONO-BLOCK SYSTEM

kV range: 40kV to 125kV (continuously variable)
mA range: 0.1 mA to 4.0 mA x-ray

Tube type: Varian fixed anode
    Tube focal spot size: 0.5 mm square
    Tube heat storage: 75 kHU

FLAT PANEL DETECTOR

Matrix layout: 1536 × 1920
Active area: 195.1mm × 243.8mm (7.76 in × 9.6 in)
Frame rate: 30 frames/sec
Spatial resolution: 0.5 lppm at 75% MTF and
    2.0 lppm at 30% MTF

IMAGE PROCESSOR

Time to first image from an acquisition: <300 mS

Courtesy Picker International; Cleveland, Ohio.

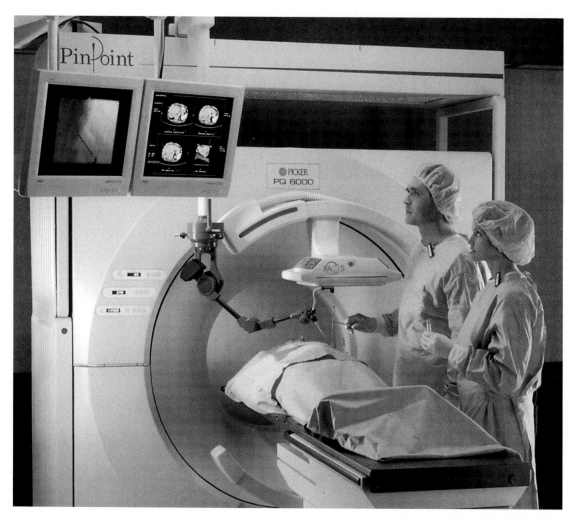

FIG. 16-9. The use of both FACTS and PinPoint in CT interventional procedures (Courtesy Picker International; Cleveland, Ohio.)

When the radiologist inserts the needle, its advancement is imaged via the CT scanner and viewed on a monitor located in the CT scan room. This means the needle's advancement can be controlled and viewed from insertion to penetration of the pathology, without leaving the patient's side. Complications are decreased and time on the table is kept to a minimum for the patient comfort, safety and throughput (Picker International 1999).

This arm is labeled *PinPoint* by Picker International. It features an articulated arm and a flat-panel monitor, both of which are mounted onto the CT gantry. Fig. 16-9 shows the use of both the frameless stereotactic arm (PinPoint) and the fluoro-assisted CT system (FACTS). The performance specifications of PinPoint are listed in the box below.

Combined Applications to Reduce Exposure (CARE)

CARE is a CT fluoroscopy system (Fig. 16-10) that consists of both hardware and software designed to provide real-time image reconstruction and display of CT fluoroscopic images at varying frame rates. The imaging system features a spiral/helical scanner using fan-beam geometry for data collection, coupled to a high-speed array processor to speed up image reconstruction of images that can be displayed on a monitor. The matrix size for image reconstruction is 256×256, the matrix size for image display is 1024×1024. Additional features of CARE are listed in the box on p. 278.

CARE can be used in many clinical applications, including drainage of cysts, abscesses, lymphoceles, hematomas, biopsy, pain therapy (injection of a drug into the spinal disk, for example, to relieve pain), CT arthrography, dynamic motion studies of the knee and elbow, and swallowing studies.

CLINICAL APPLICATIONS

As the technology for CT fluoroscopy matures, its applications in the clinical arena will likely continue to grow. Currently, the clinical application of CT fluoroscopy is widespread in a number of anatomic regions. (See Daly and Templeton [1999] for a discussion of clinical applications.) In addition, Daly and Templeton (1999) indicate that future improvements in CT fluoroscopy will be in the development of more sensitive digital detectors (to improve image quality and to reduce dose to the patient); higher image reconstruction frame rates (greater than eight frames/second); virtual reality imaging to improve visualization; and better biopsy or access needles.

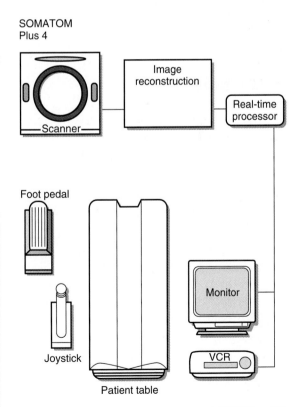

FIG. 16-10. The major components of CARE®, a CT fluoroscopy system.

THE PERFORMANCE SPECIFICATIONS OF PINPOINT™, A FRAMELESS STEREOTACTIC ARM FOR CT INTERVENTIONAL PROCEDURES

Articulated arm degree of freedom: 5 DOF
Stereotactic system accuracy: 2 mm
Arm workspace: 25 in/63.5 cm radius
Computer screen update: <1 sec
Computer display views: transverse and MPR
Laser accessory: Class II laser, 27-degree and 45-degree geometry, auto sensing
V-channel: 27-degree and 45-degree geometry, auto-sensing
LCD Monitor: 14 in/35.6 cm (20 in/50.8 cm optional)
Usage detent positions: left, center, right

Courtesy Picker International; Cleveland, Ohio.

TECHNICAL DATA AND SPECIFICATIONS OF CARE®

CARE VISION CT includes both hardware and software and provides the following features:

High quality image reconstruction/display matrix: 2562/10242

Last image hold: at the end of a CARE Vision CT run, the last image acquired is displayed on the monitor and stored to the system hard disk for future reference

Video recorder interface allows connection of a standard VCR for documentation of the fluoro run or subsequent review and archival

Continuous fluoro on time is variable up to a maximum of 100 rotations (80 sec)

Variable low dose

Imaging parameters:
- Reconstruction speed: up to 8 frames per second (fps) depending on system configuration
- Field of view: 5 to 50 cm
- Slice thickness: 1 to 10 mm
- Power: 37.5 mAs to 90 mAs at 120 kV

Multiple fluoro runs are allowed with pauses in between each run

Gantry speed:
750 ms or 100 ms per 360-degree rotation

Parameter display:
- Countdown of remaining "fluoro-on" time
- Accumulated mAs for calculation of x-ray dose during procedure

Table-side control package
(Can be used in conjunction with CARE Vision CT or Real Time Display)

In-room monitor and mobile cart for viewing images at table side while performing the procedure

Table-side joystick: user mountable on either side of table to control in-out feed during the procedure. The joystick can be covered with a sterile drape

"Fluoro on" foot pedal for hands-free control of acquisition; CARE Vision CT is "on" while pedal is engaged and turns "off" when pedal is disengaged

Table up/down pedal for hands-free control of table height during interventions

CARE Filter:
All SOMATOM Plus 4 systems are equipped with the special CARE filter, which eliminates off focal radiation, reducing unwanted dose to the patient and the physician's hands and improving image quality

Courtesy Siemens Medical Systems.

REFERENCES

Daly B, Templeton PA: Real-time CT fluoroscopy: evolution of an interventional tool, *Radiology* 211: 309-315, 1999.

Froelich JJ et al: Guidance of non-vascular interventional procedures with real-time CT-fluoroscopy, *Electromedica* 66:50-55, 1997.

Katada K et al: Guidance with real-time CT fluoroscopy: early clinical experience, *Radiology* 200:851-856, 1996.

Kato R et al: Radiation dosimetry at CT fluoroscopy: physician's hand dose and development of needle holders, *Radiology* 201:576-578, 1996.

Nawfel RD et al: Patient and personnel exposure during CT fluoroscopy–guided interventional procedures, *Radiology* 216:180-184, 2000.

Ozaki M: Development of a real-time reconstruction system for CT fluorography, *Med Rev* 53:12-17, 1995.

Toshiba America Medical Systems: *Aspire CT fluoroscopy data,* Tustin, Calif, 1999, The Association.

Wagner LK: CT fluoroscopy: another advancement with additional challenges in radiation management, *Radiology* 216:9-10, 2000.

17

Three-Dimensional Computed Tomography: Basic Concepts

Three-dimensional (3D) imaging in medicine is a method in which a set of data is collected from a 3D object such as the patient, processed by a computer, and displayed on a two-dimensional (2D) computer screen to give the illusion of depth. Depth perception causes the image to appear in 3D.

The advances in spiral/helical CT and magnetic resonance imaging (MRI) technologies have resulted in an increasing use of 3D display of sectional anatomy. As a result, 3D imaging has become commonplace in most large-scale radiology departments, and researchers continue to explore the potential of 3D applications. For example, researchers at the Brain Image Analysis Laboratory at the University of California/San Diego are using 3D models to study AIDS, Huntington's disease, and schizophrenia. At Duke University, 3D models are being used to study cardiac arrhythmias. At Radionics Software Applications in Burlington, an application called XKnife uses information from CT and MRI brain scans to show tumor shape and location for radiation treatment planning (Mahoney, 1996).

In radiology, 3D imaging has found applications in radiation therapy, craniofacial imaging for surgical planning, orthopedics, neurosurgery, cardiovascular surgery, angiography, and MRI (Wu et al, 1999; Udupa, 1999; Calhoun et al, 1999). Another use of 3D imaging has been in the visualization of ancient Egyptian mummies without destroying the plaster or bandages (Yasuda et al, 1992).

More recently, 3D imaging has created virtual endoscopy, a technique that allows the viewer to "fly through" the body in an effort to examine structures such as the brain, tracheobronchial tree, vessels, sinuses, and the colon (Vining, 1996; Rubin et al, 1996). Additionally, 3D medical reconstruction movie clips are now available on the Internet. Viewers can now "fly through" the colon, skull, brain, lung, torso, and the arteries of the heart. Additionally, 3D imaging unearthed a whole new dimension in examining contrast-filled vessels from volumetric spiral/helical CT data, CT angiography (CTA). CTA and virtual reality imaging are described in Chapters 18 and 19, respectively.

This chapter describes the fundamental concepts of 3D imaging in CT to provide technologists with the tools needed to enhance their interaction with 3D imaging systems.

RATIONALE FOR 3D IMAGING

The purpose of 3D imaging is to use the vast amounts of data collected from the patient by volume CT scanning (and other imaging modalities such as MRI, for example) to provide both qualitative and quantitative information in a wide range of clinical applications. Qualitative information is used to compare how observers perform on a specific task to demonstrate the diagnostic value of 3D imaging; quantitative information is used to assess three elements of the technique: precision (reliability), accuracy (true detection), and efficiency (feasibility) of the 3D imaging procedure (Udupa, 1999).

HISTORY

In 1970 Greenleaf et al produced a motion display of the ventricles using biplane angiography. Soon after, the commercial introduction of CT renewed

---

EARLY HISTORY OF 3D MEDICAL IMAGING

1969—Hounsfield and Cormack develop the CT Scanner.

1970—Greenleaf and colleagues report first biomedical 3D display: computer-generated oscilloscope images relating to pulmonary bloodflow.

1972—First commercial CT scanner introduced.

1975—Ledley and colleagues report first 3D rendering of anatomic structures from CT scans.

1977—Herman and Liu publish 3D reconstructions of heart and lung of a dead frog.

1979—Herman develops technique to render bone surface in CT data sets; collaborates with Hemmy to image spine disorders.

1980—A CT scanner manufactured by General Electric features optional 3D imaging software.

1980-1981—Researchers begin investigating 3D imaging of craniofacial deformities.

1983—Commercial CT scanners begin featuring built-in 3D imaging software packages.

1986—Simulation software developed for craniofacial surgery.

1987—First international conference on 3D imaging in medicine organized in Philadelphia, Pennsylvania.

1990-1991—First textbooks on 3D imaging in medicine published; atlas of craniofacial deformities illustrated by 3D CT images published.

Adapted from Schwartz B: Computerized medical imaging, *Med Devices Res Rep* 1:8-10, 1994.

interest in medical 3D images because it was clearly apparent that a stack of contiguous CT sectional images could generate 3D information. This idea resulted in the development of specialized hardware and software for the production of 3D images and the development of algorithms for 3D imaging.

Technologic developments in 3D imaging continued at a steady pace throughout the 1970s, and by the early 1980s many CT scanners featured 3D software as an optional package. In the early 1980s 3D imaging was discovered useful for clinical applications, when several researchers began using the technology in craniofacial surgery, orthopedics, radiation treatment planning, and cardiovascular imaging. The box on p. 280 summarizes the major developments in the evolution of 3D imaging to the year 1991. Today, 3D imaging has evolved as a discipline on its own, demanding an understanding of various image processing concepts such as preprocessing, visualization, manipulation, and analysis operations (Udupa, 1999).

FUNDAMENTAL 3D CONCEPTS
Coordinates and Terminology

To understand how 3D images are generated in medical imaging, it is necessary first to identify and outline four coordinate systems that relate to the CT scanner, the display device, the object, and the scene. These coordinate systems are illustrated in Fig. 17-1, and include the scanner coordinate system, *abc*; the display coordinate system, *rst*; the object coordinate system, *uvw*; and the scene coordinate system, *xyz*. Each of these is defined in Table 17-1.

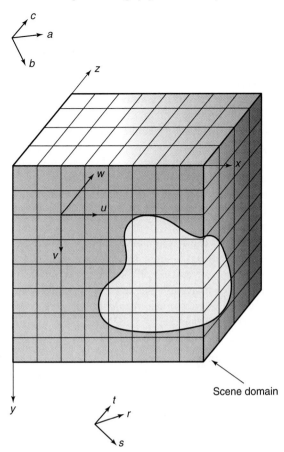

FIG. 17-1. Drawing provides graphic representation of the four coordinates used in 3D imaging: *abc*, scanner coordinate system; *rst*, display coordinate system; *uvw*, object coordinate system; *xyz*, scene coordinate system.

TABLE 17-1

Frequently Used Terms in 3D Medical Imaging

TERM	DEFINITION
Scene	Multidimensional image; rectangular array of voxels with assigned values
Scene domain	Anatomic region represented by the scene
Scene intensity	Values assigned to the voxels in a scene
Pixel size	Length of a side of the square cross section of a voxel
Scanner coordinate system	Origin and orthogonal axes system affixed to the imaging device
Scene coordinate system	Origin and orthogonal axes system affixed to the scene (origin usually assumed to be upper left corner to first section of scene, axes are edges of scene domain that converge at the origin)
Object coordinate system	Origin and orthogonal axes system affixed to the object or object system
Display coordinate system	Origin and orthogonal axes system affixed to the display device
Rendition	2D image depicting the object information captured in a scene or object system

From Udupa J: Three-dimensional visualization and analysis methodologies: a current perspective, *Radiographics* 19:783-806, 1999.

The most familiar system is the xyz, the scene or Cartesian coordinate system, as it is commonly called. In this system, the x, y, and z axes are positioned at right angles (orthogonal) to one another. The width of an object is described by the x axis, whereas the height is described by the y axis. The z axis, on the other hand, describes the dimension of depth and adds perspective realism to the image.

Use of the coordinate system allows description of an object by measuring distances from the point of intersection, or zero point. Distances can be positive or negative from the zero point, and images can be manipulated to rotate about the three axes. This rotation occurs in what is referred to as *3D space* and computer software helps the observer to view 3D space by displaying the front, back, top, and bottom of the object, providing a perspective from the observer's vantage point. The technique is known as *computer-aided visualization* or *3D visualization*, and the application of 3D visualization in medicine is called *3D medical imaging*.

In medicine, 3D imaging uses a right-handed x, y, and z coordinate system (Udupa, 1999) because images are displayed on a computer screen. The x, y, and z coordinates define a space in which multidimensional data (a set of slices) are represented. This space is called the *3D space* or *scene space*. The coordinate system helps to define the voxels (volume elements) in 3D space and allows use of the voxel information such as CT numbers or signal intensities in MRI to reconstruct 3D images.

Transforming 3D Space

Generally, 3D space can be subjected to a series of common 3D transformations (Fig. 17-2). The radiologic technologist can manipulate scene, structure, geometric, and projective transformations, as well as control image processing and image analysis. The technologist may transform 3D space in four ways (Table 17-2).

Modeling

The generation of a 3D object using computer software is called modeling. Modeling uses mathematics to describe physical properties of an object. According to one definition, modeling is "a computer simulation of a physical object in which length, width, and depth are real attributes. A model, with x, y, and z axes can be rotated for viewing from different angles" (Microsoft Press, 1999).

Several modeling techniques are used. In extrusion, one of the most common techniques, computer software is used to transform a 2D profile into a 3D object. In Fig. 17-3, for example, a square is changed into a box. Extrusion can also generate a wireframe model from a 2D profile. The wireframe is made up of triangles or polygons often referred to as *polygonal mesh*. Wireframes were common during the early development of 3D display in medi-

TABLE 17-2

Transforming 3D Space

SPACE DESIRED	TASK REQUIRED
Image space	Translate, rotate, or scale scenes, objects, or surfaces
Object space	Extract structural information about the object from the 3D space
Parameter space	Take measurements from the image's view space on the computer screen
View space	View the 2D screen of the computer monitor

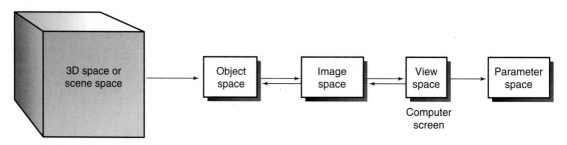

FIG. 17-2. Sequence of transformations characteristic of 3D imaging.

cine, and they are still being used today in other applications.

During the next step of modeling, a surface is added to the object by placing a layer of pixels (image mapping) and patterns (procedural textures) on top of the wireframes. The radiologic technologist can control various attributes of the surface, such as its texture.

Shading and Lighting

Shading and lighting also add realism to the 3D object. There are several shading algorithms, including wireframe shading, flat shading, Gouraud shading, and Phong shading. Each technique has its own set of advantages and disadvantages; however, a full discussion of shading algorithms is outside the scope of this chapter.

Although shading determines the final appearance of surfaces of the 3D object, lighting helps us to see the shape and texture of the object (Fig. 17-4). Various lighting techniques are available to enhance the appearance of the 3D image; one of the most common is called *ray tracing*, which is described later in this chapter.

Rendering

Rendering is the final step in the process of generating a 3D object. It involves the creation of the simulated 3D image from data collected from the object space. More specifically, *rendering* is a computer program that converts the anatomic data collected from the patient into the 3D image seen on the computer screen. With most 3D software, the object must be rendered before the effects of lighting and other attributes can be observed. Rendering therefore adds lighting, texture, and color to the final 3D image.

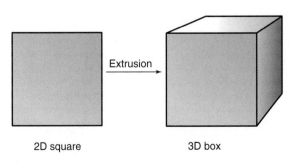

2D square   **3D box**

FIG. 17-3. Extrusion is a modeling technique that generates a 3D object from a 2D profile on a computer screen.

Two types of 3D rendering algorithms are used in radiology: surface rendering and volume rendering. Surface rendering uses only contour data from the set of slices in 3D space, whereas volume rendering makes use of the entire data set in 3D space. Because it uses more information, volume rendering produces a better image than surface rendering, but it takes longer and requires a more powerful computer.

CLASSIFICATION OF 3D IMAGING APPROACHES

Udupa and Herman (1991) have identified three classes of 3D imaging approaches: slice imaging, projective imaging, and volume imaging.

Slice Imaging

Slice imaging is the simplest method of 3D imaging. In 1975 Glenn and colleagues generated and displayed coronal and sagittal images from the CT axial data set. This technique is known as *multiplanar reconstruction* (MPR). Other researchers such as Herman and Liu (1977), Marvilla (1978), and Rhodes, Glenn and Azzawi (1980) also used slice imaging to produce coronal, sagittal, and paraxial images from the transaxial scans. Today, MPR is available on all CT and MRI scanners. However, MPR does not produce true 3D images but rather 2D images displayed on a flat computer screen

Projective Imaging

Projective imaging is the most popular 3D imaging approach. However, it still does not offer a true 3D mode; it produces a "2.5D" mode of visualization, an effect somewhere between 2D and 3D. As Udupa and Herman (1991) explain:

> *Projective imaging* deals with techniques for extracting multidimensional information from the given image data and for depicting such information in the 2D viewspace via a process of projection. Surface rendering and volume rendering are two major classes of approaches available under projective imaging.

The technique of projection is illustrated in Fig. 17-5. The contiguous axial sections represent the volume image data. Information from this volume image data is projected at various angles into the 2D view space.

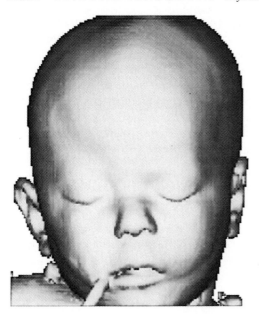
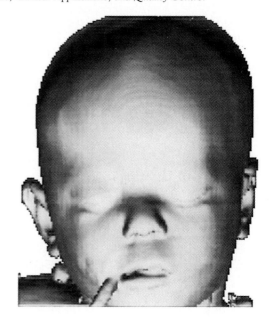
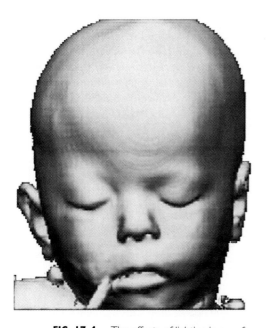
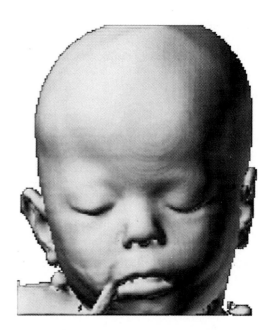

FIG. 17-4. The effects of lighting in a surface-rendered 3D image. As the light source is moved to different locations, various features of the image become clearly apparent.

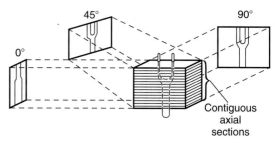

FIG. 17-5. The technique of projection used in 3D imaging. This is a major characteristic of projective imaging (one class of 3D imaging techniques).

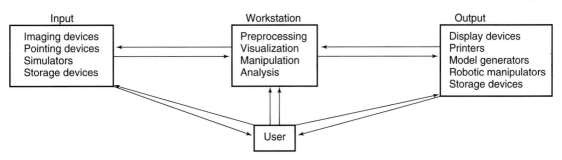

FIG. 17-6. A typical 3D imaging system consists of four major components: input, workstation, output, and the user.

Volume Imaging

Volume imaging must not be confused with volume rendering. Volume rendering belongs to the class of projective imaging, whereas volume imaging produces a true 3D visualization mode. Volume imaging methods include holography, stereoscopic displays, anaglyphic methods, varifocal mirrors, synthalyzers, and rotating multidiode arrays (Budinger, 1983).

GENERIC 3D IMAGING SYSTEM

In a recent article describing the current perspective of 3D imaging, Udupa (1999) provides a framework for a typical 3D imaging system (Fig. 17-6). Four major elements are noted: input, workstation, output, and the user. *Input* refers to devices that acquire data. Imaging input devices, for example, would include CT and MR scanners. The acquired data are sent to the workstation, which is the heart of the system. This powerful computer can handle various 3D imaging operations. These operations include preprocessing, visualization, manipulation, and analysis. Once processing is completed, the results are displayed for viewing and recording onto output devices. Finally, the user can interact with each of the three components—input, workstation, and output—to optimize use of the system.

The goals of each of the four major 3D imaging operations and the commonly used processing techniques are summarized in Table 17-3.

TECHNICAL ASPECTS OF 3D IMAGING IN RADIOLOGY
Definition of 3D Medical Imaging

Dr. Gabor Herman of the Medical Image Processing Group at the University of Pennsylvania defines 3D medical imaging as "the process that starts with a stack of sectional slices collected by some medical imaging device and results in computer-synthesized displays that facilitate the visualization of underlying spatial relationships" (Herman, 1993). Additionally, Udupa (1999) emphasize that the term *3D imaging* can also refer to the four categories of 3D operations: preprocessing, visualization, manipulation, and analysis.

Four steps are needed to create 3D images (Fig. 17-7):

1. Data acquisition. Slices, or sectional images, of the patient's anatomy are produced. Methods of data acquisition in radiology include CT, MRI, ultrasound, positron emission tomography (PET), single photon emission tomography (SPECT), and digital radiography and fluoroscopy.
2. Creation of 3D space or scene space. The voxel information from the sectional images is stored in the computer.
3. Processing for 3D image display. This is a function of the workstation and includes the four operations listed above.
4. 3D image display. The simulated 3D image is displayed on the 2D computer screen.

These four steps vary slightly depending on which imaging modality is used to acquire the data. Each of the four steps is described in detail below, using CT as the method of data acquisition.

Data Acquisition

In CT, data are collected from the patient using x-rays and special electronic detectors. Data can be acquired slice-by-slice with a conventional CT scanner or in a volume with a spiral/helical CT scanner. During *slice-by-slice acquisition*, the x-ray tube and detectors rotate to collect data from the first slice of the anatomic area of interest, which then is sent to the computer for image reconstruction. After the first slice is scanned, the tube and

TABLE 17-3

Goals of Various Operations for 3D Medical Imaging

CLASSES OF 3D OPERATIONS	GOALS	COMMONLY USED OPERATIONS	GOALS
Preprocessing	To take a set of scenes and output computer object models or another set of scenes from the given set, which facilitates the creation of computer object models	Volume of interest	To reduce the amount of data by specifying a region of interest and a range of intensities of interest
		Filtering	To enhance wanted (object) information and suppress unwanted (noise) background, other object information in the output scene
		Interpolation	To change the level of discretization (sampling) of the input scene
		Registration	Takes two scenes or objects as input and outputs a transformation that when applied to the second scene or object, matches it as closely as possible to the first
		Segmentation	To identify and delineate objects
Visualization	To create renditions from a given set of scenes or objects that facilitate the visual perception of object information	Scene-based Visualization • Section mode • Volume mode	To create renditions from scenes
		Object-based Visualization • Surface rendering • Volume rendering	To create renditions from defined objects
Manipulation	To create a second object system from a given object system by changing objects or their relations	Rigid manipulation	Operations to cut, separate, add, subtract, move, or mirror objects and their components
		Deformable manipulation	Operations to stretch, compress, bend, and so on
Analysis	To generate a quantitative description of the morphology, architecture, and function of the object system from a given set of scenes or object system	Scene-based analysis	Quantitative descriptions obtained from scenes to provide ROI statistics and measurements of density, activity, perfusion, and flow
		Object-based analysis	Quantitative descriptions obtained from objects on the basis of morphology, architecture, change over time, relationships with other objects in the system, and changes in these relationships

Modified from Udupa J: Three-dimensional visualization and analysis methodologies: a current perspective, *Radiographics* 19:783-806, 1999.

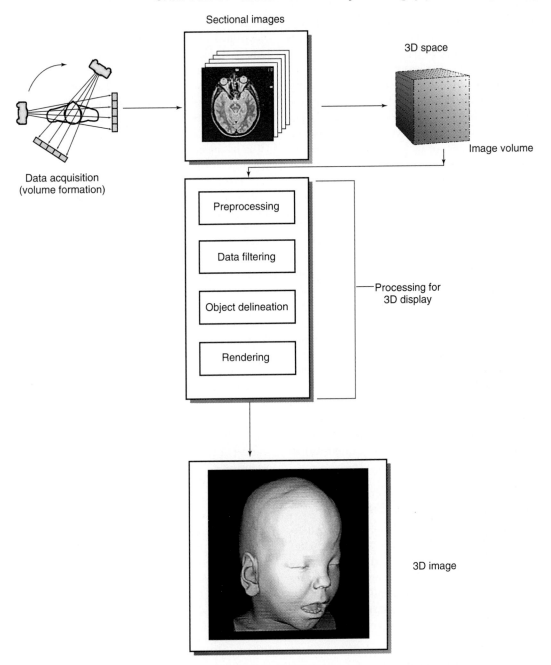

FIG. 17-7. The major steps in creating 3D images. First, data are collected from the patient and reconstructed as sectional images, which form 3D space or scene space. Secondly, 3D space can be processed to generate simulated 3D images displayed on a computer screen.

detectors stop, the patient is moved into position for the second slice, and scanning continues. The data from the second slice is transferred to the computer for image reconstruction. This "stop-and-go" technique continues until the last slice has been scanned.

One of the fundamental problems of slice-by-slice CT scanning is that certain portions of the anatomy may be missed because motion caused by the patient's respiration can interfere with scanning or be inconsistent from scan to scan. This problem can lead to inaccurate generation of 3D and multiplanar images. The final 3D image can have the appearance of steplike contours known as the *stair-step artifact* (see Fig. 13-5).

In volume data acquisition, a volume of tissue rather than a slice is scanned during a single breath-hold. This means that more data are sent to the computer for image reconstruction. Volume scanning is achieved because the x-ray tube rotates continuously as the patient moves through the gantry. One advantage of this technique is that more data are available for 3D processing, improving the quality of the resultant 3D image (see Fig. 13-5).

Creation of 3D Space or Scene Space

All information collected from the voxels that compose each of the scanned slices goes to the computer for image reconstruction. The voxel information is a CT number calculated from tissue attenuation within the voxel. In MRI the voxel information is the signal intensity from the tissue within the voxel. The result of image reconstruction is the creation of 3D space, where all image data are stored (Fig. 17-7).

Data in 3D space are systematically organized so that each point in 3D space has a specific address. Each point in 3D space represents the information (CT number or MRI signal intensity) of the voxels within the slice.

Processing for 3D Image Display

Processing is a major step in the creation of simulated 3D images for display on a 2D computer screen and is accomplished on the workstation. Although it is not within the scope of this chapter to address these operations in detail, it is important that technologists have an understanding of how sectional images are transformed into 3D images.

Mankovich, Robertson, and Cheeseman (1990) identified two classes of processing to explain 3D image display: voxel-based processing and object-based processing. *Voxel-based processing* "makes determinations about each voxel and decides to what degree each should contribute to the final 3D display," whereas *object-based processing* "uses voxel information to transform the images into a collection of objects with subsequent processing concentrating on the display of the objects."

Voxel-based processing was used as early as 1975 as a means of generating coronal, sagittal, and oblique images from the stack of contiguous transverse axial set of images—the technique of *multiplanar reconstruction*. Although MPR is not a true 3D display technique, it does provide additional information to enhance our understanding of 3D anatomy (Mankovich, Robertson, and Cheeseman, 1990). In MPR, the computer scans the 3D space and locates all voxels in a particular plane to produce that particular image (see Fig. 17-8).

Object-based processing involves several processing methods to produce a model (called an *object model* or *object representation*) from the 3D space and transforms it into a 3D image displayed on a computer screen. The processing of an object model into a simulated 3D image involves four steps:

1. Segmentation is a processing technique used to identify the structure of interest in a given scene (Udupa and Herman, 1991). It determines which voxels are a part of the object and should be displayed and which are not and should be discarded (Mankovich, Robertson and Cheeseman, 1990).

2. Thresholding is a method of classifying the types of tissues, such as say bone, soft tissue,

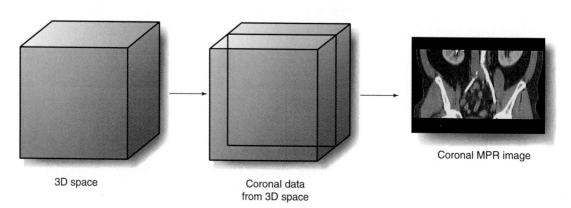

3D space   Coronal data from 3D space   Coronal MPR image

FIG. 17-8. The basic concept of multiplanar reconstruction (MPR).

or fat, represented by each of the voxels. The CT number is used for assigning thresholds to tissues.

3. Object delineation is portraying an object by drawing it. It involves boundary and volume extraction and detection methods. Although boundary extraction methods search the 3D space for only those voxels that define the outer or inner border or surface of the object called the object contour, volume extraction methods find all the voxels in 3D space and its surface (Mankovich, Robertson, and Cheeseman, 1990).

4. Rendering is the stage when an image in 3D space is transformed into a simulated 3D image to be displayed on a 2D computer monitor. Rendering is a computer display technology-based approach (computer program) and therefore requires specific hardware and software to deal with millions of points identified in 3D space.

RENDERING TECHNIQUES

Two classes of rendering techniques are common in radiology: surface rendering and volume rendering (Udupa, 1999; Calhoun et al, 1999).

Surface Rendering

Surface rendering, or shaded surface display (SSD), has evolved through the years with significant improvements in image quality (Fig. 17-9). In surface rendering, the computer creates "an internal representation of surfaces that will be visible in the displayed image. It then 'lights' them according to a standard protocol, and displays an image according to its calculation of how the light rays would be reflected to the viewer's eye" (Schwartz, 1994).

According to Udupa (1999), surface rendering involves essentially two steps: surface formation and depiction on a computer screen (rendering) (see the box below. Surface formation involves the operation of contouring. Rendering follows surface formation and is intended to add photorealism and create the illusion of depth in an image, making it appear 3D on a 2D computer screen. A simulated light source can be positioned at different locations to enhance features of the displayed 3D image (see Fig.17-4).

STEPS FOR SURFACE RENDERING

1. Scan the 3D space or scene space for all voxel information relating to the object to be displayed.
2. Create the surface of the object using contour information (segmentation) obtained by thresholding. The threshold setting determines whether skin or bone surfaces will be displayed. The 3D images of the skull shown in Fig. 17-9 are examples of surface rendering.
3. Select the viewing orientation to be processed for 3D image display and assign the position of one or more lighting sources. A standard set of views is shown in Fig. 17-10.
4. Surface rendering begins. The pixels of the object to be displayed are shaded for photorealism and particularly to give the illusion of depth. Those pixels farthest away from the viewer are darker than those closer to the viewer.

A   B   C

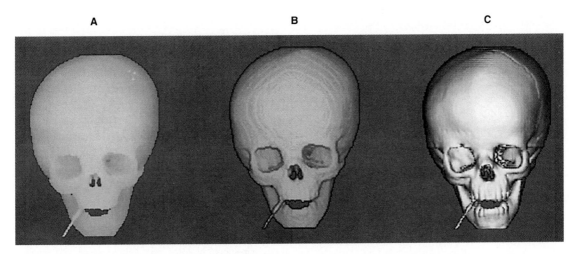

FIG. 17-9. The evolution of surface rendering technique, demonstrating the improvement in image quality. **A,** Older processing methods; **B,** recent methods; **C,** current techniques.

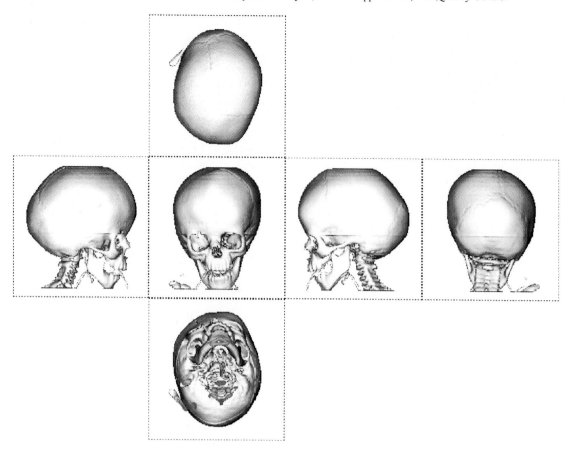

FIG. 17-10. Examples of several views selected by the CT operator for 3D display.

The advantage of surface rendering techniques is that they do not require a lot of computing power because they do not use all the voxel information in 3D space to create the 3D image. Only contour information is used. However, this results in poor image information content.

Heath et al (1995) demonstrated this disadvantage when they used surface rendering to image the liver. They reported that

no information about structures inside or behind the surface such as vessels within the liver capsule or thrombus within a vessel is displayed. In medical volume data, which are affected by volume averaging because of finite voxel size, clear-cut edges and surfaces are often difficult or impossible to define. Many voxels necessarily contain multiple tissue types and classifying them as being totally not part of a given tissue introduces artifacts into the image. Surface renderings are very sensitive to changes in threshold, and it is often difficult to determine which threshold yields the most accurate depiction of the actual anatomic structures.

Fig. 17-11 illustrates surface rendering numerically. Numbers represent the voxel values for a sample 2D data set. An algorithm is applied to locate a "surface" within the data set at the margin of the region of voxels with intensities ranging from 6 to 9. Standard computer graphics techniques are then used to generate a surface that represents the defined region of voxel values (Heath et al, 1995).

Volume Rendering

Volume rendering is a more sophisticated technique and produces 3D images that have a better image quality and provide more information compared with surface rendering techniques. Volume rendering overcomes several of the limitations of surface rendering because it uses the entire data set from 3D space. Because of this, volume rendering requires more computing power and is more expensive than surface rendering.

Udupa and Herman (1991) describe the conceptual framework of volume rendering:

the scene is considered to represent blocks of translucent colored jelly whose color and opacity (degree of transparency) are different for different tissue regions. The goal of rendering is to compute

Threshold range (6 to 9) with subvoxel surface

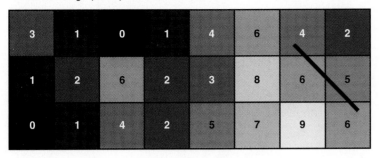

Displayed
surface

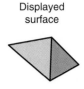

FIG. 17-11. Surface rendering (or SSD) technique.

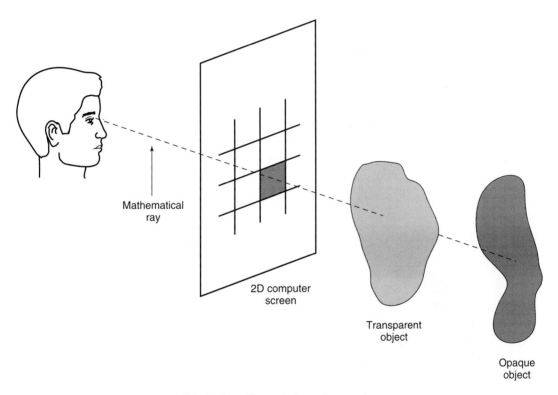

FIG. 17-12. The technique of ray tracing.

images that depict the appearance of this block from various angles, simulating the transmission of light through the block as well as its reflection at tissue interfaces through careful selection of color and opacity.

The two stages to volume rendering are preprocessing the volume and rendering.

Preprocessing involves several image processing operations including segmentation, also referred to as *classification,* to determine the tissue types contained in each voxel, and to assign different brightness levels or color. In addition, a partial transparency (0% to 100%) is also assigned to different tissues that make up 3D space. Three tissue types—fat, soft tissue, and bone—are used for voxel classification.

Rendering is stage two of the volume rendering technique. It involves image projection to form the simulated 3D image. One popular method of image projection is ray tracing illustrated in Fig. 17-12. During *ray tracing,* a mathematical ray is sent from the observer's eye through the 2D computer screen to pass through the 3D volume that contains opaque and transparent objects. The pixel intensity on the screen for that single ray is the average of the intensities of all the voxels

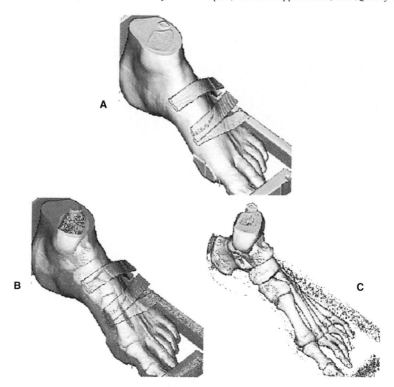

FIG. 17-13.   A, A surface-rendered image. **B,** An example of volume rendering, in which the soft tissues have been made transparent and allows the viewer to see both the skin and bone surfaces at the same time. **C,** The entire surface is removed.

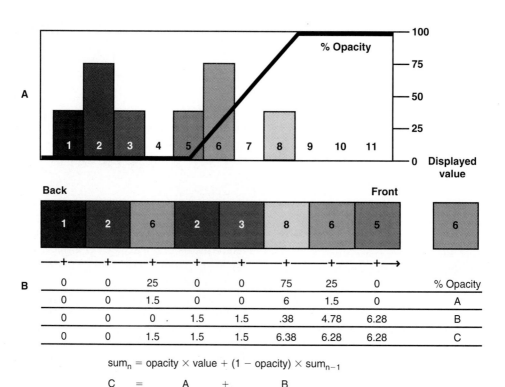

$$\text{sum}_n = \text{opacity} \times \text{value} + (1 - \text{opacity}) \times \text{sum}_{n-1}$$

$$C = A + B$$

FIG. 17-14.   Diagram illustrates volume rendering technique. A histogram of the voxel values (**A**) in the data "ray" (**B**).

through which the ray travels. As Mankovich, Robertson, and Cheeseman (1990) explain, "If all objects are opaque, only the nearest object is considered, and the ray is then traced back to the light source for calculation of the reflected intensity. If the nearest object is transparent, the ray is diminished and possibly refracted to the next nearest object and so on until the light is traced back to the source."

Unlike surface rendering, volume rendering offers the advantage of seeing through surfaces allowing the viewer to examine both external and internal structures (Fig. 17-13). A numeric illustration of how this is accomplished is shown in Fig. 17-14. An opacity of 0% and 100% are assigned for values of 5 or lower and 9 or higher, respectively. The resulting intermediate opacities for values 6, 7, and 8 are 25%, 50%, and 75%, respectively. The lower portion of the diagram shows the equation and progressive computational results used to determine weighted summation along the "ray" through the volume. The resulting displayed value (6) is affected by both opacity (as determined in the graph at the top) and the value of underlying voxels (Calhoun et al, 1999).

Alternatively, volume rendering can be explained by examining the flow of volume data from the CT scanner to the computer monitor for image display. A detailed description of such implementation of 3D volume rendering is given in a recent paper by Calhoun et al (1999).

Maximum Intensity Projection

Maximum intensity projection (MIP) is a volume rendering 3D technique that originated in magnetic resonance angiography (MRA) and is now used frequently in computed tomography angiography (CTA). MIP does not require sophisticated computer hardware because, like surface rendering, it makes use of less than 10% of the data in 3D space (Heath et al, 1995).

Fig. 17-15 details the underlying concept of MIP. Essentially, the MIP computer program renders a 2D image on a computer screen from a 3D data set (slices) as follows:

1. A mathematical ray (similar to the one in ray tracing) is projected from the viewer's eye through the 3D space (data set).
2. This ray passes through a set of voxels in its path.
3. The MIP program allows only the voxel with the maximum intensity (brightest value) to be selected.

4. The selected voxel intensity is then assigned to the corresponding pixel in the displayed MIP image.
5. The MIP image is displayed for viewing (Fig. 17-16).

Fig. 17-17 numerically illustrates the MIP technique.

MIP images can also be displayed in rapid sequence to allow the observer to view an image that can be rotated continuously back and forth to enhance 3D visualization of complex structures, us-

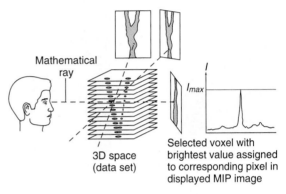

FIG. 17-15. Maximum intensity projection (MIP). The intensity, *I*, is plotted as function of slice number.

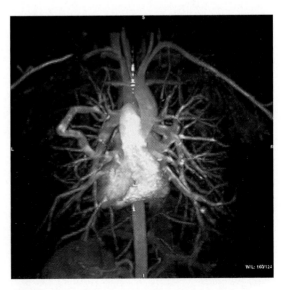

FIG. 17-16. Example of an MIP image. (Courtesy Vital Images; Minneapolis, Minnesota.)

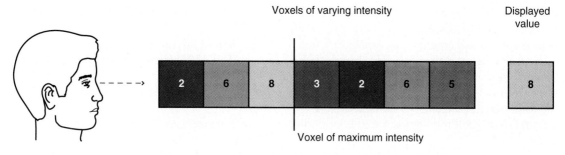

FIG. 17-17. Numerical representation of the MIP rendering technique.

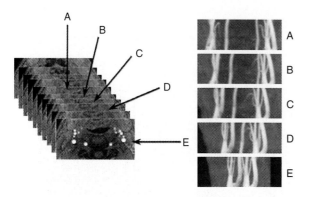

FIG. 17-18. A complete projection image at different viewing angles. Postprocessing of the 3D data set can generate different views to allow the observers to rotate the image back and forth to enhance the perception of 3D relationships in the vessels. (From Laub G et al: Magnetic resonance angiography techniques, *Electromedica* 66:68-75, 1998.)

ing postprocessing techniques. Fig. 17-18 shows multiple projections that vary only slightly in degree increments.

One of the basic problems with the MIP technique is that "images are three-dimensionally ambiguous unless depth cues are provided" (Heath et al, 1995). To solve this problem, a depth-weighted MIP can be used to deal with the intensity of the brightest voxel, depending on its distance from the viewer. Other limitations include the inability of the MIP program to show superimposed structures because only one voxel (the one with the maximum intensity) in the set of voxels traversed by a ray is used in the MIP image display. Additionally, MIP generates a "string of beads" artifact because of volume averaging problems with tissues that have lower intensity values (Heath et al, 1995),

and artifacts arising from pulsating vessels and respiratory motion, (Prokop et al, 1997).

A significant advantage of the MIP algorithm is that it has become the most popular rendering technique in CTA (Prokop et al, 1997) and MRA because vessels containing contrast medium are clearly seen. Additionally, because MIP uses less than 10% of the volume data in 3D space, it takes less time to produce 3D simulated images than volume-rendering algorithms.

Comparison of 3D Rendering Techniques

One comprehensive comparison of surface and volume rendering techniques was performed in 1991 by Udupa, Hung, and Chuang. They concluded that the surface method had a minor advantage over the volume methods with respect to display ability, clarity of the display, smoothness of ridges and silhouettes, computational time, and storage requirements. It had a significant advantage with its time and storage requirements.

In 1995 Heath et al (1995) compared surface rendering, volume rendering, and maximum intensity projection using spiral/helical CT during arterial portography. They compared the techniques with respect to seven parameters: depiction of 3D relationships, edge delineation, demonstration of overlapping structures, depiction of vessel lumen, percentage of data used, artifacts, and computational cost. Their results are summarized in Table 17-4. It is clearly apparent that volume rendering is superior in all parameters compared; however, it has the highest computational cost. In addition, 3D volume rendering has been shown to be useful in a wide range of applications (Calhoun et al, 1999), including the thoracic aorta (Christine

TABLE 17-4

Comparison of 3D Rendering Techniques in Medical Imaging

	SURFACE RENDERING	MIP	VOLUME RENDERING
Depiction of 3D relationships	Good	Fair	Good
Edge delineation	Good	Good	Fair
Demonstration of overlapping structures	No	No	Yes
Depiction of vessel lumen	No	Depicts section that is 1 pixel thick	Yes
Percentage of data used	Typically <10%	Typically <10%	Up to 100%
Artifacts present in medical images	Many false surfaces	MIP artifact and background enhancement	Few if properly segemented
Computational cost	Low	Low	High

From Heath DG et al: Three-dimensional spiral CT during arterial portography: comparison of three rendering techniques, *Radiographics* 15:1001-1011, 1995.

et al, 1999), and in evaluating carotid artery stenosis (Leclerc et al, 1999).

EQUIPMENT

Equipment for 3D image processing falls into two categories: the CT or MRI scanner console and stand-alone computer workstations.

Both types of equipment use software designed to perform several image processing operations, such as interactive visualization, multi-image display, analysis and measurement, and 3D rendering. Most processing for 3D imaging is done on stand-alone workstations, which are becoming more popular as their costs decrease.

Stand-Alone Workstations

Picker, Siemens, General Electric, and several other manufacturers provide 3D packages for their CT and MRI scanners, and many are offering both 3D hardware and software packages for use in radiology. Although the technical specifications of each workstation vary depending on the manufacturer, typical 3D processing features include the following:

- Multiplanar reconstruction (MPR). Fig. 17-19 shows both routine and curved MPR images. Curved MPR takes views from any curved plane and displays curved anatomy such as arteries, spinal cord, or the pancreas
- Surface rendering (Fig. 17-20)

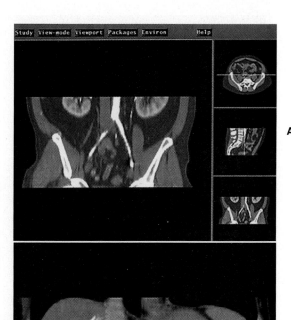

FIG. 17-19. Routine and curved MPR images. (Courtesy Picker International; Cleveland, Ohio.)

- Slice plane mapping (Fig. 17-21). This technique allows two tissue types to be viewed at the same time.
- Slice cube cuts (Fig. 17-22). This is a processing technique that allows the operator

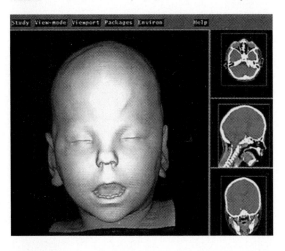

FIG. 17-20. A surface rendered image. (Courtesy Picker International; Cleveland, Ohio.)

to slice through any plane to demonstrate internal anatomy.

- Transparency visualization (Fig. 17-23). This processing technique allows the operator to view both surface and internal structures at the same time.
- Maximum intensity projection (see Fig. 17-16)
- 4-D angiography. This technique shows bone, soft tissue, and blood vessels at the same time and allows the viewer to see tortuous vessels with respect to bone (Fig. 17-24).
- Disarticulation. This shaded surface display technique allows the viewer to enhance the visualization of certain structures by removing others (Fig. 17-25).

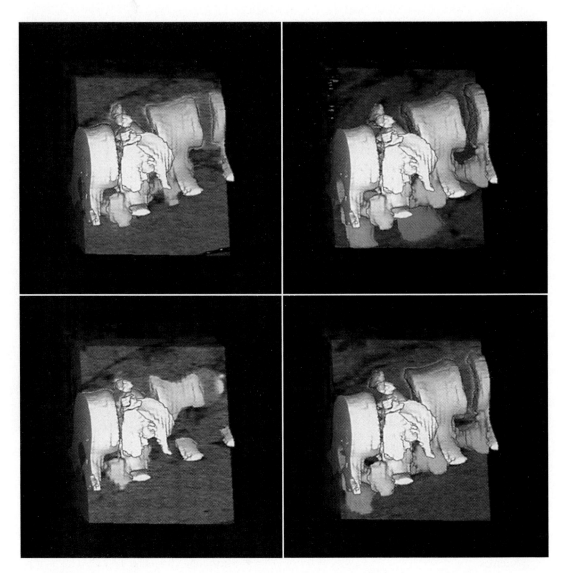

FIG. 17-21. Slice plane mapping allows two types of tissues to be seen at the same time. (Courtesy Picker International; Cleveland, Ohio.)

- Virtual reality imaging. Some workstations are also capable of virtual endoscopy, a processing technique that allows the viewer to look into the lumen of the bronchus and colon for example. It is also possible for the viewer to "fly through" the 3D data set. Virtual CT endoscopy is described Chapter 19.

CLINICAL APPLICATIONS OF 3D IMAGING

One of the major motivating factors for the development and application of 3D imaging in medicine is to improve the communication gap between the radiologist and surgeon. According to Zonneveld and Fukuta (1994), 3D imaging can help radiologists locate the pathology and identify the best way to reach it. Interestingly, craniofacial surgery was one of the first clinical applications of 3D medical imaging. Today, 3D medical imaging is used for applications ranging from orthopedics to radiation therapy (Udupa and Herman, 1991; Fishman et al, 1992; Zonneveld and Fukuta, 1994; Calhoun et al, 1999).

The applications of 3D imaging in CT, MRI, nuclear medicine, and ultrasonography continue to evolve at a rapid rate, with most of the work being done in CT and MRI. For example, the most recent clinical application of 3D imaging is in the area of endoscopic imaging, where the viewer can

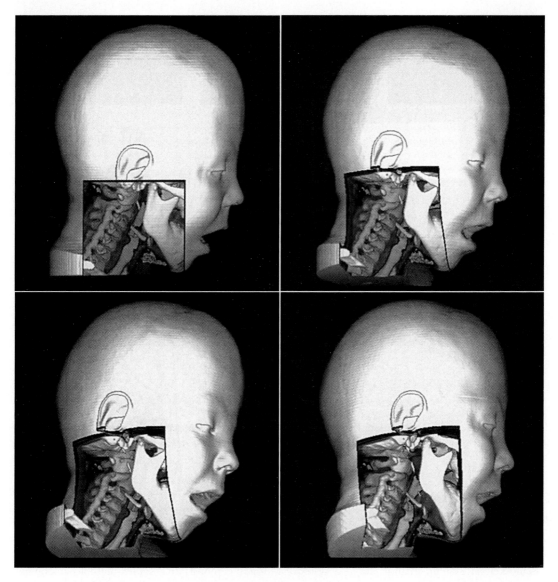

FIG. 17-22. Examples of slice cube cuts. (Courtesy Picker International; Cleveland, Ohio.)

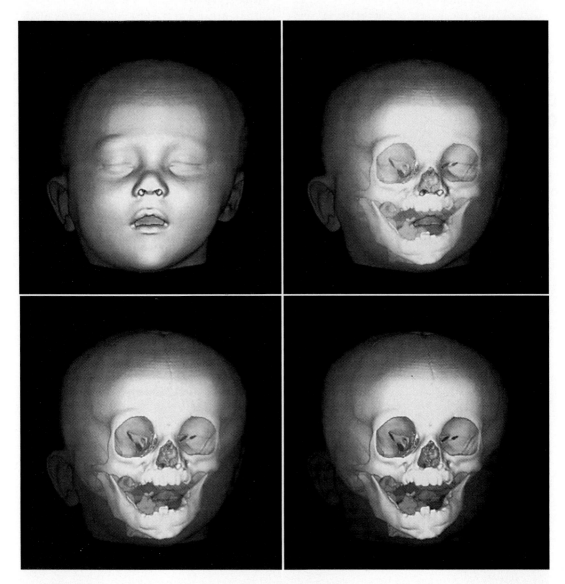

FIG. 17-23. Transparency visualization, a 3D processing technique allows the viewer to look at both surface and internal structures at the same time. (Courtesy Picker International; Cleveland, Ohio.)

"fly through" CT and MRI data sets with the goal of performing "virtual endoscopy" (Rubin et al, 1996).

Clinical Applications of 3D Imaging in CT

To date, clinical applications of 3D imaging in CT have been in the craniomaxillofacial complex, musculoskeletal system, central nervous system, cardiovascular system, pulmonary system, gastroin-

testinal (GI) system, and genitourinary (GU) system, as well as in radiation treatment planning for therapy. In the craniomaxillofacial complex, for example, 3D has been used to evaluate congenital and developmental deformity (shape of the deformed skull and the extent of suture ossification) and to assess trauma (bone fragment displacement and fractures).

In 1984, Totty and Vannier applied 3D imaging to demonstrate complex musculoskeletal anatomy. Subsequently, other workers applied 3D

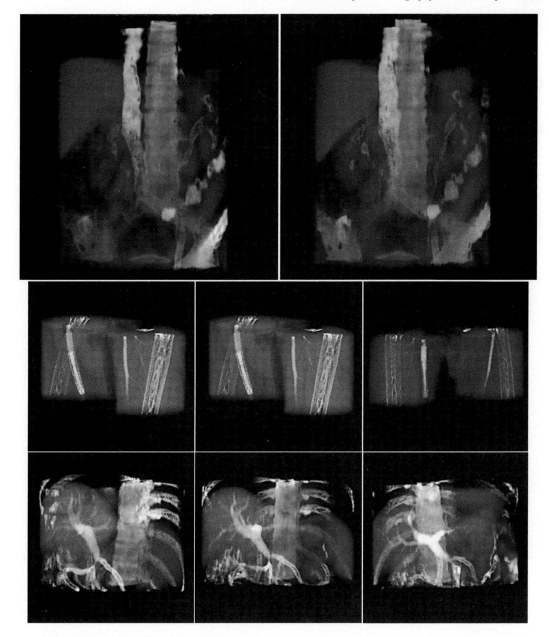

FIG. 17-24. 4-D angiography images processed on the workstation. (Courtesy Picker International; Cleveland, Ohio.)

imaging to study acetabular and calcaneal trauma, muscle atrophy, spinal pathology, and trauma of the spine, knee, carpal bones, and shoulder.

The development of CTA opened up additional avenues for the use of 3D imaging in the evaluation of cerebral aneurysms and arteriovenous malformations. It has been applied in CT of the GI system, primarily imaging the liver (Heath et al, 1995), and GU systems, primarily in kidney and bladder assessment. Recent reports by Wu et al (1999) and by Leclerc et al (1999) indicate that 3D volume rendering provides accurate evaluation of the thoracic aorta, and internal carotid artery stenosis, respectively.

In radiation therapy the purpose of 3D imaging is especially "to reconstruct isodose surfaces and display these in conjunction with anatomical surfaces" (Zonneveld and Fukuta, 1994).

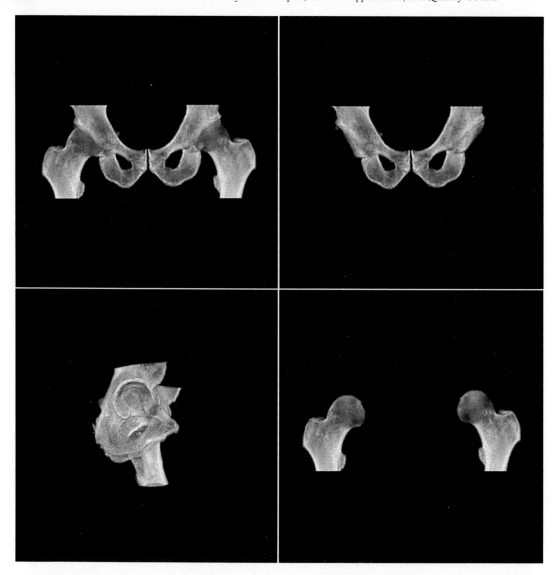

FIG. 17-25. Examples of disarticulation with surface shading. (Courtesy Picker International; Cleveland, Ohio.)

Clinical Applications of 3D Imaging in MRI

The clinical applications of 3D imaging in MRI have been limited because of the continuing developments in the technology, but MRI has the same potential for 3D imaging as CT. For example, in the musculoskeletal region, MRI has been used to assess hip subluxation and acetabular coverage. According to Zonneveld and Fukuta (1994) this technique has the potential to assess the extent of femoral head necrosis, disruption of cartilagious structures such as meniscal tears, tendons, and ligaments, such as the cruciate ligaments and tendons of the foot and ankle, and the distribution of joint fluid. Other potential includes outlining pannus formation and joint effusion in rheumatoid arthritis.

Recently, 3D imaging has become popular in MR angiography (MRA). In particular, the maximum intensity projection algorithm is now used extensively in the study of the vasculature of tissues (Saloner, 1995; Laub et al, 1998).

THE FUTURE OF 3D IMAGING

The first two decades of 3D imaging have generated a new and vast knowledge base on the technology of 3D imaging and on its clinical role in medicine. It has provided additional information that has helped in the diagnostic interpretation of images and enhanced the communication between radiologists and surgeons and other physicians.

As research and development in 3D imaging continue, experts predict promising gains for radiology. In the area of new computer hardware technology, we will see advances in user-interface technology, such as 3D joysticks, data gloves, voice-control and head-mounted displays (Zonneveld and Fukuta, 1994). Additionally, we can expect to see developments in computer architecture that will boost processing power and speed. Software developments will include improvements in segmentation techniques, for example. In addition, morphing techniques (Sorenson, 1992) and 3D-animation (MacNicol, 1993) and robot-assisted surgery (Calhoun et al, 1999) will become available. Also the cost of dedicated computer hardware and software will decrease, and personal computer-based workstations will become available. Limited 3D rendering is now possible on the Internet.

As the technology for 3D imaging becomes increasingly sophisticated and better refined, clinical applications will expand and 3D imaging will be applied to other areas of the body. Applications in CT, MRI, and other imaging modalities will expand with the goal of providing additional information to support and validate diagnostic interpretation. For example, the technique of "virtual endoscopy," which a few workstations already offer, will soon become commonplace.

Researchers are now investigating 4D imaging. According to Grangeat and Amans (1996), "4-D reconstruction for time-varying objects is beginning to be explored such as angiography, to study abdominal blood flow circulation between arteries and veins or in cardiac-gated SPECT, to reduce the blurring caused by the heart motion, or in 4-D image reconstruction of functional images."

THE ROLE OF THE RADIOLOGIC TECHNOLOGIST

As 3D imaging technology expands, it is likely that radiologic technologists will play an increasing role in image processing and analysis techniques. Radiologic technologists may need to expand their knowledge base to include a basic understanding of 3D imaging concepts, and the curricula of educational programs in the radiologic sciences may need to offer courses that prepare students to perform 3D imaging.

To perform quality 3D medical imaging, the technologist and the radiologist must work as a team. Technical ability in performing CT or MRI examinations and an understanding of the 3D imaging process are equally important. In addition, effective communication between the technologist and radiologist is vital in performing 3D medical imaging and will become even more important as the technology expands into new clinical applications (Udupa, 1999; Calhoun et al, 1999).

REFERENCES

Budinger T: 3D image displays bring scans to life, *Diagnostic Imaging* 2:54; 1983.

Calhoun PS et al: Three-dimensional volume rendering of spiral CT data. Theory and method, *Radiographics* 19:745-764, 1999.

Fishman EK et al: Three-dimensional imaging, Radiology 181:321-337, 1991.

Grangeat P, Amans, J-L, editors: *Three-dimensional image reconstruction in radiology and nuclear medicine,* Boston, 1996, Kluwer.

Heath DG et al: Three-dimensional spiral CT during arterial portography: comparison of three rendering techniques, *Radiographics* 15:1001-1011, 1995.

Herman GT, Liu HK: Display of three-dimensional information in computed tomography, *J Comput Assist Tomogr* 1:155-160, 1977.

Herman GT: 3D display: a survey from theory to applications, *Comput Med Imag Graph* 17:131-142, 1993.

Laub G et al: Magnetic resonance angiography techniques, *Electromedica* 66:68-75, 1998.

Leclerc X et al: Internal carotid artery stenosis: CT angiography with volume rendering, *Radiology* 210: 673-682, 1999.

MacNicol G: 3D animation is expensive and effective, *Comput Graph World* 16:37-44, 1993.

Mahoney DP: The art and science of medical visualization, *Comput Graph World* 14:25-32, 1996.

Mankovich NJ, Robertson DR, Cheeseman AM: Three-dimensional image display in medicine, *J Digit Imaging* 3:69-80, 1990.

Marvilla KR: Computer reconstructed sagittal and coronal computed tomography head scans. Clinical applications, *J Comput Assist Tomogr* 2:120-123, 1978.

Microsoft Press: *Computer dictionary,* Redmond, Wash, 1999, Microsoft Press.

Prokop M et al: Use of maximum intensity projections in CT angiography : a basic review, *Radiographics* 17:433-451, 1997.

Rhodes ML, Glenn WV, Azzawi VM: Extracting oblique planes from serial CT sections, *J Comput Assist Tomogr* 4:649-657, 1980.

Rubin GD et al: Perspective volume rendering of CT and MR images. Applications for endoscopic imaging, *Radiology* 199:321-330, 1996.

Saloner D: An introduction to MR angiography, *Radiographics* 15:453-465, 1995.

Schwartz B: 3D Computerized medical imaging, *Medical Device Research Report* 1:8-10, 1994.

Seeram E: *Computed tomography: physical principles, clinical applications and quality control*, Philadelphia, 1994, WB Saunders.

Sorenson P: Morphing magic, *Comput Graph World* 15:36-42, 1992.

Totty WG, Vannier MW: Complex musculoskeletal anatomy: analysis using three-dimensional surface reconstruction, *Radiology* 150:173-177, 1984.

Udupa JK: Three-dimensional visualization and analysis methodologies: A current perspective, *Radiographics* 19:783-803, 1999.

Udupa JK, Herman GT, editors: *3D imaging in medicine*, Boca Raton, Fla, 1991, CRC Press.

Vining DJ: Virtual endoscopy flies viewer through the body, *Diagn Imaging* 3:127-129, 1996.

Wu CM et al: Spiral CT of the thoracic aorta with 3D volume rendering: a pictorial review, *Cardiaovasc Intervent Radiol* 22:159-167, 1999.

Yasuda T et al: 3D visualization of an ancient Egyptian mummy, *IEEE Comput Graphics Appl* 2:13-17, 1992.

Zonneveld FW, Fukuta K: A decade of clinical three-dimensional imaging: a review. Part 2: Clinical applications, *Invest Radiol* 29:574-589, 1994.

BIBLIOGRAPHY

Bushong S: *Magnetic resonance imaging*, ed 2, St Louis, 1996, Mosby.

Crass JR et al: Radiological applications of three-dimensional imaging systems, *Semin Ultrasound CT MRI* 13:94-101, 1992.

Glenn W et al: Image generation and display techniques from CT scan data. Transverse and reconstructed coronal and sagittal planes, *Invest Radiol* 10:403-416, 1975.

Hemmy DC: Future directions in three-dimensional imaging. In Udupa JK, Herman GT: *3D imaging in medicine*, Boca Raton, FL, 1991, CRC Press.

Udupa JK, Hung HM, Chuang KS: Surface and volume rendering in three-dimensional imaging: a comparison, *J Digit Imaging* 4:159-168, 1991.

18

Computed Tomography Angiography: Technical Considerations

Chapter 14 introduced computed tomography angiography (CTA) as one the advances of volume scanning. This chapter elaborates on the technical requirements for CTA, including patient preparation, acquisition parameters, and contrast media administration. Secondly, the chapter addresses several 3D visualization tools for use in CTA. These tools are described in detail in Chapter 17.

DEFINITION

A significant advantage of spiral/helical CT data acquisition is its application to 3D imaging of vascular structures with an intravenous injection of contrast medium. This application, *CT angiography*, is defined as "any CT image of a blood vessel that has been opacified by a contrast medium" (Kalender, 1995).

During spiral/helical data acquisition, the entire area of interest can be scanned during the injection of contrast. Images can be captured when vessels are fully opacified to demonstrate either arterial or venous phase enhancement through the acquisition of both data sets (arterial and venous). CTA has been applied successfully to a number of examinations investigating vascular anatomy, problems, and disease. In particular, CTA techniques have proved useful in imaging the neurovasculature, the abdominal and thoracic aorta, renal vasculature, and in evaluating the vasculature of the abdominal viscera (Fishman and Jeffrey, 1998).

CTA is based on 3D imaging to display images of the vasculature through intravenous administration of contrast, differing from conventional intraarterial angiography. The advantages of CTA over conventional angiography are provided in Table 18-1. A major disadvantage of CTA is that of its poor spatial resolution (Rawlings, 1995).

REQUIREMENTS

At least four major steps are crucial to carrying out a CTA examination. Careful execution of these steps will serve to optimize the examination and produce high-quality images that will aid the radiologist in making an accurate diagnosis. These steps include the following:

1. Patient preparation
2. Acquisition parameters
3. Contrast medium administration
4. Postprocessing techniques

Patient Preparation

A successful CTA examination depends on careful preparation of the patient before the examination. Such preparation requires that both the technologist and radiologist work together to obtain the appropriate and correct information from the patient and to ensure that the patient understands the procedure, particularly breath-holding techniques. A number of patient preparation schemes are described by several investigators for a wide range of CTA applications (Raymond, Zwiebel, and Swartz, 1998). Smith and Fishman (1998) describe a scheme pertinent to 3D-CTA in renal applications:

> Preceding the 3D-CTA, a patient history should be obtained to identify patients with histories of iodine allergy, renal dysfunction, cardiac disease, and asthma. Steroid premedication should be administered to those patients with a history of iodine allergy or previous reaction to iodinated contrast agents. Patients with a history of renal dysfunction should be further evaluated with creatinine level and blood urea nitrogen level assessed before the procedure. Water (750 ml total) is administered as a negative contrast agent before the examination. Positive contrast agents are not administered because they can produce streak artifacts and interfere with the evaluation of the 3D-CTA. Patients are instructed on breath-holding techniques, and practicing with the patient, before the examination, will help provide a successful motion-free examination. Hyperventilation performed immediately before the examination facilitates patient breath-holding ability. Secure placement of a 20-gauge catheter in an antecubital vein provides safe intravenous access for a bolus administration of an intravenous contrast agent.

Acquisition Parameters

In general, a routine CT examination precedes a CTA examination. The routine examination provides some evidence of the range of anatomy to be scanned. Once the scan distance or scan range, R (mm), has been determined, a number of parameters must be carefully chosen to optimize both the quality of the 3D images and the accuracy of the CTA examination. These parameters include the total spiral/helical scan time, T (sec); the slice thickness, S (mm); and the speed of the patient through the gantry, that is, the table speed, d (mm/sec) (Kalender, 1995).

TABLE 18-1

Comparison of the Advantages of CT Angiography and Conventional Angiography

CONVENTIONAL ANGIOGRAPHY	CT ANGIOGRAPHY
Biplane systems can acquire at most two view angles of a given vascular structure per contrast injection. When required, alternate views and examination of additional structures require added x-ray exposure and contrast media.	CTA acquires an entire volume of 3D data using a single injection of contrast agent. Thus arbitrary views can be retrospectively targeted and reconstructed without the need for additional iodine or x-ray exposure.
Because an arterial puncture is made, patients must recover from the procedure with close nursing observation and strict bedrest for a minimum of 6 to 8 hrs. An overnight hospital stay may also be required. Thus recovery time adds significantly to the cost of the examination.	Peripheral intravenous injections permit a true outpatient examination with minimal postprocedure observation.
Serious complications from angiography can include reactions to contrast media, and thromboembolic complications from catheterization of arteries that can lead to infarctions, strokes, arterial dissections, pseudoaneurysms, and arterial bleeding. Using cerebral angiography as an example, the risk of a neurologic complication such as a transient ischemic attack or stroke is about 4% and the risk of developing a permanent neurologic deficit from a disabling stroke is about 1%.	Though the contrast agent is the same, peripheral IV injections significantly reduce the risk of thromboembolic complications.
Conventional angiography is a projection imaging technique that produces 2D images of 3D structures. Therefore blood vessels and other structures that overlap in the direction of the projection may obscure the site of interest.	CTA is a 3D examination. Overlying structures may be eliminated by postprocessing.
Conventional angiography is an intraluminal technique and as such does not display mural abnormalities or true mural dimensions, making percent stenosis and aneurysm size measurements difficult.	CT is a cross-sectional imaging modality that exhibits excellent soft tissue discrimination. As such, it has utility for depicting mural thrombus, calcifications, and true mural dimensions.

From Napel SA: Principles and techniques of 3D spiral CT Angiography. In Fishman EK and Jeffrey RB Jr, editors: *Spiral CT: principles, techniques and clinical applications,* New York, 1995, Raven Press.

The table speed can be calculated using Equation 18-1 or 18-2.

(Kalender, 1995):

$$d = R/T \qquad (18\text{-}1)$$

$$d = S \times P/t \qquad (18\text{-}2)$$

where s = slice collimation
  p = pitch
  t = scan time (secs) per 360 degrees rotation

Collimation influences spatial resolution (z-axis or longitudinal resolution). A collimation of 1 mm (used when the Circle of Willis is of interest) results in tube heating before the completion of a specified scan length. A solution to this problem is using lower mA values than those used in conventional CT, keeping in mind the trade-off between noise and contrast resolution. A 3-mm collimation is generally used in abdominal CTA for demonstrating the celiac, superior mesenteric, and renal arteries (Jeffrey, 1998).

The pitch is the ratio of the distance the table travels per 360 degrees rotation to the collimation width. As the pitch increases, volume coverage increases, but spatial resolution decreases (the slice-sensitivity profile broadens). In this regard, Kuszyk and Fishman (1998) suggest that a pitch of up to 2 provides acceptable coverage of the area of interest and increases the effective slice thickness minimally, compared with a pitch of 1 with 180-degree linear interpolation.

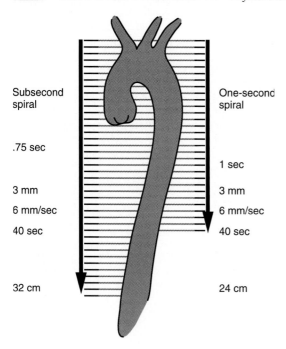

Subsecond
spiral

.75 sec

3 mm

6 mm/sec

40 sec

32 cm

One-second
spiral

1 sec

3 mm

6 mm/sec

40 sec

24 cm

FIG. 18-1. In CTA, a subsecond spiral/helical scanner increases volume coverage without a loss of image quality, compared with its counterpart 1 second spiral/helical scanner. (From Kuszyk BS, Fishman EK: Technical aspects of CT angiography. In Raymond HW, Zwiebel WJ, Swartz JD, editors: *Semin Ultrasound CT MRI.* 19(5), 1998.)

Also influencing the quality of the CTA examination is careful selection of kVp and mA values and the image reconstruction intervals. The selection of kVp and mA used in CTA examinations is usually determined by the size of the patient and the level of noise in the images. To maintain a good signal-to-noise ratio, mA and kVp must be adjusted accordingly. In this respect, Kalender (1995) points out that although 120 kVp is commonly used, the mA values selected are based on the size of the patient's body section to be examined. Noise also affects of the mA values. Kalender (1995) also notes that it is not necessary to increase these values for spiral CTA examinations compared with standard spiral examinations of the same body part.

The image reconstruction interval refers to the spacing between the center of the slices. Reconstruction intervals are important because they play a role in the quality of the 3D-CTA images. Overlapping reconstructions improve the 3D image quality and several investigators report that a minimum of 50% overlap with reconstructing intervals of 1 mm optimizes image quality in 3D-CTA ex-

aminations (Smith and Fishman, 1998; Kuszyk and Fishman, 1998).

Another important acquisition parameter that is of significance in CTA and is facilitated by modern state-of-the-art CT scanners is subsecond spiral/helical scanning. These scanners provide increased volume coverage (Fig. 18-1) without a loss of image quality. In general, these scanners can provide about 33% increased performance compared with 1 sec scanners; 33% more volume coverage; 33% faster scanning for the same volume (improved temporal resolution); and 33% thinner slices (for the same volume), which provides improved spatial resolution, as well as better 3D images. In addition, subsecond spiral/helical scanning reduces artifacts resulting from motion.

Contrast Medium Administration

Imaging the contrast while it is in the vascular area of interest during the CTA examination is a critical step in the acquisition of images. Contrast injection techniques take into consideration the volume of contrast needed to opacify vascular regions; the contrast injection rate; and the timing between the start of contrast medium injection and the start of the spiral/helical scan. Measuring the contrast circulation times for different patients is important in CTA to ensure that images are recorded when flow-in of contrast is optimum in the vessels. To help with this task, various automated systems such as SmartPrep (GE Medical Systems), Siemens Combined Applications to Reduce Exposure (CARE Bolus), and Toshiba's SureStart are available commercially. These products ensure optimized contrast monitoring in CTA. Fig. 18-2 demonstrates such optimization using Toshiba's SureStart package. The change in CT number on the image, which is displayed in real time, is monitored by the monitoring scan. When the contrast reaches a set value (threshold), the monitoring scan ends, and the main scan (helical scan) starts automatically, to provide images when contrast flow in the vessels is optimum. Fig. 18-3 details the essential steps for operating SureStart.

Consideration must be given to the size of the needle and the site of the injection. Various-size intravenous angiocatheters, such as 18- or 20-gauge or 20- or 22-gauge, are commonly inserted into a medial antecubital vein, using volumes of about 20 ml of nonionic contrast injected at rates that vary from 3 to 4 ml/sec to 5 ml/sec. Parameters for neurovascular applications of CTA are given in Table 18-2.

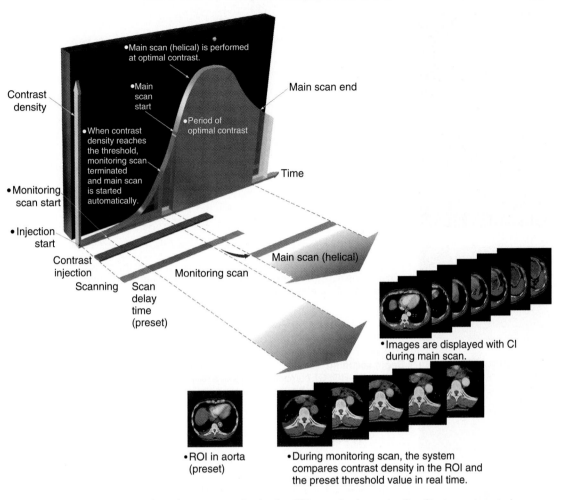

FIG. 18-2. Optimization of contrast monitoring for CTA examinations using SureStart, an automated package for optimal scan control for contrast studies. (Courtesy Toshiba America Medical Systems; Tustin, Calif.)

TABLE 18-2

CT Angiography Parameters for Extracranial Carotid Artery and Intracranial Circulation

	EXTRACRANIAL CAROTID	INTRACRANIAL CIRCULATION
Collimation	1-2 mm	1-2 mm
Table speed (pitch)	2-4 mm/sec (2)	2-3 mm/sec (1.5)
Reconstruction interval	1 mm	1 mm
Gantry rotation time	0.75-1 sec	0.75-1 sec
Contrast		
Rate	3 ml/sec	3 ml/sec
Volume	120 ml	120 ml
Delay	12 sec	15 sec
Volume of interest	C6-7 → C2-3	Circle of Willis
Rendering algorithm	VRT, MIP, Multiplanar	VRT, Surface

From Kuszyk BS, Beauchamp NJ, Fishman EK: Neurovascular applications of CT angiography. In Raymond HW, Zwiebel WJ, Swartz JD, editors: *Semin ultrasound CT MRI,* 19(5), 1998.

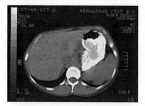

1 Observe the target vessel
The operator views an axial image which includes the structure to be monitored for contrast arrival.

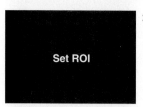

2 Define an ROI and set target threshold
A threshold CT value is assigned to the ROI for automatic initiation of the scan. SureStart operating techniques and preset delay times may be selected at this time.

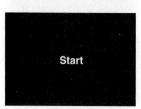

3 Begin SureStart
SureStart preparation is selected from the touch panel of the console. The contrast injection is begun, and the START key is pressed. SureStart imaging commences at the end of a pre-set delay.

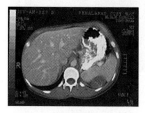

4 Begin scanning
When the ROI CT number matches or exceeds the threshold value, or when the NEXT SCAN key is hit, the next scan in the exam plan sequence is initiated.

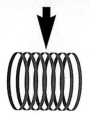

NOTE: SureStart is a selectable element which can be included in any exam plan, and can be followed by helical or dynamic acquisition. SureStart may be interrupted at any time using the ABORT KEY.

FIG. 18-3. The four essential steps to operating SureStart, Toshiba's automated system for optimized contrast monitoring in CTA. (Courtesy Toshiba America Medical Systems; Tustin, Calif.)

Another CTA parameter that is essential for optimum image quality is the orientation of the vessel under study with respect to the axial direction. Such orientation influences the accuracy of luminal measurements (Kuszyk and Fishman, 1998). Vessels perpendicular to the scan plane (axial plane) are imaged at a better resolution than vessels parallel to the scan plane. In the latter situation, the spatial resolution is a function of the collimation width instead of the pixel size (Huppert et al, 1994). Yee (1995) also indicates that a collimation of 3 mm will result in volume averaging, which affects the visualization of vessels smaller than 3 mm in size. Also, vessel edges might be seen as bigger than they really are, particularly if the vessel is oriented to the scan plane. This of course leads to an artifact that Charnsangavej et al (1994) called *blooming*.

POSTPROCESSING TECHNIQUES: VISUALIZATION TOOLS

The algorithms used to display 3D images from the axial data set were described in detail earlier. These algorithms are postprocessing techniques or visualization tools, which are used quite exten-

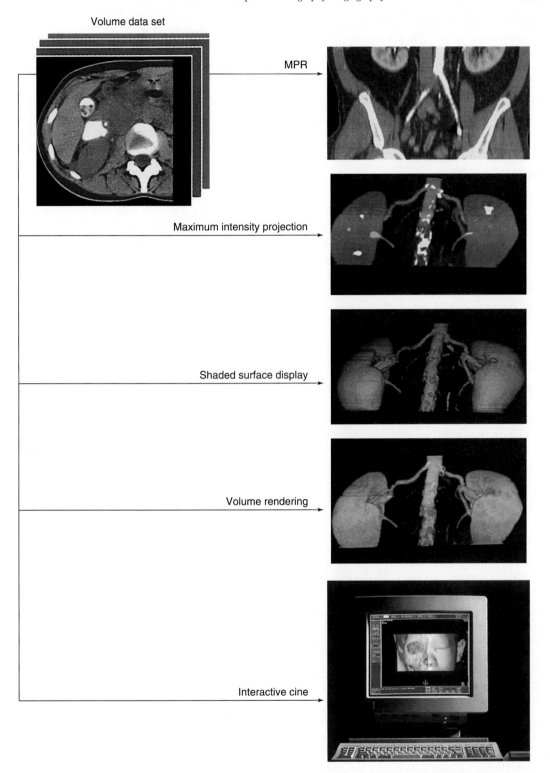

FIG. 18-4. Five 3D visualization tools for use in CTA. Each of the tools uses data from the axial images to produce 3D images and allows the user to interact with the data to facilitate viewing a set of images in real-time. (Courtesy Picker International; Cleveland, Ohio; courtesy Toshiba America Medical Systems; Tustin, Calif.)

sively in CTA. Currently, the following techniques are commonplace in CTA (Fig. 18-4):

1. Multiplanar reconstruction (MPR) including curved MPR
2. Maximum intensity projection (MIP)
3. Shaded surface display (SSD)
4. Volume rendering (VR)
5. Interactive cine

Multiplanar Reconstruction

MPR is the first visualization tool for use in CTA. It is simple and faster to reconstruct than any other 3D technique and enables visualization of the volume data set in any plane including curved planes. However, MPR is less useful in a number of applications, such as visualization of complex vessels (Circle of Willis) and intracranial AVMs. In addition, no editing is required when using MPR in CTA examinations.

Shaded Surface Display

The SSD visualization tool requires little editing to remove overlapping structures obscuring the vessels. It is faster than VR because it uses only a small fraction of the total axial data set. This characteristic can result in artifact generation and images that are not very accurate. SSD images are useful in the display of vascular relationships, vessel origins, and the surface contours of vessels.

Maximum Intensity Projection

The MIP visualization tool is the most frequently used in CTA examinations to display the structure of vessels. It is popular in CT and MRI and is more accurate than SSD (Kuszyk and Fishman, 1998). Although MIP has proved useful in CTA, it requires editing to remove unwanted structures, such as bone and calcified plaques, that prevent the observer from viewing intravascular detail. Additionally, the MIP algorithm can produce what Napel (1995) refers to as the *beading* or *stair-step artifact* (belonging to the category of "aliasing" artifacts, related to data sampling frequency). This can be reduced by overlapping reconstruction intervals. The MIP can be used successfully to separate out vascular calcifications, lumen thrombus, and intravascular thrombus (Oldendorf and Weber, 1997).

An example of the application of these visualization tools, MPR, SSD and MIP, to various clinical situations is presented in the following box.

Volume Rendering

Another postprocessing 3D visualization tool that is becoming more and more popular for use in CTA is volume rendering (Kuszyk and Fishman, 1998; Kuszyk et al, 1998; Johnson et al, 1998; and Leclerc et al, 1995). Volume rendering uses all of the information in the axial data set to display internal structures (soft tissues, vascular and bony anatomy), as well as provide accurate vessel diameters and 3D vascular relationships. In the past, volume rendering was performed only on powerful workstations, and not only was it expensive but also time consuming. Today, volume rendering can be performed "at real-time frame rates (5 to 10 frames per second) using relatively inexpensive workstations" (Kuszyk and Fishman, 1998). Fig. 18-5 provides an example of clinical images generated by using three 3D visualization tools in CTA, for the abdominal aorta.

SSD and MIP processing techniques use data from surface and voxel intensities respectively. However, volume rendering uses all the data in the

---

APPLICATION OF VISUALIZATION TOOLS TO VARIOUS CLINICAL AND MEDICAL CONDITIONS

MPR
- The fastest postprocessing modality
- Simple handling
- Useful for all problem-solving tasks
- Display of arteries and veins by means of different contrasts
- Thrombotic parts in aneurysms
- Calcifications in aneurysms
- Dissections
- Tumor-vessel topography

3D SURFACE DISPLAY
- Vessel anatomy
- Vessel-bone relationship
- No information about free vessel lumen
- Osseous destruction in tumor patients

MIP
- 2D angiographic display of vessels rotating in all spatial axes
- Pathologic vessel calcifications
- Parallel display of arteries and veins
- Therapeutic planning: PTA, stent, operation
- Postoperative checking of vessel interventions

From Oldendorf M, Weber P: Postprocessing techniques in CT angiography, *Electromedica* 65:21-26, 1997.

axial volume data set. Therefore all voxel information is used in the processing. Developments in computer graphics hardware now make it possible to process volume rendering images at higher speeds and higher frame rates (5 to 20 frames/sec), thus resulting in real-time rendering.

Kuszyk and Fishman (1998) describe four volume-rendering (VR) parameters intended to enhance the "accuracy and the practicality of CT angiography." These parameters include windowing (window width and window level), opacity, brightness, and accuracy. Although windowing allows observers to alter the image contrast and density to suit their viewing needs, opacity

refers to the degree that structures close to the user obscure structures which are further away. Opacity can be varied from 0% to 100%. Higher opacity values produce an appearance similar to surface rendering, which helps to display complex 3D relationships. Lower opacity values allow the user to "see through" structures and can be very useful for such applications as seeing a free-floating thrombus within the lumen of a vein or evaluating bony abnormalities such as tumors that are located below the cortical surface (Kuszyk and Fishman, 1998).

Brightness, on the other hand, provides the observer with the ability to alter the image appearance from 0% to 100%. Kuszyk and Fishman (1998) report that a brightness setting of 100% is useful for a wide range of examinations. Finally, the volume rendering provides more accurate results for a number of vascular problems (stenosis, for example) than SSD and MIP 3D visualization tools (Kuszyk et al, 1997; Johnson et al, 1997). However, Ebert et al (1998) have shown that VR is not without problems. One such problem is that of *inter-observer variability*. Currently, techniques are being developed that will help to maintain consistency in diagnostic interpretation (Kuszyk and Fishman, 1998).

These 3D visualization tools are described in detail in Chapter 17.

Interactive Cine

The developments in image processing and display of 3D images have led to interactive cine viewing and display. *Interactive cine* refers to the viewing and evaluation of the images in the axial data set by panning through the set of images. Because

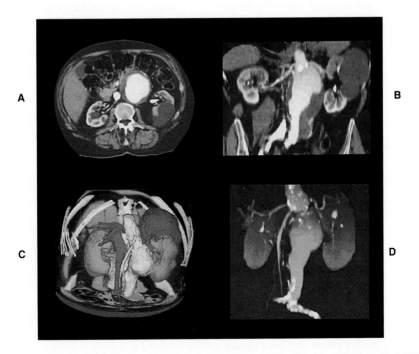

FIG. 18-5. The use of three 3D visualization tools: **B,** Curved MPR; **C,** 3D multitissue; **D,** MIP. These are used to produce 3D images from the 2D axial data set for abdominal aorta CTA examination. (Courtesy Elscint; Hackensack, NJ.)

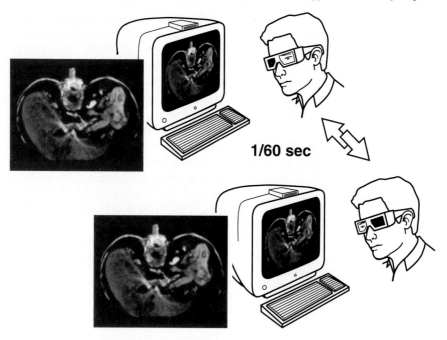

FIG. 18-6. Stereoscopic display technique uses shutters in viewing glasses to show images from slightly different perspectives to the right and left eyes. This technique is relatively inexpensive and greatly enhances the 3D effect of the volume rendered images. (From Kuszyk BS, Fishman EK: Technical aspects of CT angiography. In Raymond HW, Zwiebel WJ, Swartz, JD, editors: *Seminars in Ultrasound, CT and MRI*, 19(5), 1998.)

each of these images is separated only slightly in time, the rapid display of the set of axial images provide the effect of motion (much like a cine film). Johnson et al (1998) notes that although axial images can be used to provide a diagnosis, 3D images help to demonstrate anatomic relationships and show vessels that run along the z axis.

Stereoscopic Viewing

Another display technique used to enhance the viewing of 3D images in CTA is stereoscopic viewing (Fig. 18-6). This is an experimental technique (not used routinely as yet) described by Kuszyk and Fishman (1998) to enhance the different 3D relationships among various structures. The investigators explain *stereoscopic display* as techniques that

> Convey perspective and depth cues by providing slightly different images to the left and right eyes. This effect can be achieved by slightly altering the perspective of alternating images and using shutter devices incorporated into viewing eye wear which open and close to alternate frames between the left and right eyes. Head motion parallax allows the

viewer to see an object from different angles as his or her head moves with respect to the display...preliminary experiments in our laboratory show that both radiologists and non-radiologists prefer the stereoscopic display to conventional displays. We routinely view 3D medical images using both conventional and stereoscopic displays.

REFERENCES

Charnsangavej C et al: Artifacts in Helical CT angiography with MPR and MIP: experimental evaluation (abstract), *Radiology* 193:138, 1994.

Ebert DS, Heath DG, Kuszyk BS: Evaluating the potential and problems of three-dimensional computed tomography measurements of arterial stenosis, *J Dig Imag* 11:1-8, 1998.

Fishman E, Jeffrey RB Jr: CT Angiography. In Raymond HW, Zwiebel WJ, Swartz JD, editors: *Seminars in Ultrasound, CT and MRI*, Vol 19, No 5. Oct. 1998.

Huppert PE et al: Small-vessel spiral CT angiography: experimental evaluation of acquisition and reconstruction parameters (abstract), *Radiology* 193:139, 1994.

Johnson PT et al: Interactive three-dimensional volume rendering of spiral CT data, current applications in the thorax, *Radiographics* 18:165-1987, 1998.

Kalender WA: Spiral CT angiography. In Goldman LW and Fowlkes JB, editors: *Medical CT and Ultrasound*, New London, Connecticut, 1995, American Association of Physicists in Medicine.

Kuszyk BS, Beauchamp NJ, Fishman EK: Neurovascular applications of CT angiography, *Semin Ultrasound CT MRI* 19(5):394-404, 1998.

Kuszyk BS, Fishman EK: Technical aspects of CT angiography. In Raymond HW, Zwiebel WJ, Swartz JD, editors: *Semin Ultrasound CT MRI*, 19(5), 1998.

Leclerc X et al: Carotid artery stenosis, *Stroke* 26(9): 1577-1581, 1995.

Napel SA: Principles and techniques of 3D spiral CT angiography. In Fishman EK, editor: *Spiral CT: principles, techniques and clinical applications*, New York, 1995, Raven Press.

Oldendorf M, Weber P: Postprocessing techniques in CT angiography, *Electromedica* 65:21-26, 1997.

Rawlings LH: Non-invasive cardiovascular imaging: focus on spiral CT angiography, *Appl Radiol* March 1995, pp 28-32.

Yee D: Small-vessel CT angiography, *Appl Radiol* March 1995, pp 21-27.

Virtual Reality Imaging

2D DATA SETS

The increasing size of data sets (2D axial images) obtained from spiral/helical CT scanners has created a range of applications including CT fluoroscopy, CT angiography (CTA), 3D imaging and, most recently, CT virtual reality imaging.

Spiral/helical single-slice and multislice CT scanners produce very large 2D contiguous data sets of the anatomy under investigation. Hundreds of images can be obtained and presented to the radiologist for interpretation and diagnosis. In general, these images are examined one at a time, and observers must rely on their mental reconstruction abilities to visualize the anatomy in three dimensions using the 2D images. The perception of 3D anatomy from 2D images often is difficult for some individuals because of the complexity of the structures in terms of their geometric shapes. One solution is a 3D image processing technique, referred to as *virtual reality imaging*.

OVERVIEW OF VIRTUAL REALITY IMAGING

Virtual reality is a branch of computer science that immerses users in a computer-generated environment and allows them to interact with 3D scenes. The use of virtual reality concepts to the creation of inner views of tubular structures is called *virtual endoscopy* (Vining, 1996). As explained by Higgins et al (1998):

> A virtual endoscope is a graphics-based software system used for simulating endoscopic exploration inside a 3D image. In virtual endoscopy, a 3D image acts as a 'copy' or virtual environment, representing the scanned anatomy. With the use of computer-

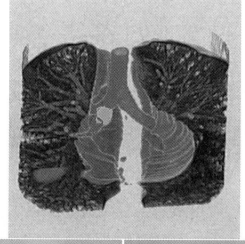

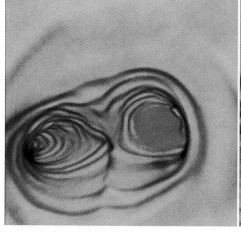
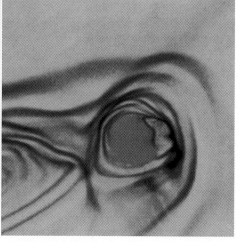

FIG. 19-1. The appearance of CT virtual endoscopy images of the bronchus. **A,** Holographic projection helps the observer to localize exact position and shows the "flow in flight path." **B** and **C,** Virtual endoscopic images. (Courtesy Picker International; Cleveland, Ohio.)

based rendering tools, a virtual endoscope produces endoluminal surface views inside the virtual environment similar to those from a real endoscope. A virtual endoscope permits essentially unrestricted exploration because it cannot traumatize the virtual environment.

A real endoscope uses optical video-assisted technology to help physicians interactively examine the inside of tubular anatomic structures. Because of the nature of the physical device, the patient may experience some discomfort, and other risks may also exist.

APPLICATIONS OF VIRTUAL ENDOSCOPY

Virtual endoscopy is evolving into a clinical tool with a wide range of applications. It has been used to evaluate the colon (virtual colonoscopy) (Vining, 1999), airways (virtual bronchoscopy) (Hooper, 1999), paranasal sinuses, bladder, spinal canal, and, more recently, the pancreatic and common bile ducts (virtual cholangiopancreatoscopy) (Prassopoulos et al, 1998) and the inner ear (virtual labyrinthoscopy) (Tomandl et al, 2000). Fig. 19-1 shows an example of images from CT virtual endoscopy of the bronchus.

ADVANTAGES AND LIMITATIONS

The various features of virtual endoscopy and real endoscopy have been described in the literature (Hooper, 1999; Vining, 1999; Higgins et al, 1998; Blezek and Robb, 1997). Early results indicate that virtual endoscopy offers unique features and advantages for gathering both endoluminal and extraluminal information. (Table 19-1 presents a comparison of the features of virtual and real bronchoscopy.) Virtual endoscopy can also reduce complications (e.g., infection and perforation) that could arise from real endoscopy.

Virtual endoscopy is not without disadvantages, such as its high cost, lack of texture and quantitative data of the anatomy under study, and problems with interactive exploration (Higgins et al, 1998).

TECHNICAL CONSIDERATIONS

Several technical requirements must be taken into account when considering CT virtual endoscopy. The four fundamental requirements are data acquisition, image preprocessing, 3D rendering, and image display and analysis (Fig. 19-2).

Data Acquisition

The first step in virtual endoscopy imaging is careful selection of the scan parameters to be used for creating the data set. These parameters, which optimize image display while reducing the radiation dose to the patient, include slice thickness, spiral/helical pitch, slice reconstruction overlap, and the scanning exposure technique (i.e., kVp, mA/revolution, and scan time/revolution).

TABLE 19-1

Comparison of Features of Virtual and Real Bronchoscopy

VIRTUAL BRONCHOSCOPY	REAL BRONCHOSCOPY
Imaging environment is a virtual environment as captured in a 3D CT image.	Imaging environment is illuminated in vivo endoluminal regions.
Awareness is enhanced by the many display tools.	Video is the only display. tool.
Many quantitative measurements can be taken.	Quantitation is limited.
Viewing direction is unrestricted.	Only frontal views are possible.
Views inside and outside solid structures are possible.	Only endoluminal views are possible.
Viewing geometry is controllable.	Perspective is fixed.
User can track 3D position during navigation.	User must remember position of scope.
Multiple simultaneous views are possible.	User can see only one view at a time.
Cine sequences can be recorded.	High-quality video can be recorded.
No information on the mucosal surface can be obtained.	Detailed information on the mucosal surface can be obtained.
Performance of interventional procedures with views is not possible without linkage to a real bronchoscope.	Real intervention is possible.
View quality is limited by image resolution.	High-resolution video is used.

From Hooper KD: CT bronchoscopy, *Semin Ultrasound, CT, MR* 20(1):10-15, 1999.

The selection of these parameters has been discussed in the literature for several virtual endoscopic examinations. For CT bronchoscopy, for example, Hooper (1999) reports that a 2-mm slice thickness, a pitch of 1, and a 75% slice reconstruction overlap produce significantly better virtual images than a slice thickness of 4 to 8 mm, a pitch of 1.5 to 2, and a 25% to 50% slice overlap.

The imaging parameters represent a trade-off between radiation dose and image quality. The effect of slice thickness, for example, on image quality is demonstrated in Fig. 19-3. Table 19-2 presents suggested techniques for virtual studies in bronchoscopy, colonoscopy, and angioscopy.

Image Preprocessing

Preprocessing of image data is the next step after data acquisition, and it is intended to optimize the images before they are subject to further processing and analysis. Preprocessing involves the use of various noise filtering algorithms, image segmentation, defining paths through tubular structures, and other tools, such as classification, "cropping," and "cutting."

Image segmentation is another important step in the creation of virtual reality images in CT. Segmentation can be performed by the operator (semiautomatic), or it can be done automatically. In the semiautomatic mode, the user selects objects to include the data set through the use of windowing. These objects are then prepared for rendering. For bronchoscopy the result of this procedure defines a 3D image mask that, as Higgins et al (1998) explained, "excludes voxels not belonging to the lungs or major airways. All mediastinal structures, bones, and other extraneous structures are removed."

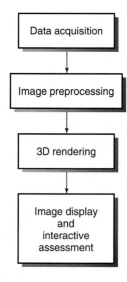

FIG. 19-2. Technical requirements for CT virtual endoscopy.

3D Rendering

Two rendering techniques used in virtual CT endoscopy are surface rendering and volume rendering. Both have been used in various virtual CT examinations, but most experts agree that surface rendering is not best suited for use in CT VR imaging (Fleiter et al, 1997; Higgins et al, 1998) because of problems such as the production of partial volume averaging artifacts.

Volume rendering provides the best results because it produces optimum visualization of the anatomy (e.g., mucosal patterns and lesions), minimizes partial volume averaging artifacts, and adds lifelike reality to images (Hooper, 1999, 2000; Vining, 1996; Tomandl, 2000). Hybrid rendering, or techniques that combine features of both surface and volume rendering algorithms, are under investigation (Vining, 1999).

TABLE 19-2

Suggested Techniques for Three Types of CT Virtual Endoscopic Studies*

STUDY	kVp	mA/REVOLUTIONS	SCAN TIME/ REVOLUTION	PITCH FACTOR	COLLIMATED SLICE THICKNESS (mm)	IMAGE INDEX (mm)
Bronchoscopy	120	150 mA/30 rev	1 sec/rev	1	5	1
Colonoscopy	110	100 mA/45 rev	1 sec/rev	1.25	5	2
Angioscopy	12	150 mA/30 rev	1 sec/rev	1.25	5	2

Courtesy Picker International; Cleveland, Ohio.
*Maximum z axis spiral spatial resolution (each frame)   15 Lp/cm
Maximum length of single-run organ coverage (1.5 pitch factor)   105 cm
Reformatting capability (compositing)   4D angiography
Reformatting time   <1 sec/view
Study acquisition/preparation time (movie loop)   10 min

Image Display and Analysis

Because of the nature of the visualizations and interactivity needed for optimum viewing and evaluation of images, image display and analysis in CT virtual reality imaging require powerful computer workstations. As an alternative, some CT consoles may also facilitate virtual endoscopy. The console in Fig. 19-4 can handle both data acquisition and advanced visualization processing operations.

Virtual CT endoscopy includes image analysis techniques that allow the user to assess images interactively using a wide range of software

A   B   C

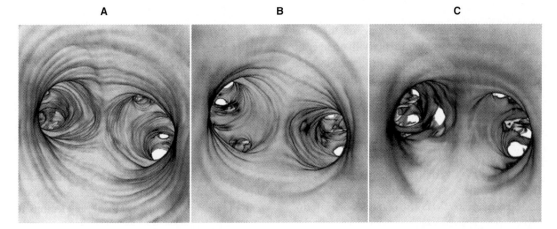

FIG. 19-3. The effect of slice thickness on image quality in CT virtual endoscopy. Thin (2 mm) slices produce sharper images (**A**) compared with 4-mm (**B**) and 8-mm (**C**) thick slices. These images were obtained with 50% reconstruction overlap using a pitch of 1. (From Hooper KD: CT bronchoscopy, *Semin US, CT, MRI* 20(1):10-15, 1999.)

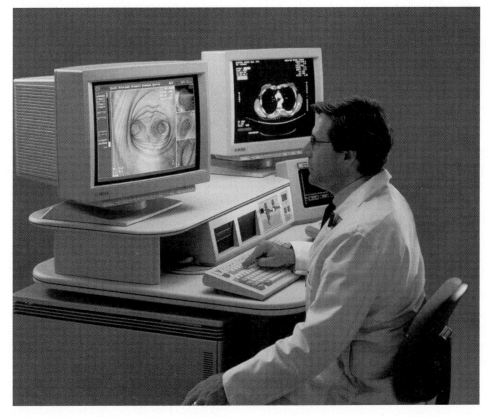

FIG. 19-4. A workstation for CT virtual reality image display and analysis. (Courtesy Picker International; Cleveland, Ohio.)

tools. With these tools the user can do the following:

- Pan through a stack of 2D images (axial CT display mode)
- "Fly through" the 3D-rendered anatomic models (virtual endoscopic mode)
- Navigate the 3D anatomic models using automated flight path programs
- Split or unfold anatomic models
- Identify pathologic conditions through computer-aided detection
- Depict topography of inner colonic surfaces as flattened structures (panoramic endoscopic display mode)

In a recent study conducted by Beaulieu et al (1999), the researchers found that panoramic endoscopy is more sensitive than virtual endoscopy for detection of polyps.

SOFTWARE FOR INTERACTIVE IMAGE ASSESSMENT

A wide range of software tools for interactive image assessment is available. All these packages feature a variety of visual and quantitative tools specifically for use in virtual endoscopy imaging in CT and MRI. For example, Higgins et al, (1998) used QUICKSEE and VIDA in their virtual bronchoscopy studies; Blezek and Robb (1997) used ANALYZE software, developed and used at The Mayo Clinic in Rochester, Minnesota. Several features of two popular advanced visualization tools, Voyager (Picker International) and 3D Navigator (General Electric Medical Systems) are discussed here.

Voyager

Voyager is a CT virtual endoscopy advanced visualization package that can provide real time "fly through" within and around tubular anatomy in the same manner that a real endoscope is used. Voyager features an intuitive user interface that provides considerable flexibility in interactive image assessment. For example, mouse technology is used to guide the user through the anatomy. In addition, Voyager can provide movie loop presentations, which can be recorded on videotape and used for remote communications.

A unique feature of Voyager is compositing (a volumetric imaging technique that displays bone, soft tissues, and vessels at the same time), also called 4D angiography, which provides 3D images with a fourth dimension, opacity. Other features of the Voyager visualization package are listed in the box on this page.

FEATURES OF THE VOYAGER VISUALIZATION TOOL

- Voyager 4D angiographic reformations allow visualization of soft tissue and organ surface.
- Color can be automatically assigned to various tissues or structures to enhance presentation and communication.
- Perspective reformatting with cut screen options provide versatility in viewing modes.
- CSD technology provides dose efficiency, superior spatial resolution, and continuous detector calibration, necessary ingredients for extended 3D reformations.
- PQ-Series CT scanner can acquire long, single-acquisition data sets with an extended pitch, increasing speed and coverage capabilities while maintaining z axis resolution and increasing CT endoscopy capabilities.
- Voyager can create images using shaded surface display (SSD).
- AutoNavigation automatically determines the center of the organ examined and plots an appropriate path down the structure of interest
- AutoAlert automatically prevents traversal of an organ wall during routine navigation, ensuring a course through the center of the structure.

Courtesy Picker International; Cleveland, Ohio.

Voyager can be used in a wide range of clinical applications including preendoscopic evaluation of lesion screening and planning of endoscopic or surgical procedures. It also can be used to explore hollow anatomic structures such as the bronchus, colon, stomach, blood vessels, upper respiratory tract and larynx, paranasal sinuses, bladder, and spinal canal. Examples of Voyager images are shown in Figs. 19-1 and 19-5.

3D Navigator

The 3D Navigator advanced visualization software provides a single icon-driven interface for ease of use and interaction with virtual endoscopic images. For example, it allows real-time navigation of structures, unique "fly through" of tubular structures, enhanced visualization capabilities for viewing inside cavities, smooth or edge detail viewing, and endoluminal viewing of 3D surface-rendered abnormalities of tubular structures (e.g., polyps, tumors, clots, vascular strictures or aneurysms, and blockages). The 3D Navigator also allows the user to "fly around" the outside of the anatomy such as the circle of Willis.

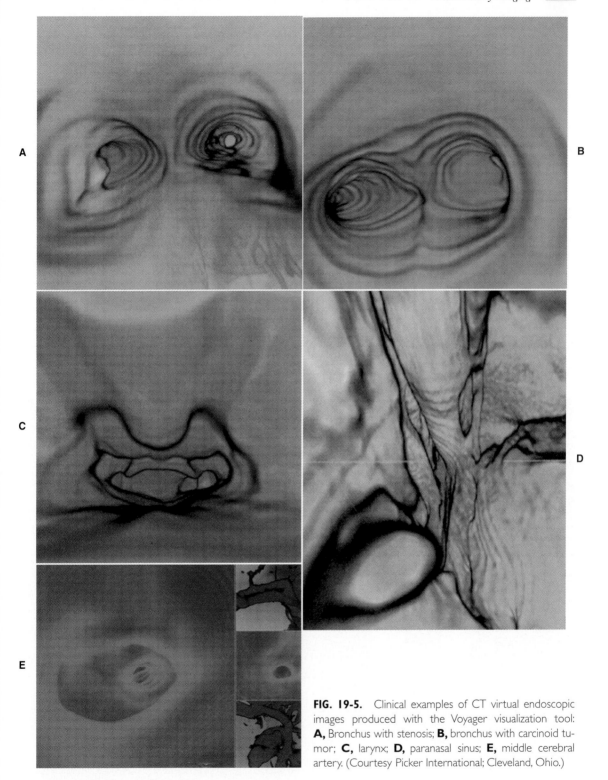

FIG. 19-5. Clinical examples of CT virtual endoscopic images produced with the Voyager visualization tool: **A,** Bronchus with stenosis; **B,** bronchus with carcinoid tumor; **C,** larynx; **D,** paranasal sinus; **E,** middle cerebral artery. (Courtesy Picker International; Cleveland, Ohio.)

FLIGHT PATH PLANNING

Fig. 19-6 shows the difference between surface-rendered and volume-rendered images in CT virtual endoscopy. Fig. 19-7 shows the use of the navigation tool, one of the visualization tools of

Voyager. Three orthogonal projections are created from the image data set sent to the computer workstation to assist the user in navigating through the anatomy. First, the navigation path is outlined by placing markers along the anatomy to be exam-

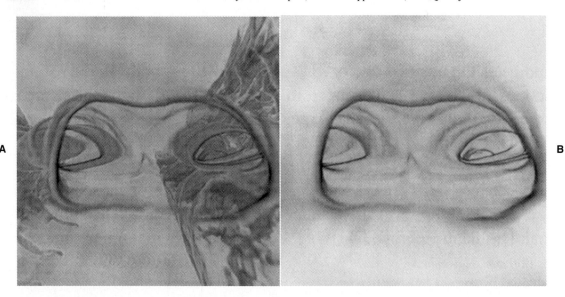

FIG. 19-6. Visual comparison of a surface-rendered image (**A**) and a volume-rendered image (**B**) in CT virtual endoscopy. Volume rendering not only improves image quality but also reduces artifacts caused by partial volume averaging. (From Hooper KD: CT bronchoscopy, *Semin Ultrasound, CT, MR* 20(1):10-15, 1999.)

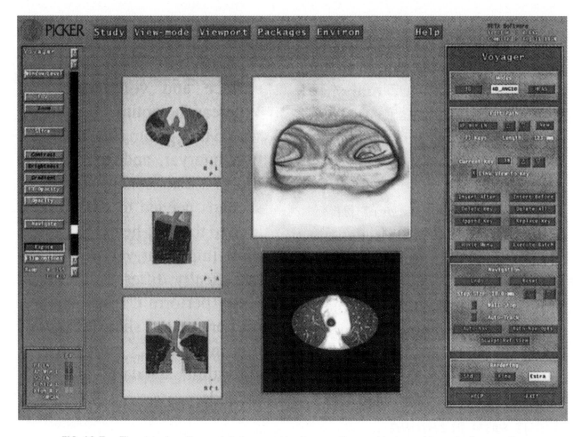

FIG. 19-7. The virtual reality workstation provides three orthogonal holographic projections on the left to localize the observer's exact position and "flown flight path." The central color working screen shows the current image. The bottom middle image shows a reconstructed slice through the observer's position and can be provided in the sagittal, coronal, oblique, or parallel to field of view plane. (From Hooper KD: CT bronchoscopy, *Semin Ultrasound, CT, MRI* 20(1):10-15, 1999.)

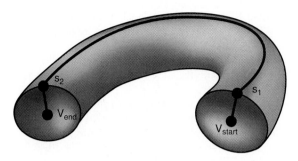

FIG. 19-8. An example of planning a flight path in virtual endoscopy. (Paik DS et al: Automated flight path planning for virtual endoscopy, *Med Phys* 25(5):629-637, 1998.)

ined. This is followed by a "fly through" of the path. The active virtual image is shown in the middle of the screen.

Navigation

Successful navigation within the hollow anatomic region is essential so that structures of interest can be located and examined; such navigation depends on flight path algorithms. Because manual planning of flight paths can be time-consuming, algorithms have been developed that plan the flight paths automatically.

One such algorithm, described by Paik et al (1998), uses a virtual "camera" to fly through the anatomy. First, the camera's position and orientation (straight pointing and angled pointing) are defined. Then a sequence of views along a path can be rendered as a sequence of frames to make a virtual endoscopic movie. Fig. 19-8 presents an example of flight path planning. It shows a portion of a hollow anatomic structure in which a path has been defined. The path has three segments: start voxel (V_{start}) to S_1 segment, a segment from S_1 to S_2, and a segment from S_2 to an end voxel (V_{end}). The authors, Paik et al (1998), explain this initial path selection as follows:

> Our algorithm determines the voxel on the surface that is closest to the start voxel, S_1, and the voxel closest to the end voxel, S_2. With a goal voxel of V_{start}, the algorithm computes a Euclidean distance map for the union of the surface and the voxels in the V_{start} to S_1 line segment and the S_2 to V_{end} line segment. This distance map is computed by assigning the goal voxel a distance of zero and iteratively assigning neighbor voxels the minimum Euclidean distance along a voxel path back to the goal voxel in a breadth first traversal until all voxels are reached. The algorithm follows the shallowest descent to find a path connecting V_{end} to V_{start}.

THE FUTURE OF CT VIRTUAL ENDOSCOPY

CT virtual endoscopy is an evolving diagnostic imaging tool that is still in its infancy. Investigators involved in research and practical applications of virtual endoscopy have noted that its future is promising. It has great potential as a diagnostic tool for providing better visualization of various anatomic structures such as the colon, airways, and other tubular structures, from both outside and inside perspectives.

Developments in the technology for virtual endoscopy, such as digital image processing and computer visualization tools and automated techniques, can only lead to improvement of virtual endoscopy as a clinically useful tool. Multislice CT technology will have a significant impact on the accuracy of virtual endoscopy. The vast amount of data sets collected from a multislice CT scanner will generate much better virtual endoscopic images than those obtained with single-slice data sets (Kopecky, 1999).

Already, studies are under way to validate the clinical usefulness of CT virtual endoscopy in a wide range of applications including colonoscopy and bronchoscopy, which have received more attention in the literature because of the prevalence of colorectal and bronchogenic carcinoma (Vining, 1999; Hooper, 1999; Higgins et al, 1998). Some of these studies have shown that compared with real endoscopy, virtual endoscopy is much cheaper and risk free and causes the patient less discomfort.

As noted by Vining (1999), other factors must be considered before the use of virtual endoscopy becomes commonplace such as:

- It must be better than real endoscopy in detecting various anatomic structures and pathologic conditions.
- It should be easy to perform on patients and easy for technologists and radiologists to use.
- It should be available on all spiral/helical CT and MRI scanners.
- It must be accepted by primary care physicians and insurance companies.
- It must be accepted by the public.

VIRTUAL ENDOSCOPY ON THE INTERNET

The Internet currently offers a number of sites that provide not only 3D images but also virtual endoscopic images. More important, these sites offer the opportunity for "fly through" explorations of various anatomic regions. For example, the Wake Forest University School of Medicine website features a virtual endoscopy center that allows users to examine the school's "Free Flight" software, a virtual endoscopic system, and a virtual endoscopic image gallery (http://www.vec.bgsm.edu).

REFERENCES

Beaulieu CF et al: Display modes for CT colonography, *Radiology* 212:203-212, 1999.

Blezek DJ, Robb RA: Evaluating virtual endoscopy for clinical use, *J Digit Imaging* 10(3):51-55, 1997.

Fleiter T et al: Comparison of real-time virtual and fiberoptic bronchoscopy in patients with bronchial carcinoma: opportunities and limitations, *Am J Roentgenol* 169:1591-1595, 1997.

Higgins WE et al: Virtual bronchoscopy for three dimensional pulmonary image assessment: state of the art and future needs, *Radiographics* 18:761-778, 1998.

Hooper KD: CT bronchoscopy, *Semin Ultrasound, CT, MR* 20(1):10-15, 1999.

Hooper KD et al: Mucosal detail at CT virtual reality: Surface versus volume rendering, *Radiology* 214:517-522, 2000.

Kopecky KK: Multislice CT spirals past single-slice CT in diagnostic efficiency. *Diagn Imaging* 21(4): 36-42, 1999.

Paik DS et al: Automated flight path planning for virtual endoscopy, Med Phys 25(5):629-37, 1998.

Prassopoulos P et al: Development of virtual CT cholangiopancreatoscopy, *Radiology* 209:570-574, 1998.

Tomandl BF et al: Virtual labyrinthoscopy: visualization of the inner ear with interactive direct volume rendering, *Radiographics* 20:547-558, 2000.

Vining DJ: Virtual endoscopy: is it reality? *Radiology* 200:30-31, 1996.

Vining DJ: Virtual colonoscopy, *Semin Ultrasound CT MR* 20(1):56-60, 1999.

BIBLIOGRAPHY

Stoll E et al: A new filtering algorithm for medical magnetic resonance imaging and computer tomography images, *J Digit Imaging* 12(1):23-28, 1999.

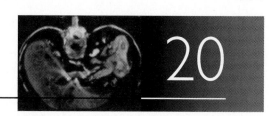

20

Computed Tomography of the Head, Neck, and Spine

R.A. NUGENT AND DONNA KEOBKE

CHAPTER *Outline*

Before the introduction of computed tomography (CT) in 1972, information about the brain generally was obtained through cerebral angiography or pneumoencephalography, and information about the spine was often obtained through myelography. These procedures were time consuming, painful for the patient, and potentially dangerous (Eisenberg, 1992). They did not provide direct information about brain substance, but rather gave only indirect information about the location of masses or the occurrence of other processes. Computed tomography revolutionized neuroradiology, providing excellent spatial and contrast resolution and allowing easy detection of intracranial abnormalities.

SECTIONAL ANATOMY

Axial or transverse images of the head or spine are viewed as though the observer were looking up at a section of the brain with the patient's right side on the viewer's left and the patient's left side on the viewer's right. Depending on the area of the body being assessed, coronal and (in some cases) oblique or even direct sagittal images can be obtained.

Head

Transverse Sections

Slices through the skull base (Fig. 20-1) give exquisite detail of the foramina, facial structures, pituitary fossa, and temporal bones. Cerebrospinal fluid (CSF) in the basal cisterns and ventricles helps define the anatomy, as does calcium in normal structures such as the choroid plexus, pineal gland, and falx cerebri. Differentiation of white and gray matter allows for definition of the basal ganglia, thalamus, and external and internal capsules.

Coronal Sections

Coronal images (Figs. 20-2 to 20-5) are particularly useful for assessing bone when the plane of the bone runs parallel to the axial slice. Coronal images therefore are valuable for scans of the floor and roof of the orbit, the skull base, and the top of

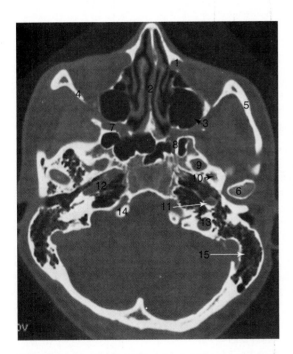

FIG. 20-1. A 1.5-mm thick axial slice through the base of the skull using the bone algorithm shows excellent spatial resolution. *1,* Opening of the nasolacrimal duct; *2,* nasal septum; *3,* maxillary sinus; *4,* lateral orbital wall; *5,* zygomatic arch; *6,* mandibular condyle; *7,* pterygopalatine fossa; *8,* vidian (pterygoid) canal; *9,* foramen ovale; *10,* foramen spinosum; *11,* ascending carotid canal; *12,* horizontal carotid canal; *13,* jugular fossa; *14,* jugular tubercle; *15,* mastoid air cells.

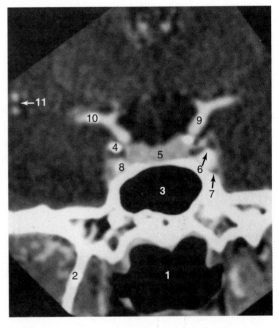

FIG. 20-2. Sella turcica. A 1.5-mm thick coronal slice through the sella turcica, obtained with intravenous contrast enhancement, demonstrates these structures: *1,* Oropharynx; *2,* lateral pterygoid plate; *3,* sphenoid sinus; *4,* anterior clinoid; *5,* pituitary gland; *6,* cranial nerve III; *7,* cranial nerve VI; *8,* cavernous portion of the internal carotid artery; *9,* supraclinoid portion of the internal carotid artery; *10,* middle cerebral artery; *11,* branches of the middle cerebral artery.

the cranial vault. The pituitary gland is well defined as a fairly rectangular structure within the sella turcica that is intersected in the midline, slightly posteriorly, by the pituitary stalk. The cranial nerves, in the cavernous sinus, can be identified on either side of the pituitary.

Coronal images of the temporal bone can highlight the relationships of the ossicles and structures along the medial wall of the middle ear, including the facial canal, oval window, and lateral semicircular canal. Coronal images intersect the tentorium and demonstrate its tentlike appearance. They help define whether a lesion is supratentorial or infratentorial, which aids in surgical planning.

A tumor that abuts a ventricle can be assessed in the coronal plane to determine whether it arises from or is extrinsic to the ventricle.

Sagittal Sections

Sagittal sections are not used routinely in most institutions. They are used only occasionally as a special procedure in which special apparatus is available to allow this positioning. Although sagittal images can demonstrate anatomy satisfactorily, they seldom provide significant information that cannot be obtained on good coronal or axial images.

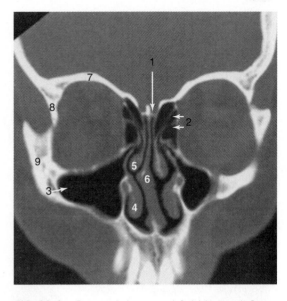

FIG. 20-4. Paranasal sinuses and facial bones. A 3-mm thick coronal image using the bone algorithm demonstrates the air-containing paranasal sinuses and nasal airway. *1,* Cribriform plate; *2,* ethmoid sinuses; *3,* maxillary sinus; *4,* inferior turbinate; *5,* middle turbinate; *6,* nasal septum; *7,* roof of the orbit; *8,* lateral orbital wall; *9,* zygoma.

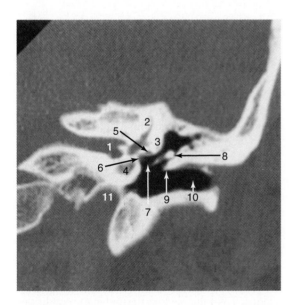

FIG. 20-3. Temporal bone. A 1-mm coronal image through the left temporal bone using the high-resolution bone algorithm is demonstrated. The thinness of the slice, as well as the smaller field of view, helps maximize the spatial resolution. *1,* Internal auditory canal; *2,* superior semicircular canal; *3,* lateral semicircular canal; *4,* cochlea; *5,* horizontal portion of the facial canal; *6,* oval window; *7,* stapes; *8,* malleus; *9,* Chausse spur; *10,* external auditory canal; *11,* carotid canal.

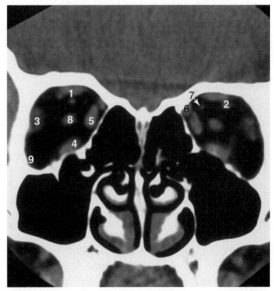

FIG. 20-5. Orbits. A 3-mm thick coronal view of the orbits, obtained without intravenous contrast enhancement, demonstrates that orbital fat produces excellent contrast, resulting in good definition of the extraocular muscles and optic nerve. *1,* Superior rectus muscle; *2,* superior ophthalmic vein; *3,* lateral rectus muscle; *4,* inferior rectus muscle; *5,* medial rectus muscle; *6,* superior oblique muscle; *7,* ophthalmic artery; *8,* optic nerve.

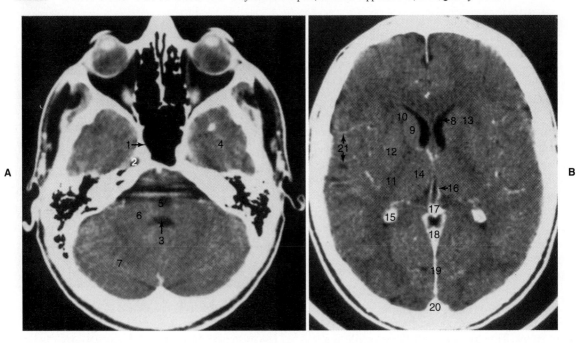

FIG. 20-6. (**A** and **B**) Brain. The normal appearance of the brain using a standard algorithm and 5-mm thick images, obtained with intravenous contrast enhancement. *1*, Sphenoid sinus; *2*, trigeminal ganglion; *3*, fourth ventricle; *4*, temporal lobe; *5*, pons (partly obscured by streak artifact); *6*, middle cerebellar peduncle; *7*, cerebellar hemisphere; *8*, frontal horn of the lateral ventricle; *9*, head of the caudate nucleus; *10*, anterior limb of the internal capsule; *11*, posterior limb of the internal capsule; *12*, lentiform nucleus; *13*, external capsule; *14*, thalamus; *15*, calcified choroid plexus; *16*, internal cerebral vein; *17*, pineal calcification; *18*, straight sinus; *19*, falx cerebri; *20*, superior sagittal sinus; *21*, branches of the middle cerebral artery. The use of a standard algorithm with a relatively narrow window (80 units) results in good contrast between white and gray matter.

Neck

When an intravenous (IV) contrast medium is used to enhance images, major vascular structures such as the carotid arteries and jugular veins can be identified. Both the superficial mucosa and the submandibular glands enhance. The parotid gland, with its high fat content, demonstrates an intermediate density between those of fat and muscle (Fig. 20-7).

Thin sections of the larynx show the relationship of the cartilages to the adjacent soft tissue. The level of the true vocal cords is defined by the position of the arytenoid cartilages (Fig. 20-8).

Spine

The sectional anatomy of the lumbar and cervical spines is illustrated in Figs. 20-9 and 20-10, respectively. Spine imaging is almost always done in the transverse plane, although the obliquity of the transverse image may be varied slightly. Coronal or sagittal images can be obtained only in small chil-

dren. Because of its contrast resolution, CT differentiates the disk from the adjacent ligamentum flavum, thecal sac, intraspinal fat, and bone. The nerve roots are easily identified as they exit through the intervertebral foramina. Epidural veins can be seen, particularly in the lumbar spine, but are better visualized with contrast medium enhancement.

INDICATIONS

Head

Because of the remarkable anatomic detail it provides, CT is valuable for assessing many conditions of the head.

Trauma

If a brain injury is suspected, CT can provide direct information about contusions (bruises) or hematomas (blood clots) of the brain, as well as hematomas outside the brain, such as epidural or subdural hematomas.

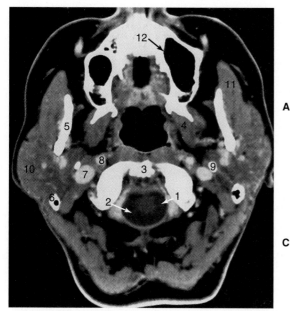

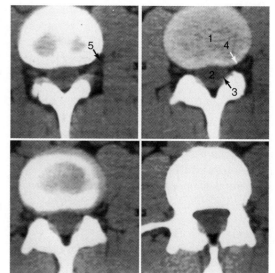

FIG. 20-7. Neck. This 3-mm thick axial slice through the upper neck was obtained with intravenous contrast enhancement. *1,* Spinal cord; *2,* cerebrospinal fluid; *3,* top of the odontoid; *4,* pterygoid muscles; *5,* mandible; *6,* tip of the mastoid; *7,* internal jugular vein; *8,* internal carotid artery; *9,* styloid process; *10,* parotid gland; *11,* masseter muscle; *12,* maxillary sinus.

FIG. 20-9. Lumbar spine. Four sections *(A-D)* through the L3-L4 disk space were obtained every 4 mm using a slice thickness of 5 mm. The disk *(1)* is slightly higher in density than the adjacent paravertebral muscle and the thecal sac *(2).* The ligamentum flavum *(3)* is also slightly more dense than the thecal sac. Fat in the spinal canal and intervertebral foramen *(4)* helps define the root sleeve *(5).*

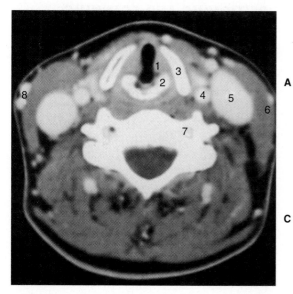

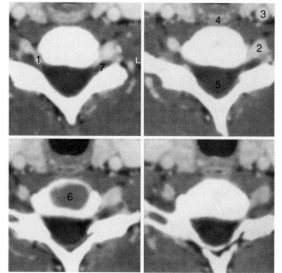

FIG. 20-8. Larynx. A 3-mm thick axial slice through the larynx obtained at the level of the vocal cords demonstrates prominent enhancement of the vascular structures. The laryngeal cartilages are better defined on the bone setting, which is not included here. *1,* True vocal cord; *2,* arytenoid cartilage; *3,* thyroid cartilage; *4,* common carotid artery; *5,* internal jugular vein; *6,* sternocleidomastoid muscle; *7,* vertebral artery; *8,* superficial veins.

FIG. 20-10. Cervical spine. Sequential 3-mm thick images *(A-D)* obtained every 2 mm through the C6-C7 disk space demonstrate prominent enhancement of the epidural veins *(1),* vertebral artery *(2),* and carotid artery *(3),* as well as the esophagus *(4),* spinal cord *(5),* and disk *(6).* The dorsal root ganglion *(7)* is outlined by the epidural veins.

Inflammatory Disease

A CT scan is essential if a cerebral abscess or inflammatory disease, such as herpes simplex encephalitis, is suspected. If meningitis is suspected, the CT scan usually does not show any abnormality; however, by confirming a lack of hydrocephalus or mass effect, it allows the physician safely to perform a lumbar puncture for CSF analysis. This procedure would not be safe if the CT scan indicated elevated intracranial pressure.

Congenital Problems

A CT scan can demonstrate most of the major congenital anomalies of the brain in babies or children.

Endocrine Disease

Suspected abnormalities of the pituitary gland are easily assessed with CT, particularly with thin-section coronal imaging.

Tumors

By providing direct anatomic information about the brain, CT allows detection of intracerebral and extracerebral cranial tumors.

Neck or Face

The indications for CT of the neck or face are as follows:

- Developmental anomalies
- Inflammation or infection (particularly evaluation of sinusitis, the spread of infection into the orbit, and infection involving the deeper structures of the neck)
- Trauma (fractures of the facial structures and foreign bodies in the orbit are easily assessed)
- Tumors (the extent of tumor involvement can be assessed before definitive treatment is begun)

Spine

CT of the spine is indicated in the following situations:

- Disk herniation suspected
- Spinal stenosis suspected
- Spinal infection suspected (disk space infection or epidural abscess)
- Intraspinal tumor suspected
- Spinal trauma with the danger of neurologic compromise

PATIENT PREPARATION

Little patient preparation is required for a CT scan, but the following points should be noted:

1. All metallic objects should be removed from the area to be studied, including such items as earrings, bobby pins, and necklaces.
2. The patient should be instructed to empty the bladder shortly before the scan is done, because use of an IV contrast medium causes the bladder to fill rapidly, and the scan should not be interrupted for a bathroom break.
3. The reason for the contrast medium should be explained to the patient and the IV line started before the scan.
4. The patient need not be fasting for the scan but should be discouraged from eating a large meal shortly before the procedure.
5. The technician should remember that patients with brain or spinal disease may suffer from memory loss, severe pain, or hearing or vision impairment. Their anxiety can be eased if technicians introduce themselves and explain the procedure briefly.
6. If the patient is comfortable on the table, the result is less motion and therefore less degradation of image quality.

POSITIONING AND SCANNING PROTOCOLS

Brain

The axial plane is used most often for brain imaging. If the plane of the scans is based on the anthropologic baseline, which joins the infraorbital point anteriorly to the superior border of the external auditory meatus (Fig. 20-11), better cross-sectional images of the orbit, sella turcica, temporal lobe, and brainstem are obtained than with a more steeply angled plane. A slice thickness of 10 mm is often used, although many sites use 5- to 8-mm slices to improve spatial resolution. Slices 3- to 5-mm thick are used through the posterior fossa to diminish beam hardening artifact and improve spatial resolution. Coronal images can be useful when lesions involve the most inferior or superior aspect of the brain and it is not entirely clear from axial images whether the abnormality affects adjacent bone or arises from the brain or meninges. Thin coronal images are the preferred technique for the pituitary gland and for assessing the internal auditory canal for an acoustic neuroma. The helical technique, which is discussed later in the

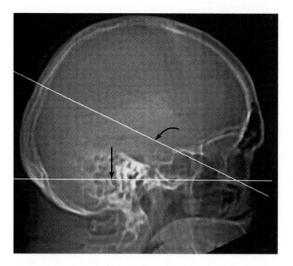

FIG. 20-11. Scanning planes. This scout view demonstrates the standard plane for head or orbital scanning *(straight arrow)* and the angled plane for scanning of the optic canal *(curved arrow)*.

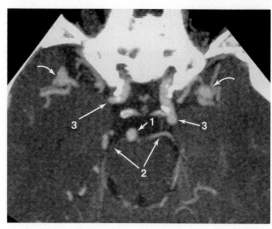

FIG. 20-12. Intracranial aneurysms. A reformatted, axial, 4-mm thick, maximum intensity projection image from a helical CT angiogram reveals bilateral middle cerebral artery aneurysms *(curved arrows)*. The basilar artery *(1)*, posterior cerebral artery *(2)*, and internal carotid arteries *(3)* are easily identified.

chapter, is used to assess vascular abnormalities, such as intracranial aneurysms (Fig. 20-12) or arteriovenous malformations.

Temporal Bone

Because of the combination of high-density bone and low-density air within the temporal bone, a wide window and a bone algorithm (discussed later in the chapter) are preferred for assessing this area. Abnormalities in the middle ear (e.g., cholesteatoma, congenital abnormalities of the ossicles, or tumors) can be assessed with 1- to 2-mm thick axial and coronal images. Soft tissue masses that lie outside the temporal bone, such as an acoustic neuroma, require brain techniques for ideal visualization.

Orbit

Thin-slice (preferably 3 mm) axial and coronal images of the orbit are preferred, because they allow assessment of soft tissue lesions and help detect any involvement of adjacent orbital bony walls. Some institutions prefer to use 1-mm axial slices with reformatting to produce coronal or sagittal images. This technique is useful when coronal images cannot be obtained; however, reformatted im-

ages tend to be of poor quality compared with direct images. If the optic canal is to be assessed specifically, the axial images should be angled appropriately in the plane of the optic canal (see Fig. 20-11). The easiest way to obtain this plane is to align the slice plane from the most anteroinferior margin of the orbit to the anterior clinoid.

Paranasal Sinuses

Thin coronal images (usually 3 mm) generally are sufficient for assessing the sinuses and represent the best view for showing the infundibulum of the maxillary sinus. These images should be obtained with the bone algorithm to achieve optimal detail of the bony septa. However, if a soft tissue lesion, such as a tumor, is suspected, axial images might also be worthwhile, and images using a standard algorithm for better soft tissue delineation are also desirable.

Base of the Skull and Temporomandibular Joint

Optimal detail of the base of the skull requires thin slices, usually 1 to 3 mm thick. Bone detail is optimal on a bone algorithm, but a standard algorithm also may be required to assess soft tissue lesions.

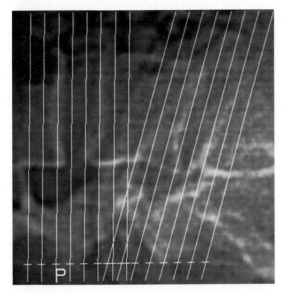

FIG. 20-13. Scanning plane for the lumbar spine. This scout view demonstrates the way the 5-mm thick slices are programmed every 4 mm in the plane of the disk spaces.

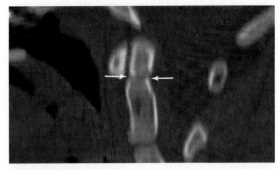

FIG. 20-14. Fractured odontoid. A reformatted sagittal image from a helical CT of the cervical spine clearly shows a transverse fracture at the base of the odontoid *(arrows)*. The fracture was very difficult to identify on the initial transverse 3-mm thick slices.

The axial images can be done in a plane parallel to the orbitomeatal line, which is slightly steeper than the anthropologic baseline. This plane more closely parallels the slope of the skull base in the middle fossa. Coronal views may be worthwhile to confirm or refute suspicion of a lesion seen on axial views. The temporomandibular joint can also be assessed using thin axial slices and appropriate coronal images.

Neck

The larynx is best assessed with axial slices obtained parallel to the plane of the vocal cords. This is approximately the same plane as the cervical disk spaces. The remainder of the neck, particularly the area of the parotid glands and nasopharynx, can be assessed with slightly oblique axial views, which allow the x-ray beam to avoid passing through dental fillings. It is particularly useful to do two sets of angled oblique images for the parotid gland to avoid scanning through the teeth.

The helical technique (discussed later) is particularly useful in the neck for assessing the carotid or vertebral arteries when dissection is suspected and for assessing the larynx when patient motion significantly degrades visualization. Patients with laryngeal trauma or tumors often have difficulty limiting motion.

Spine

Axial slices 3 mm thick are preferred in the cervical spine and should be done in the plane of the disk spaces. These should be done every 2 mm to assess for disk disease but can be done every 3 to 4 mm for trauma. In the lumbar spine the axial slices should also be done parallel to the disk spaces (Fig. 20-13). A good overall assessment of the spine can be done with 5-mm thick slices obtained every 4 mm.

Helical CT of the spine is important whenever reformatted images in other planes are desired, as is often the case with trauma (Fig. 20-14) or bone destruction caused by neoplasms.

RADIOGRAPHIC TECHNIQUE

Unlike conventional radiography, CT is governed by more than just the milliamperage (mA), kilovoltage (kV), and exposure time. Image quality depends on a number of important factors, which are discussed below.

Patient Preparation

A patient who is comfortable, both physically and emotionally, is more cooperative. This greatly increases the likelihood of acquiring a good CT study.

Patient Positioning

When positioning the patient, the technician must make sure that the anatomy in question is in the center of the gantry, both horizontally and vertically. Measuring the patient and choosing a scan field of view (FOV) that encircles the entire anatomy is essential (a small FOV is 25 cm; medium, 35 cm; and large, 48 cm). Coverings, such as blankets, should be tucked in to prevent interference with the reference detectors, which must receive air only. Poor positioning and an inadequate scan FOV lower CT numbers and produce inaccurate images.

Milliamperage, Kilovoltage, and Scan Time

The signal-to-noise ratio can be improved by increasing the mA, kV, or scan time. This is particularly important for contrast resolution of soft tissue structures, and for that reason these settings are relatively high for brain scans. With large patients, detail is reduced in spinal studies; however, increasing the mA, kV, and scan time can compensate for this factor. Increasing the scan time, however, also increases the possibility of motion artifact. As slice thickness is reduced, the mA and kV generally are increased to provide an adequate signal-to-noise ratio. For example, when a large patient is scanned for a possible lumbar disk herniation, a noisy image can be improved by increasing the scan time and slice thickness to improve the contrast resolution. Spatial resolution may be sacrificed, but this can be compensated for by overlapping the thicker slices.

Slice Thickness

Thinner slices improve spatial resolution but sacrifice signal to noise. This can be compensated for by increasing the mA, kV, and scan time. When spatial resolution is the paramount consideration, thin slices are a requirement. Thus, when imaging areas such as the middle ear or pituitary gland, a slice thickness of 1 to 2 mm usually is chosen. Thin slices through the brain provide good definition of mass lesions but poor definition of gray and white matter because contrast resolution is reduced. Conversely, 10-mm thick slices provide excellent contrast resolution of the brain but reduce spatial resolution. The radiologist chooses the slice thickness according to the diagnosis suspected.

Reconstruction Algorithms and Matrix Size

The standard algorithm, the bone algorithm, and the detail algorithm are the three basic reconstruction algorithms used in CT of the head, neck, and spine.

Standard Algorithm

The standard algorithm provides good contrast resolution and therefore is the algorithm of choice for the brain. It is also useful for soft tissue assessment in the head, face, and spine. To help maximize soft tissue resolution, a narrow window and low window levels are used with the photography.

Bone Algorithm

The bone algorithm helps optimize spatial resolution but produces poor contrast resolution. Consequently, it is used only in areas with great extremes of tissue density, such as the paranasal sinuses or temporal bones, where contrast resolution is not a factor. Wide windows and high window levels are used with this technique.

Detail Algorithm

The detail algorithm gives adequate contrast resolution with good edge definition. It therefore can be useful for obtaining better edge definition between tissue types, particularly in the neck and face. Moderate window widths and levels are used.

Matrix Size and Field of View

The scan field of view must be large enough to encompass the anatomic area to be assessed. The display FOV may be the same size or smaller; the advantage of the latter is that the pixel size is reduced, because pixel size is equal to display FOV divided by matrix size. A smaller pixel size improves spatial resolution. The matrix chosen is 256, 340, or 512, and resolution can be maximized by using a minimal display FOV with the largest matrix acceptable for that FOV. For example, spatial resolution in the temporal bone can be maximized by using a display FOV of 9.6 cm with a matrix of 512.

USE OF CONTRAST MEDIA

Intravenous contrast media are sometimes used in CT because iodine further attenuates the x-ray beam, which makes structures containing the contrast medium appear denser. In particular, normal structures with a rich vascular supply, such as the blood vessels, choroid plexus, and dura, appear denser with contrast enhancement. This is an advantage when highlighting normal anatomy in the head and neck, because it allows differentiation of vessels from lymph nodes in the neck and helps define disk herniation in the cervical spine by outlining the epidural venous plexus. In the lumbar spine, a contrast medium can be used to help distinguish scar tissue from a recurrent disk herniation because the latter generally does not enhance, whereas the scar tissue does.

A contrast medium also may be used because it increases the CT density of more vascular lesions, making them easier to see. A meningioma, for example, typically is vascular and therefore readily increases in density when an IV contrast medium is used. Intracerebral tumors, such as a glioblastoma, do not have a normal blood-brain barrier, and the contrast medium passes into the tumor but not into normal brain tissue. Thus these tumors show increased density, or "enhancement." Similarly, the wall of a cerebral abscess shows enhancement.

A standard dose of intravenous contrast medium generally is considered to be at least 30 g of iodine, which corresponds to approximately 100 ml of Conray 60. A double dose of contrast medium (60 to 80 g of iodine) has proved advantageous in some circumstances, such as differentiating scar tissue

from a recurrent disk herniation in the lumbar spine. Patients with metastatic cerebral disease can be better assessed if a double dose of contrast medium is given and scanning is delayed for 30 to 45 minutes. This allows better enhancement of metastases. The same technique can be useful with multiple sclerosis, although this disease is much better assessed with magnetic resonance imaging (MRI).

Caution must be exercised when using an IV contrast medium in some patients. In particular, a history of a significant reaction to a contrast medium, insulin-dependent diabetes, significant heart disease, and impaired renal function are serious considerations. Contrast media should not be used in patients with multiple myeloma because of the danger of associated renal impairment. The newer nonionic contrast agents have some safety advantages but are also more costly. They can be selectively used for patients in the categories mentioned above.

Intrathecal administration of a contrast medium after a lumber puncture can improve CT assessment of intraspinal abnormalities and occasionally of intracranial abnormalities. The intrathecal contrast medium allows better demonstration of the spinal cord and cauda equina.

HELICAL SCANNING

Helical scanning has greatly enhanced the diagnostic capabilities of CT. Because it provides much better definition of vascular structures, it is used to assess intracranial aneurysms (see Fig. 20-12), arteriovenous malformations, and possible carotid artery dissection in the neck. The helical technique's speed and ability to reduce motion artifact are ideal for imaging the larynx. The superior quality of reformatted images, in a variety of planes, is tremendously valuable in assessing spinal and facial trauma. Helical 3D techniques are useful for better understanding facial injuries or deformities (Fig. 20-15).

ABNORMALITIES SHOWN BY CT
Cerebral Abnormalities

Cerebral Infarction

A cerebral infarction, or stroke, initially produces edema in the area of the ischemic brain tissue, followed by necrosis or cystic change. As seen on a CT scan, the result is a low-density change in the affected area of the brain, often extending to the

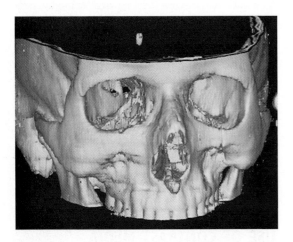

FIG. 20-15. 3D view of facial bone anatomy. An oblique frontal view of the facial bones was created from a continuous series of 1-mm thick helical images; maximum intensity projection with thresholding values was used to eliminate all soft tissues.

cortical surface and obliterating the normal gray-white distinction. Swelling may obliterate adjacent sulci. Fig. 20-16 shows a CT scan of an acute cerebral infarction.

Hemorrhage

Blood released by a recent hemorrhage contains considerable hemoglobin, which is relatively dense on CT because of its protein content. As the hematoma ages, the hemoglobin is removed and the density of the hematoma diminishes. Several types of hemorrhage can occur:

- An *acute subdural hematoma* typically produces a high-density collection of blood between the skull and adjacent brain. The collection of blood follows the contour of the brain and is associated with a variable amount of mass effect. A chronic subdural hematoma appears as low density but is otherwise similar.
- A *cerebral contusion* classically causes a mixture of edema and hemorrhage, which appears on a CT scan as mixed low density and high density in the affected area. Contusions most often affect the anterior portion of the temporal or frontal lobe.
- A *subarachnoid hemorrhage* (Fig. 20-17) most frequently is caused by a ruptured aneurysm. The CT scan shows increased density in the basal cisterns rather than the normal low density of CSF. CT is approximately 85% accurate in demonstrating subarachnoid hemorrhage when performed within 24 hours of the event. If the CT scan shows no evidence of a hemorrhage, a lumbar puncture is performed, which can produce confirmation up to 7 to 10 days after the event.

Meningioma

Meningiomas are the most common benign intracranial tumors. Meningiomas are extraaxial (lying outside the brain) and arise from dura adjacent to the inner table of the skull. These tumors typically are vascular and enhance prominently when

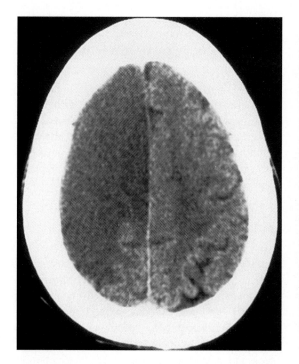

FIG. 20-16. Acute cerebral infarction. An axial slice through the upper part of the brain demonstrates a large area of low density involving the right hemisphere. The gray-white distinction is lost, as are the sulci, indicating swelling of the involved area. This appearance is typical of an acute cerebral infarction.

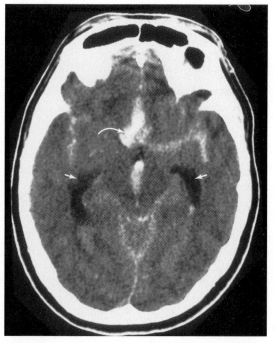

FIG. 20-17. Subarachnoid hemorrhage. Cerebrospinal fluid density is seen within the temporal horns *(short arrows)*, but a higher density relating to subarachnoid hemorrhage is seen within the basal cisterns, particularly the area adjacent to the anterior communicating artery *(curved arrow)*. This appearance is typical of subarachnoid hemorrhage that occurs secondary to rupture of an aneurysm of the anterior communicating artery.

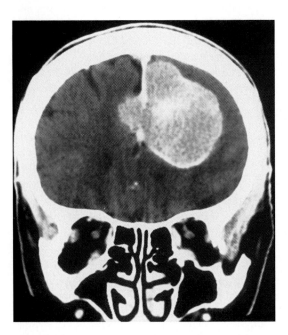

FIG. 20-18. Intracranial meningioma. A coronal image, obtained with intravenous contrast enhancement, demonstrates a large enhancing mass arising from the falx and protruding largely to the left, with a small component extending through the falx to the right of the midline. This appearance is typical of a falcine meningioma.

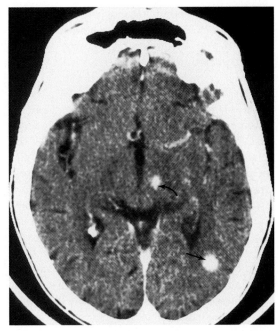

FIG. 20-19. Metastatic disease. An axial slice obtained with intravenous contrast enhancement demonstrates lesions in the left thalamus *(curved arrow)* and the gray-white junction at the posterior aspect of the left temporal lobe *(straight arrow).* The presence of two or more distinct lesions, particularly when they are round and located at the gray-white junction, is a sign of metastatic disease.

an IV contrast medium is used. A typical falcine meningioma is shown in Fig. 20-18.

Cerebral Glioblastoma

Gliobastomas are the most common primary tumor of the brain. On a CT scan, the tumor typically shows a mixture of low density and enhancing areas with mass effect. Patients with these tumors generally are over 30 years of age. The prognosis is poor, and few patients survive longer than 1 year.

Metastatic Disease

Patients with metastatic disease have multiple lesions that have arisen from a primary tumor located elsewhere, most often in the lung or breast. Typically, multiple enhancing lesions are seen, usually with adjacent edema (Fig. 20-19). The presence of two or more lesions within the brain indicates metastatic disease until it is proved otherwise.

Cerebral Abscess

The typical abscess within the brain produces a doughnut-shaped lesion with a low-density center

and a rim that enhances readily. As with many other intracerebral or extracerebral masses, this configuration may be associated with an increase in fluid within the white matter of the adjacent brain, called *vasogenic edema.* The edema appears as lower density white matter.

Spinal Abnormalities

Disk Herniation

Lumbar disk herniation (Fig. 20-20) is most common at the L4-L5 or L5-S1 disk space. Both the disks and spinal canal are large at this level, consequently disk material that extends beyond its normal boundary can be readily identified. The herniation may occur centrally, so that it abuts the thecal sac, or posterolaterally, where it can abut or displace the nerve root. More lateral herniations can extend into the foramen or even more anterolaterally to the foramen. The latter type cannot be identified on myelography, which is one reason CT is the preferred imaging study. The site of disk herniation must correlate with the clinical

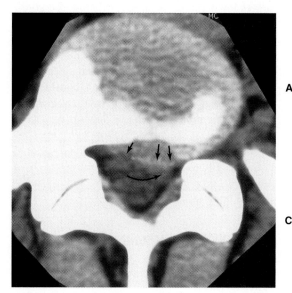

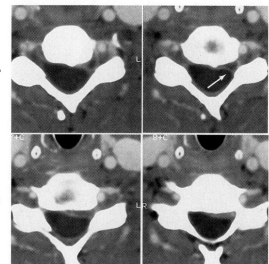

FIG. 20-20. Lumbar disk herniation. Left posterolateral disk herniation (short arrows) causes a focal change in the contour of the L5-S1 disk. The left S1 root sleeve *(curved arrow)* has been displaced posteriorly.

FIG. 20-21. Cervical disk herniation. Three-mm thick images *(A-D)* obtained every 2 mm through the C5-C6 disk space demonstrate a left posterolateral and foraminal disk herniation *(straight arrow)*. The herniation is much easier to identify because of contrast enhancement of the epidural veins, which outline the margins.

findings, because approximately 30% of asymptomatic individuals show evidence of disk herniation on CT.

Cervical disk herniations are seen most often at the C5-C6 level. Because cervical disks are much smaller than lumbar disks, herniation is better identified when an IV contrast medium is used to enhance the epidural veins, demarcating the boundaries of the disk herniation (Fig. 20-21). Thoracic disk herniations occur much less often and are usually smaller. Thin CT slices are required, and the accuracy may be improved further by using an IV or intrathecal contrast medium. The size of the disk herniation in the thoracic area often correlates poorly with the clinical manifestations.

Spinal Fractures

Displaced fracture fragments can be well assessed on CT, particularly with the helical technique, which can provide high-quality reformatted images in the sagittal and coronal planes. Encroachment on the spinal canal and cord is easily identified.

Neck and Laryngeal Abnormalities

Nasopharyngeal Cancer

Soft tissue masses in the nasopharynx can be assessed with thin slices (usually 3 mm). Use of a high dose of contrast medium is helpful for assessing soft tissue lesions in the neck because it allows differentiation of vessels, lymph nodes, and most tumors. Nasopharyngeal cancer has a tendency to spread into the base of the skull, therefore coronal views with bone detail may be a useful adjunct.

Parotid Gland Tumors

Parotid gland tumors are the most common salivary gland tumors. Most are benign and well defined and enhance readily (Fig. 20-22). CT can be helpful in planning surgery for these tumors, because these should be completely removed.

Laryngeal Cancer

Because deep extension of laryngeal tumors below the mucosal surface is poorly assessed clinically, CT is essential before treatment. Thin slices are mandatory for obtaining good anatomic detail of

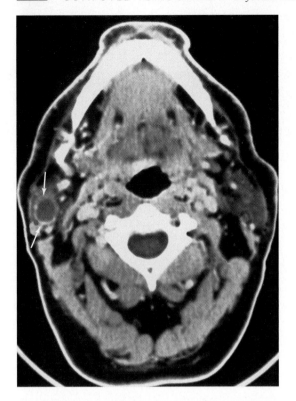

FIG. 20-22. Parotid gland tumor. A contrast medium–enhanced, 3-mm thick axial slice through the neck demonstrates a rounded mass in the right parotid gland *(arrows)* that has a ring-enhancing appearance.

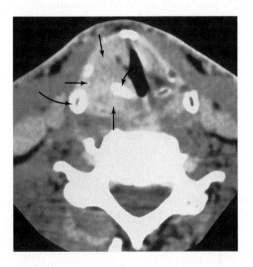

FIG. 20-23. Laryngeal cancer. A 3-mm thick axial slice through the larynx, obtained with intravenous contrast enhancement, demonstrates an enhancing soft tissue mass *(straight arrows)* involving the right larynx at the level of the vocal cord. This mass is causing sclerosis, with reactive change in the right arytenoid cartilage *(short curved arrow)* and some bony change in the inferior cornu of the right thyroid cartilage *(long curved arrow).*

the larynx. Good detail around the true vocal cords is particularly important for assessing whether tumors have extended above or below the cords, because this can change the surgical plan. Also, good bone detail can be useful for assessing the possibility of tumor infiltration of the laryngeal cartilages. One difficulty is that the degree of calcification in the cartilages varies considerably from person to person, and a lack of calcification makes tumor infiltration more difficult to define. Fig. 20-23 shows an enhancing soft tissue mass involving the right larynx. Patient motion associated with difficulty swallowing or breathing can be a significant problem, therefore the helical technique is often useful.

Orbital and Facial Abnormalities

Orbital Tumors

A hemangioma is the most common primary mass within the orbit. It typically appears on a CT scan as a well-defined, round mass posterior to the globe and lying within the extraocular muscles (i.e., an "intraconal" lesion). The mass enhances readily, although the enhancement may not be homogeneous. It particularly tends to mold to the back of the globe and may displace adjacent muscles or the optic nerve without causing any invasion.

Another common lesion of the orbit is the sphenoid wing meningioma. This benign tumor produces thickening and sclerosis of the sphenoid wing, often associated with an enhancing soft tissue tumor in the orbit, middle fossa, or temporal fossa (Fig. 20-24).

Chronic Sinusitis

Chronic sinusitis typically causes mucosal thickening or sometimes complete opacification of the affected paranasal sinus. Also, the bone tends to thicken and become denser over time because of the inflammatory response. On CT it is useful to assess the extent of involvement, particularly the areas of drainage (e.g., the hiatus semilunaris area of the maxillary sinuses).

CT VERSUS OTHER IMAGING TECHNIQUES
Angiography

Angiography provides exquisite detail of vascular structures and therefore is much more sensitive than CT in detecting abnormalities that primarily affect vessels, such as aneurysms or vasculitis.

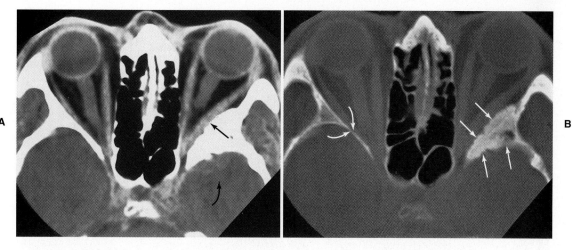

FIG. 20.24. Orbital meningioma. **A,** The standard setting demonstrates abnormal enhancement immediately posterior to the greater sphenoid wing *(curved arrow)* and thickening of the lateral rectus muscle *(straight arrow).* **B,** The bone setting demonstrates abnormal thickening of the left sphenoid wing *(straight arrows)* more definitively compared with the normal appearance of the sphenoid wing on the right *(curved arrows).* The bony changes are characteristic of meningioma and help distinguish this lesion from metastatic disease.

However, angiography no longer plays a role in the detection of mass lesions because CT is far more sensitive for this purpose. Also, angiography is invasive and is associated with rare but significant complications.

Myelography

CT is more sensitive and precise than myelography for the assessment of disk herniation, particularly because a far lateral disk herniation does not show on a myelogram. In addition, because of the larger anterior epidural space at L5-S1, a disk herniation in that area may not be revealed on a myelogram. Degenerative changes involving the facet joints are also much better shown on CT. However, intrathecal abnormalities, such as lesions of the cord or cauda equina, may be better seen on a myelogram, particularly as compared with a CT scan unaided by an IV contrast medium. Myelography is useful for lesions of the cervicothoracic junction, because CT quality is poor when scanning through the shoulders.

Plain Films

Plain radiographic films offer high resolution of bone but do not provide soft tissue detail. Therefore CT has a vast advantage for the assessment of the brain or soft tissue structures in the neck or spine. Plain films may serve as a useful screening test for bony abnormalities, such as degenerative disease or fractures involving the spine or skull.

Magnetic Resonance Imaging

A CT scan can be performed faster and is less susceptible to motion artifact than an MRI study. It also offers exquisite bone detail and is excellent for showing acute hemorrhage. For these reasons, CT is the preferred study for acute injuries, such intracranial hemorrhage or trauma to the head or spine. MRI is very sensitive for identifying edema within the brain or spinal cord and therefore is more accurate in disorders of the spinal cord, inflammatory conditions of the brain (e.g., encephalitis), and multiple sclerosis. MRI has a definite advantage with lesions in the posterior fossa, because beam-hardening artifact on a CT scan can obscure subtle lesions in this area (Fig. 20-25). An old hemorrhage, manifested by the presence of hemosiderin, is readily detected by MRI. CT, on the other hand, is much better at detecting calcification. Therefore a subtle meningioma with calcification extending along the sheath of the optic nerve may be revealed by CT but go unidentified with MRI, although the latter is better for assessing the optic nerve within the optic canal.

MRI also has the advantage of allowing multiplanar imaging without moving the patient. How-

FIG. 20-25.   A, A CT slice through the posterior fossa demonstrates a mild mass effect on the anterior aspect of the fourth ventricle *(arrow)*. No definite mass is seen in the pons, partly because of streak artifact. **B,** A magnetic resonance imaging (MRI) study through the same area demonstrates high intensity in the pons, outlining the extent of the tumor. Better definition of posterior fossa abnormalities is a major advantage of MRI studies over CT scans.

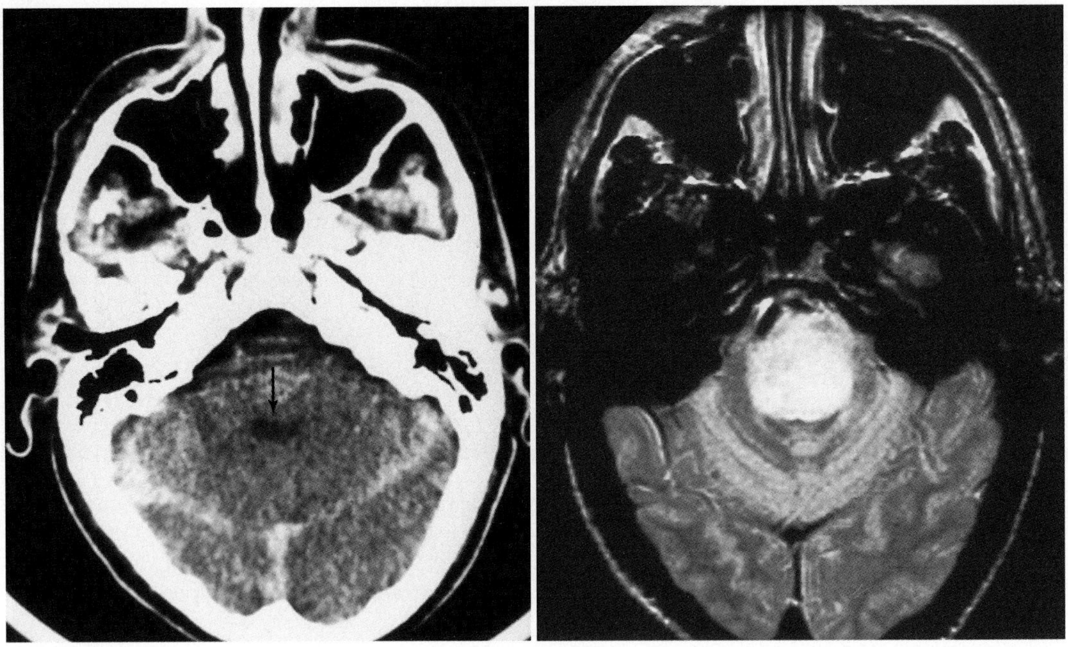

ever, MRI is contraindicated in patients with cardiac pacemakers, metallic orbital foreign bodies, and most intracranial aneurysm clips.

REFERENCE

Eisenberg RL: *Radiology: an illustrated history,* St Louis, 1992, Mosby.

BIBLIOGRAPHY

Potts G: Radiology of the skull and brain. In Newton TN, Potts DG, eds: *Radiology of the skull and brain,* St Louis, 1971, Mosby.

Som PM, Curtin HD: *Head and neck imaging,* St Louis, 1996, Mosby.

21

Computed Tomography of the Body

BORYS FLAK, DAVID K.B. LI, AND LOIS DOODY

CHAPTER *Outline*

In the early years of computed tomography (CT), many were skeptical about its usefulness outside the central nervous system. Earlier scanners were unsuitable for examining the body because of the image degradation that occurred with patient motion and movement of internal organs during the 2 to 5 minutes required for a single slice. Within a few years, however, astonishing technologic advances reduced scan times to 1 to 5 seconds per slice. CT of the body has fulfilled the expectations of its early supporters and has become an important means of evaluating many pathologic conditions. Although magnetic resonance imaging (MRI) has replaced CT as the primary method of investigation for most diseases of the cranium and spinal column and is extremely valuable for many diseases of the musculoskeletal system, CT is still superior to MRI for most clinical indications in the chest and abdomen.

CLINICAL INDICATIONS

In addition to CT, a wide variety of radiologic techniques are available for studying diseases of the body including plain radiographs, barium studies, angiography, nuclear medicine, ultrasonography, and MRI. Clinicians are faced with the dilemma of which imaging method or methods to use and in what order. Often too many examinations are requested or studies are performed in the wrong sequence before a diagnosis is reached. For these reasons, the use of algorithms or flowcharts has become popular. The suggested approach, however, may not be the most appropriate for the individual institution when the limitations of available equipment and expertise are considered. The radiologist, acting as a consultant, should discuss the clinical problem with the referring physician and choose the most expeditious and cost-effective method or methods for answering the clinician's questions. This chapter presents the major indications for CT of the body.

Chest and Mediastinum

Almost all mediastinal abnormalities detected on chest radiographs or suspected from clinical evidence can be confirmed with CT (Gamsu, 1992). CT is most commonly used to detect lymphadenopathy in patients suspected of having bronchogenic carcinoma, lymphoma, or other malignancies (Fig. 21-1). Although highly sensitive, CT and MRI have some limitations; they are less efficient at detecting tumors within normal-size nodes or differentiating between enlarged hyperplastic nodes without a tumor and tumor-containing nodes. CT is also useful in patients known to have or suspected of having bronchogenic carcinoma; in these cases CT is used to determine the extent of invasion of the chest wall, mediastinum, and diaphragm and to detect extrathoracic metastases in the liver and adrenal glands. MRI may be marginally better for demonstrating chest wall invasion and is more accurate in detecting mediastinal invasion and staging apical tumors (Manfredi et al, 1996).

With enhancement of vascular structures in the mediastinum using intravenous (IV) contrast medium, an aneurysm can be differentiated from other mediastinal masses (Posniak, Demos, and Marsan, 1989) (Figs. 21-2 and 21-3). CT is highly accurate and comparable to MRI and transesophageal echo in detecting and defining the extent of traumatic aortic ruptures and aortic dissections (Sommer et al, 1996).

In patients with myasthenia gravis, CT can detect thymic masses not evident on chest radiographs (Fon et al, 1982). Cysts and fatty deposits are distinguished by their characteristic CT numbers. A specific diagnosis cannot be made with

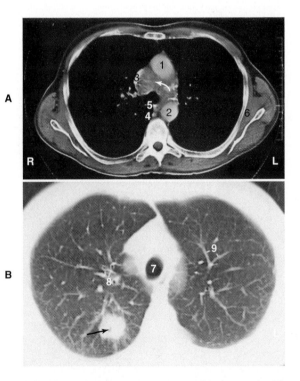

FIG. 21-1. Bronchogenic carcinoma *(black arrows)* with pretracheal mediastinal lymphadenopathy *(white arrow)*. *1,* Ascending aorta; *2,* descending aorta; *3,* superior vena cava; *4,* azygos vein; *5,* esophagus; *6,* subscapular muscle; *7,* trachea; *8,* segmental bronchi; *9,* pulmonary vessels.

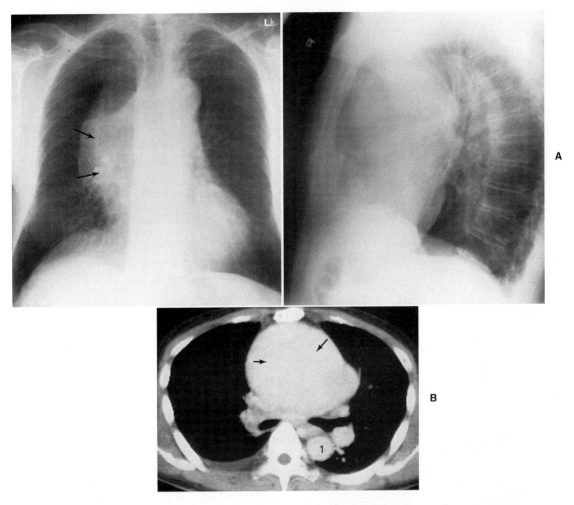

FIG. 21-2. Dissecting aneurysm of the ascending aorta *(arrows). 1*, Descending aorta.

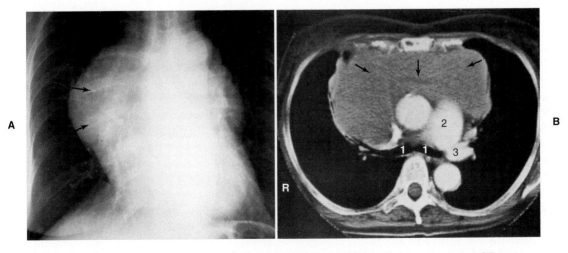

FIG. 21-3. Lymphoma seen as an anterior mediastinal mass involving the thymus on helical CT scan *(arrows). 1*, Right and left main stem bronchi; *2*, main pulmonary artery; *3*, left pulmonary artery.

A 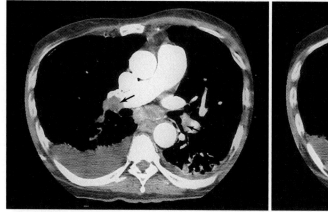 B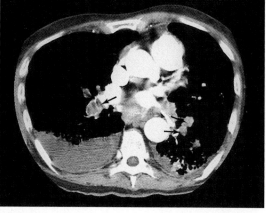

FIG. 21-4. Multiple filling defects caused by pulmonary emboli in the pulmonary arteries of both lungs *(arrows).*

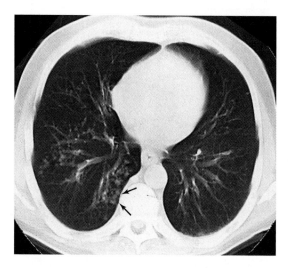

FIG. 21-5. Multiple pulmonary nodules caused by interstitial lung disease of unknown etiology *(arrows).*

most other masses, but the relationship of the mass to surrounding structures and its extension within the mediastinum can be readily defined.

CT is the most sensitive technique for detecting pulmonary metastases (Muhm et al, 1978; Schaner et al, 1978). However, the increased sensitivity is achieved at the price of decreased specificity. Benign lesions such as subpleural lymph nodes and granulomas can be detected, as well as a greater number of metastatic lesions. CT therefore is most useful in patients being evaluated for resection of metastatic pulmonary nodules, such as patients with osteogenic sarcoma. In the appropriate clinical setting, high-resolution CT (HRCT) can be diagnostic for lymphangitic carcinomatosis

(Munk, Muller, and Miller, 1988). CT also can be used to detect occult primary lung tumors in patients who show malignant cells on sputum cytologic studies but who have normal chest x-ray films. Some investigators have used nodule densitometry (Zerhouni et al, 1986) or the degree of contrast enhancement (Swensen et al, 1996) on CT to evaluate solitary pulmonary nodules that are indeterminate for malignancy on conventional radiographs.

Helical CT is more sensitive than ventilation/perfusion (V/Q) scans and of equal specificity in detecting pulmonary emboli (Mayo et al, 1997). Emboli are seen as filling defects in the enhanced pulmonary arteries (Fig. 21-4). CT will miss clots in the smaller subsegmental branches, but this may not be clinically significant unless the patient has severe underlying cardiac or pulmonary disease (Stein, Henry, and Relyea, 1995).

HRCT has become the established method for evaluating diffuse lung diseases (Muller, 1991) (Fig. 21-5). When the CT findings are analyzed in the context of the clinical history, physical findings, pulmonary function tests, and laboratory data, characteristic HRCT findings may allow a confident diagnosis in conditions such as asbestosis, silicosis, and idiopathic pulmonary fibrosis. In some cases such as allergic alveolitis HRCT findings may preclude the need for lung biopsy, or it can be used as a guide in selecting the best site for a biopsy. HRCT is more sensitive than chest radiography for detecting emphysema (Fig. 21-6), and it has replaced bronchography as the definitive method for detecting bronchiectasis (Pang, Hamilton-Wood, and Metreweli, 1989).

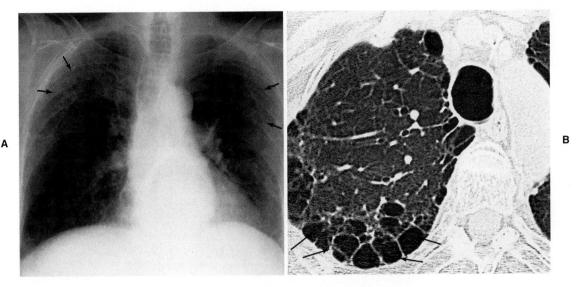

FIG. 21-6. Additional interstitial changes *(arrows)* on plain films (**A**) are shown to have occurred secondary to paraseptal emphysema on high-resolution thin sections (**B**).

Liver and Spleen

In our institution, mainly because of the large number of patients, ultrasonography remains the method of choice for initial screening for focal lesions. Although CT is more sensitive, it is used only when ultrasound results have been inconclusive or when more detailed localization and characterization of lesions are required (Fig. 21-7).

Proper use of an IV contrast medium is important for detecting focal masses in the liver. Helical CT used with power injections of boluses of contrast medium, with or without the help of bolus-tracking software, allows a so-called *biphasic examination* of the liver, one series during the early arterial phase and a second during the venous phase. Dynamic CT, which involves multiple repeat scans at the same level or several selected levels, is helpful for demonstrating the characteristic contrast medium–enhancement pattern seen with hemangiomas (Freeny and Marks, 1986) (Fig. 21-8). CT hepatic angiography and CT arterial portography are probably still the most sensitive methods available for detecting additional tumor nodules (Hori et al, 1998) and are especially useful for planning hepatic resection. The introduction of multidetector scanners, however, has allowed the use of very thin scans (e.g., 2.5 mm collimation through the entire liver), and a study by Weg, Scheer, and Gabor (1998) confirmed higher rates of detection and improved conspicuity of small liver lesions (less than 10 mm) compared with 5- to 10-mm collimation.

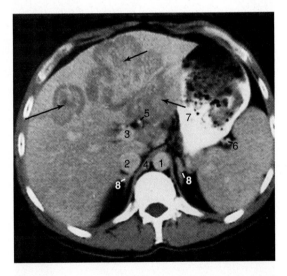

FIG. 21-7. Hepatoma *(arrows)* involving the lateral and medial segments of the left lobe of the liver. *1,* Aorta; *2,* inferior vena cava; *3,* portal vein; *4,* crus; *5,* hepatic artery; *6,* splenic artery; *7,* stomach; *8,* adrenals.

With a few exceptions, diffuse liver disease cannot be diagnosed by CT. Hemachromatosis, amiodarone therapy, and some glycogen storage diseases are associated with dense livers on CT (Goldman et al, 1985), whereas fatty infiltration is evidenced by a liver that is less attenuating than the spleen on unenhanced scans (Alpern et al, 1986).

CT and ultrasonography are equally accurate in demonstrating intrahepatic and extrahepatic

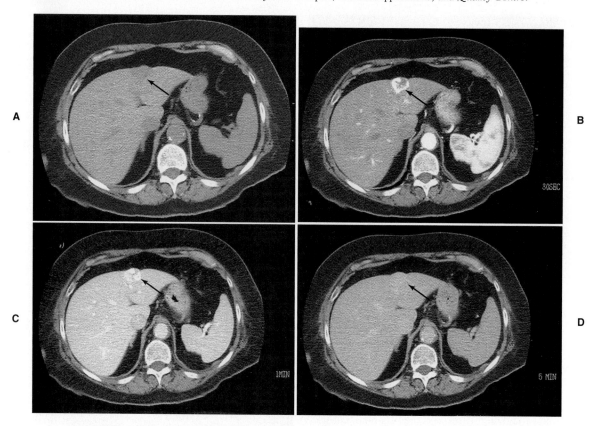

FIG. 21-8. Hemangioma of the liver. **A,** Low-density mass in the left lobe *(arrow).* **B,** Arterial phase study demonstrates dense, lobulated peripheral enhancement *(arrow).* **C,** Venous phase study demonstrates that the lesion is filling in with the contrast medium *(arrow).* **D,** Delayed scan demonstrates complete filling in of the lesion, which is nearly isodense *(arrow).*

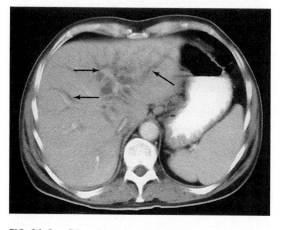

FIG. 21-9. Dilated intrahepatic ducts *(arrows)* in a jaundiced patient known to have cholangiocarcinoma.

bile ducts in jaundiced patients (Baron et al, 1982) (Fig. 21-9). At our institution, CT is performed only if the ultrasound technique is unsuccessful. If dilated ducts are demonstrated and the obstructing lesion is not delineated, the next investigation

usually is direct cholangiography (transhepatic cholangiography or endoscopic retrograde cholangiopancreatography) or MRI cholangiography.

Although focal masses can be seen in the spleen with both CT and ultrasonography, the results of spleen assessment in patients with lymphoma has unfortunately remained poor for both methods (Castellino et al, 1984). CT, however, is probably the best method for screening for splenic injury after blunt abdominal trauma (Wing et al, 1985).

Bowel

Although barium studies and endoscopy traditionally have been the mainstays of alimentary tract investigation, CT is assuming an ever-increasing role because of its ability to delineate not only the lumen but also the bowel wall and adjacent structures. Virtual colonoscopy, or CT colography, is a new development in gastrointestinal (GI) radiology that is challenging the barium enema and even colonoscopy in the detection of colonic polyps

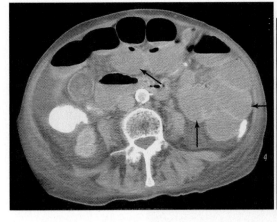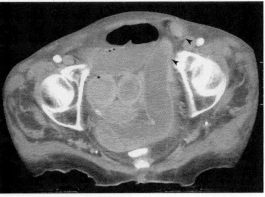

A

B

FIG. 21-10. **A,** Small bowel obstruction as evidenced by the multiple dilated loops of proximal small bowel *(arrows)*; **B,** and a herniated loop in the left groin *(arrowheads)*.

(Hara et al, 1997). This technique involves cleansing the colon with a standard bowel preparation, insufflating the colon with air or carbon dioxide (or both), performing thin-section helical scans (typically 5 mm with overlapping reconstruction in both the supine and prone positions), and subsequently reviewing the images in cine or movie mode, as well as performing multiplanar reconstructions. The data also can be volume rendered and displayed in a "fly through" navigation mode simulating colonoscopy (Fenlon et al, 1998). The results of preliminary studies have been extremely encouraging, rivaling or surpassing those of conventional methods.

Although CT has proved not very accurate for staging of GI malignancies, it is still widely used for this purpose, primarily to prevent unnecessary surgery in cases that demonstrate strong evidence of unresectability because of local invasion or distant metastases, such as to the liver (Davies et al, 1997). Plain radiographs are diagnostic in only about 50% to 60% of small bowel obstructions, equivocal in 20% to 30%, and normal or nonspecific in 10% to 20% (Mucha, 1987). CT can confirm an obstruction, determine the level and perhaps the cause, and often indicate if vascular compromise is present in uncertain cases (Fig. 21-10) (Balthazar, 1994).

Barium studies remain the primary procedure for evaluating patients with inflammatory bowel disease, but CT is the key to studying the mural extent and detecting any extraintestinal involvement or complications such as phlegmons, abscesses, sinus tracts, and fistulas (Gore et al, 1996).

In approximately 20% to 33% of patients suspected of having appendicitis, the clinical presentation is atypical (Berry et al, 1984), requiring imaging. We prefer to perform graded compression

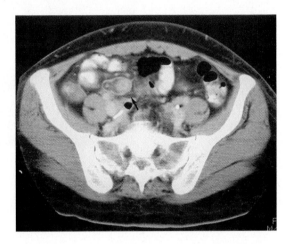

FIG. 21-11. Thickened, inflamed appendix *(arrow)* in the right lower quadrant

sonography as the initial test; however, a number of studies have demonstrated greater accuracy with CT and therefore this should be considered an alternative, especially in obese patients or if the sonogram is inconclusive (Lane et al, 1997) (Fig. 21-11). Clinically, patients with diverticulitis typically have a fever and a tender mass in the left lower quadrant. CT can accurately determine the severity of involvement and whether a complicating abscess is present (Androsetti, Grossholz, and Becker, 1997).

Retroperitoneum

Pancreas. Previously the pancreas was a difficult organ to evaluate, clinically or with routine radiologic studies. Cross-sectional imaging methods such as ultrasonography, CT, and MRI now permit

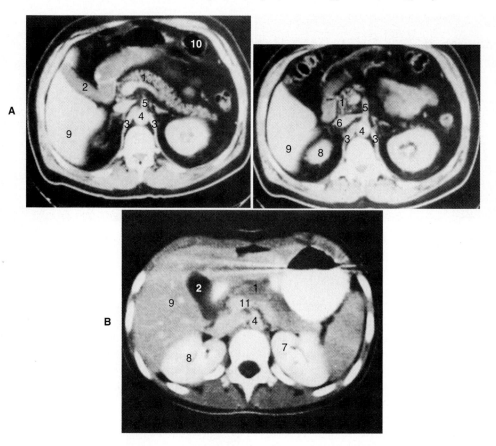

FIG. 21-12. Normal pancreas in patient with abundant (**A**) and little (**B**) intraabdominal fat. *1*, Pancreas; *2*, gallbladder; *3*, crus of the diaphragm; *4*, aorta; *5*, superior mesenteric artery; *6*, inferior vena cava with left renal vein; *7*, left kidney; *8*, right kidney; *9*, liver; *10*, bowel; *11*, splenoportal confluence.

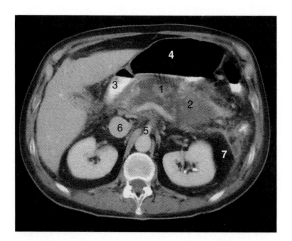

FIG. 21-13. Acute pancreatitis. Necrotic pancreas *(1)* surrounded by fluid *(2)*, duodenum *(3)*, air-filled stomach *(4)*, superior mesenteric artery *(5)*, inferior vena cava *(6)*, and perirenal fat *(7)*.

direct demonstration of the pancreas. The role of MRI in the diagnosis of pancreatic disorders is still questionable, and the technique probably offers no significant advantages over CT. When the pancreas is well visualized on a sonogram, the accuracy is comparable to that of CT. In general, the success rate for delineating the entire pancreas is much higher with CT than with ultrasonography because bowel gas often obscures part or all of the pancreas (Hessel et al, 1982) (Fig. 21-12).

Acute pancreatitis is a clinical diagnosis, and normally neither CT nor ultrasonography is necessary. Imaging should be performed only when the diagnosis is in doubt, when complications are suspected (Siegelman et al, 1980), or when the clinical course is severe or unexpected. With acute pancreatitis CT is preferred mainly because of the high incidence of associated paralytic ileus, which obscures visualization of the pancreatic region by

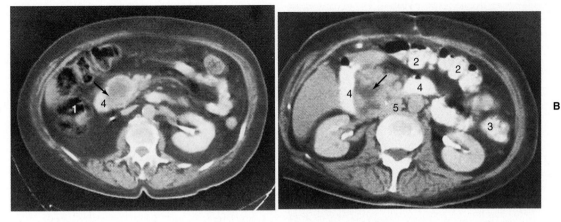

FIG. 21-14. Enlargement of the head of the pancreas *(arrows)* caused by carcinoma (**A**) and pancreatitis that has occurred secondary to a perforated ulcer (**B**). *1,* Ascending colon; *2,* transverse colon; *3,* descending colon; *4,* duodenum; *5,* inferior vena cava.

sonogram (Fig. 21-13). Larger pseudocysts can be monitored with ultrasonography, although CT generally provides a more graphic and complete delineation of the extent of involvement, and smaller changes in size and extent can be appreciated. A specific diagnosis of chronic pancreatitis can be made with CT if pancreatic calcification (often not seen on plain films) and pancreatic ductal dilation are noted.

Solid pancreatic masses may be caused by a tumor (Fig. 21-14) or by focal inflammation, and differentiation may be difficult unless an ancillary finding such as liver metastases is also present. In most cases percutaneous aspiration or core needle biopsy for cytologic and histologic diagnosis is extremely useful (Sundaram, Wolverson, and Heiberg, 1982) (Fig. 21-15). Islet cell tumors often are small and may be difficult to identify with CT (Rossi, Baert, and Passariello, 1985). However, because they are hypervascular, detection may be improved if biphasic, rapid helical scanning is done after bolus injection of a contrast agent.

Kidneys. Renal ultrasonography and excretory urography (or intravenous pyelography) traditionally have been the primary means of investigating the kidney, but CT is rapidly gaining ground. The investigation of renal colic, which was the exclusive domain of intravenous pyelography, now is more effectively and rapidly diagnosed with noncontrast CT (Chen, 1999) (Fig. 21-16). CT is more sensitive in detecting stones (Smith et al, 1995), can delineate signs associated with obstruction (Smith et al, 1996), and aids in treatment planning primarily by

determining stone size and location (Fielding et al, 1998). Although this study can certainly identify other causes of abdominal pain that may mimic renal colic, it is a limited examination because no contrast is administered and significant pathologic conditions such as renal tumors may be missed. Another concern is the radiation dosage, especially if repeated studies might be needed.

In most cases, ultrasonography can distinguish a cystic from a solid mass. When a solid lesion is identified, CT is useful for preoperative staging (Johnson et al, 1987). It is also useful for detecting local recurrence after a nephrectomy. Bowel loops and displaced normal organs make ultrasound evaluation difficult. In patients with polycystic kidneys, the demonstration of cysts with higher attenuation is consistent with a diagnosis of an infected cyst or bleeding into a cyst (Levine and Grantham, 1985). Angiomyolipomas have a characteristic CT appearance (Totty, McClennan, and Melson, 1981). Occasionally calculi may appear as filling defects in the renal pelvis, mimicking tumors or blood clots on pyelography. In these cases CT may be useful for differentiating a tumor (Fig. 21-17) from a faintly calcified stone, a distinction that may not be evident on plain film (Pollack et al, 1981).

Adrenal Glands. CT has made it possible to delineate normal adrenal glands easily and reliably, except when the patient is extremely thin (Abrams et al, 1982). If clinical and biochemical evidence of hyperfunction is present, CT usually is the only imaging method necessary. Pheochromocytomas and tumors causing Cushing's and Conn's

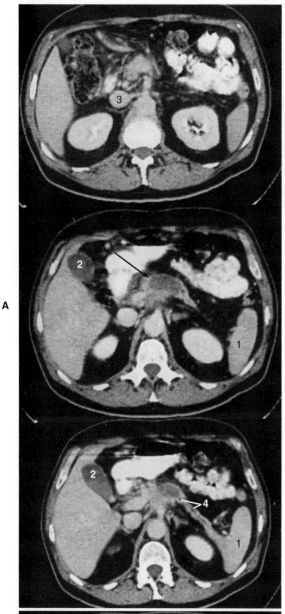

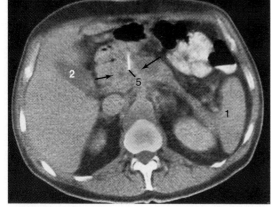

syndromes that are larger than 1 cm are consistently demonstrated on CT. In adrenal hyperplasia, the adrenals may appear normal in size or may be slightly enlarged. Because small aldosteronomas may be missed on CT, adrenal venous sampling and venography are still important (Geisinger, Zelch, and Bravo, 1983). Adrenal metastases, most commonly seen with bronchogenic and breast carcinomas, are readily demonstrated on CT and can be confirmed by biopsy.

A common clinical problem is the incidentally discovered, nonfunctioning small adrenal mass. These masses most often are nonfunctioning adenomas with a high lipid content. Recent studies have concluded that if the attenuation coefficient of the mass is low (18 or lower), a confident diagnosis of adenoma can be made (Korobkin et al, 1996) (Fig. 21-18).

Miscellaneous. The other main indications for imaging of the retroperitoneum are detection of lymphomatous or metastatic lymph nodes (Fig. 21-19) and assessment of abdominal aortic aneurysms.

The retroperitoneum often is obscured on a sonogram because of bowel gas, fat, and bony structures. CT therefore is the superior and obvious imaging method of choice. Because the main criterion for abnormality is lymph node enlargement, false-negative CT results may occur when the internal architecture of the lymph node is distorted without any associated enlargement.

Ultrasonography is adequate for sizing and following up on abdominal aortic aneurysms. Preoperative assessment, however, generally requires CT (Siegel et al, 1994) or MRI (Prince et al, 1995) to determine the relationship of the aneurysm to the renal arteries, to precisely size the entire aneurysm, and to assess the iliac arteries, especially if endovascular grafting is considered. CT is also more useful when complications are suspected, such as rupture of an aneurysm (Fig. 21-20).

FIG. 21-15.   A, Carcinoma of the neck of the pancreas *(arrows)* with associated atrophy and dilation of the pancreatic duct. **B,** Aspiration biopsy of the mass with a 22-gauge needle. *1,* Spleen; *2,* gallbladder; *3,* inferior vena cava with left renal vein; *4,* dilated pancreatic duct with cystic changes; *5,* needle tip.

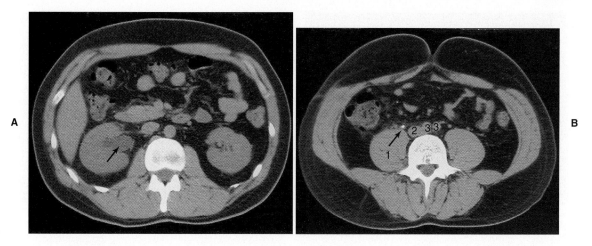

FIG. 21-16. **A,** Dilated right renal pelvis *(arrow)*. **B,** Calculus *(arrow)* in the right ureter. *1,* Psoas muscle; *2,* inferior vena cava; *3,* iliac arteries.

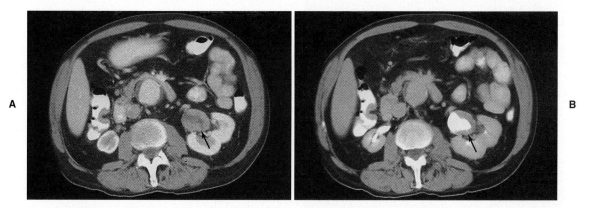

FIG. 21-17. Solid mass in the renal pelvis *(arrow)* before (**A**) and after (**B**) contrast opacification of the renal pelvis.

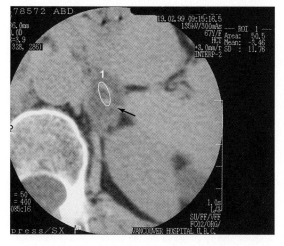

FIG. 21-18. Region of interest within an adrenal mass *(arrow)* indicating a negative Hounsfield number; confirming the diagnosis of adenoma. *1,* Left kidney; *2,* aorta.

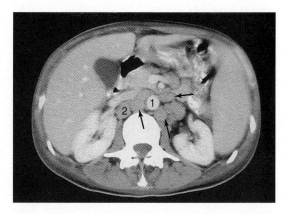

FIG. 21-19 Enlarged paraaortic and paracaval lymph nodes *(arrows)*. *1,* Aorta; *2,* inferior vena cava.

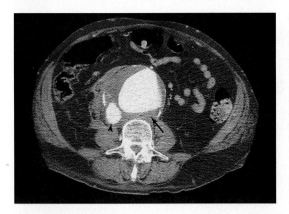

FIG. 21-20. Large abdominal aortic aneurysm *(arrow)* that has ruptured into the inferior vena cava (IVC) *(arrowhead)*, resulting in abnormally dense contrast within the IVC.

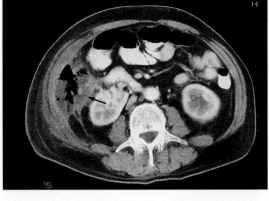

FIG. 21-22. Abnormal localized collection of gas and fluid *(arrow)* in a right flank abscess that occurred secondary to a ruptured appendix.

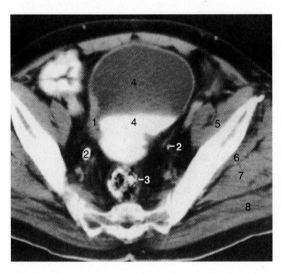

FIG. 21-21. Thickening of the bladder wall without evidence of extension into the perivesical fat (proven amyloidosis). *1*, Thickened bladder wall; *2*, ureters; *3*, sigmoid colon; *4*, urine and contrast medium in the bladder; *5*, iliac muscle; *6*, gluteus minimus; *7*, gluteus medius; *8*, gluteus maximus.

Primary retroperitoneal tumors tend to be large when first suspected clinically. When masses are large enough to be detected on physical examination, an ultrasound examination can differentiate a cystic lesion from a solid one. CT is often performed, however, because it can provide additional information about the extent of disease and the relationship to normal structures.

Pelvis

Ultrasonography remains the primary means of pelvic assessment The main role of CT in the pelvis, apart from assessment of the bowel, remains staging the extent of tumor involvement of the bladder (Fig. 21-21), prostate, uterus, and ovaries and documenting any change after treatment. However, MRI, because of its superior soft tissue contrast and multiplanar capability, is assuming a greater role in staging pelvic neoplasms.

Trauma

Because of its high sensitivity, specificity, negative predictive value, and ability to provide information about extraabdominal injuries such as pelvic and spinal fractures, pulmonary contusions, and pneumothorax, CT has become an integral component of the assessment of blunt abdominal trauma, especially in specialized trauma centers (Shuman, 1997). It has largely replaced other imaging methods and considerably reduced the need for exploratory laparotomies. The so-called *FAST ultrasonography* (focused abdominal sonogram in trauma), which is useful in screening for free intraperitoneal fluid, sometimes is performed first to identify patients more likely to have a positive CT result. However, FAST ultrasonography has a limited ability to define the extent and site of injury and cannot assess the retroperitoneal structures thoroughly (Molina, Warshauer, and Lee, 1998).

Abscess and Drainage

Unlike many neoplasms, an abscess is a potentially curable condition. Because the morbidity and mortality associated with an undrained abscess are high, it is important to use whatever means avail-

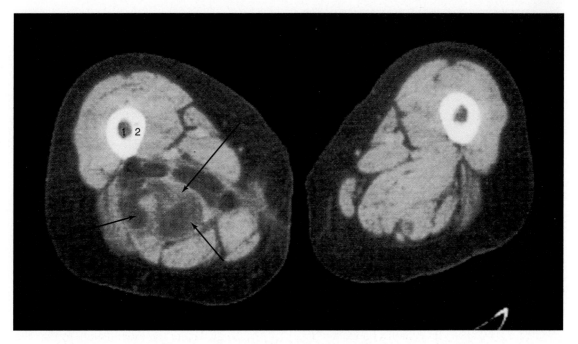

FIG. 21-23. Liposarcoma *(arrows)* involving the right adductor magnus muscle. *1,* Medullary canal; *2,* cortex.

able to localize the abscess accurately and institute prompt treatment (Callen, 1979; Halber, Daffner, and Morgan, 1979). The advantage of CT over ultrasonography is that it is not limited by wounds, drains, ostomies, bandages, or bowel gas associated with paralytic ileus, which postoperative patients commonly have. Extraluminal gas, although not always present, is the most specific CT sign of an abscess (Fig. 21-22). This may be missed on a sonogram because differentiation from normal bowel gas can be extremely difficult.

CT is also extremely useful as a guide for percutaneous drainage of abdominal abscesses and other fluid collections (Gerzof, Spira, and Robbins, 1981). The ability to determine the relationship of adjacent structures, including bowel loops, is especially useful in choosing a safe route for placing larger caliber needles and catheters.

Biopsy

Cytologic aspiration biopsy and core biopsy have proved to be effective, safe, and simple techniques for establishing a cytologic or histologic diagnosis for masses anywhere in the body (Ferrucci et al, 1980). The exact location of the needle tip relative to the tumor (see Fig. 21-15, *B*) can be displayed on CT, therefore even small lesions deep in the abdomen can be approached. This capability

was enhanced by the recent introduction of CT fluoroscopy, which allows the radiologist to directly monitor the position of the needle tip by continuous scanning at six frames per second, nearly real time. The biopsy thus can be performed under direct vision rather than using the conventional "blind" approach of advancing the needle and then determining its location. Problems arising from erratic patient breathing are diminished, the procedure time is reduced, and the patient's safety and comfort are improved.

Musculoskeletal System

CT generally is a problem-solving technique. It is often carried out after plain films or radionuclide bone scans have already been used. Conventional tomography and arteriography, which formerly were used to determine the extent of disease, are now rarely used. With bony tumors, CT is useful in showing the location of the tumor in the bone, evaluating cortical integrity, articular involvement, and intermedullary extent, and defining extraosseous extension (Schreiman et al, 1986). When soft tissues are involved, the relationship of these masses to important neurovascular structures can be determined (Fig. 21-23). However, because of its superior soft tissue contrast resolution and multiplanar capabilities (Petasnik et al, 1986;

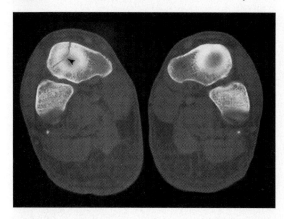

FIG. 21-24. Stress fracture of the right navicular bone *(arrow).*

Boyko et al, 1987), MRI has replaced CT for many musculoskeletal applications.

Skeletal trauma generally can be studied by standard radiographs. In complex anatomic regions, however, such as the pelvis, shoulder, foot (Fig. 21-24), and ankle, more precise information about the presence, location, orientation, and relationship of fracture fragments can be obtained with CT (Guyer et al, 1985; Lange and Alter, 1980). In this regard, multiplanar reformations and 3D reconstructions can be extremely useful.

EXAMINATION PREPARATION
Planning

After the radiologist has determined that a CT scan is clinically indicated, the radiologist and technologist must plan the patient preparation, the use of oral and intravenous contrast media, and the scanning protocol to be used. This can be done verbally or by written instructions. The use of standard protocol sheets may be helpful. When these instructions are different from those routinely followed, it is important for the technologist to discuss the case individually with the radiologist so that the examination can be tailored specifically to the clinical problem. This is even more crucial with helical scanners, which have a myriad of new and very specialized protocols. After reviewing the initial scans, the radiologist may extend, modify, or terminate the examination.

Patient Information

The "high tech" aspect of CT does not diminish the importance of establishing good rapport with the patient. Patient cooperation can mean the dif-

ference between a poor-quality examination and a high-quality result. It is essential that the technologist explain procedures clearly before and during the CT study. The explanations should be brief and given in "lay" terms so that patients know what to expect and what is expected of them. A patient information sheet may be helpful, and pictures of scans may be of interest to the person.

Before the examination, the technologist should:

1. Briefly explain the process of CT.
2. Describe the examination to be performed including the area of the body to be studied and give an estimate of the duration of the examination.
3. Emphasize the importance of keeping still because of the image degradation that occurs with motion.
4. Give appropriate breathing instructions.
5. Have the patient empty the bladder immediately before the examination, so that the patient is more comfortable and less likely to move, especially if the study involves use of an IV contrast medium.
6. If a contrast medium is to be used, explain the reason for its use and question the patient about allergies. A description of any unpleasant sensations the patient may feel from injection of the contrast material also should be given (this is especially important when mechanical power injectors are used).
7. Reassure the patient that the technologist, although not in the room, will be able to see and talk to the patient.

The patient should always be encouraged to ask questions about the examination. If the questions are more medical in nature, the patient should speak directly with the radiologist. It is important to remember that although the examination is routine to the staff, it is not for the patient. In addition to being anxious and worried about the results of the examination, patients are fearful and concerned about the examination itself. The staff should try to make the "high tech" study a "high touch" experience and constantly be sensitive to the patient's feelings.

Oral Contrast Media

The use of dilute oral contrast material to opacify the GI tract is absolutely necessary in the abdomen so that homogeneous, fluid-filled bowel loops are not mistaken for masses (Fig. 21-25) or gas-filled loops of bowel for abscesses. Proper opacification of the GI tract is especially valuable in very thin patients who lack the amount of intraabdominal fat necessary to outline various structures (see Fig. 21-12, *B*).

Dilute barium sulfate solution (e.g., 1% weight to volume, E-Z-CAT) and water-soluble iodinated contrast solutions (e.g., Gastrografin, diluted 1:25 with juice or water) are the most commonly used positive contrast agents for abdominal and pelvic CT scans. Barium sulfate suspension should not be used for patients suspected of having a GI perforation. However, when there is concern about a contrast reaction to iodinated compounds, barium sulfate solution should be used instead.

If the primary purpose of the examination is to study the stomach, the patient is given 350 to 500 ml of contrast medium to drink immediately before the examination. For assessment of gastric neoplasms, water alone with gas (see below) may be given instead of a positive contrast medium to distend the stomach. If the examination extends to the remainder of the upper abdomen, the entire small bowel should be opacified and the patient given an additional drink of contrast material 1 to 2 hours before the examination.

When the distal small bowel and colon must be opacified for examination of the pelvis, some radiologists have the patient drink oral contrast material the evening before or at least 4 to 6 hours before the examination. This ensures that every loop of bowel, including the colon, is opacified. Failure to give the patient the first dose, however, is not a reason to cancel or postpone the procedure; a small-volume contrast enema (150 to 250 ml) can be given to opacify the rectum and distal large bowel. The enema also distends the colon, whereas perioral techniques do not.

Some investigators distend the stomach with air or gas. An effervescent agent similar to that used in double-contrast upper GI examinations can be administered. Water-soluble iodinated contrast medium can also be mixed with a carbonated soft drink. This method allows good visualization of the gastric wall. If a patient cannot drink the oral contrast medium because of nausea and vomiting, it can be introduced through a nasogastric tube. However, the radiopaque markers used in nasogastric tubes to indicate their position on conventional radiographs can produce artifacts on CT, therefore these should be removed before the examination, if possible, or at least replaced by ones that are not radiopaque. Similarly, if the patient has had a recent barium examination of the GI tract, sufficient time should be allowed for elimi-

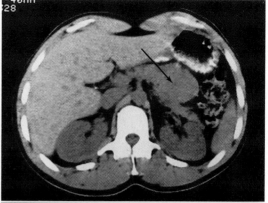

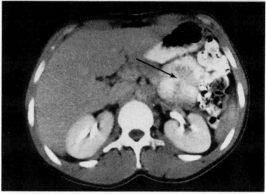

FIG. 21-25. **A,** An apparent mass of the body of the pancreas *(arrow).* **B,** When an oral contrast medium is used, the mass is revealed to be multiple small bowel loops *(arrow).*

nation of the contrast medium, or the colon can be cleansed of residual barium. Residual barium can result in considerable image degradation caused by streak artifacts.

Intravenous Contrast Agents

Intravenous contrast material is used for several purposes. The initial vascular opacification may be useful for anatomic localization, distinguishing vessels from a mass, determining the extent of vascular displacement or invasion by a tumor, assessing specific vascular disease such as aneurysms, stenoses, or loss of vascular integrity resulting in extravasation of the contrast medium. The subsequent extravascular distribution of contrast medium into various tissues helps confirm an intact blood supply of body organs and, to a limited extent, provides some functional assessment such as in opacification of the urinary tract. Often tumors and normal parenchyma do not enhance to the same extent or at the same time. This differential enhancement, which increases the attenuation difference between normal and abnormal tissue (Fig. 21-26), can be used to advantage to maximize lesion detectability. However, the timing of the scans and the contrast injection protocols must be chosen carefully because some lesions may be masked by tissue enhancement.

The degree of contrast medium enhancement is the result of a combination of complex factors, including the rate, amount and concentration of contrast material administered, the speed of injection, the timing of the scans, cardiac output, plasma expansion, extravascular redistribution, and renal filtration and excretion of the contrast material. Various approaches to IV administration of contrast material have been used, reflecting the inadequacies of any one method (Nelson, 1991). Drip infusion of contrast medium usually does not result in ideal enhancement because of inconsistent flow rates, which result in too slow a rise in the plasma iodine concentration. This method has largely been replaced by bolus injections, with some notable exceptions such as routine contrast medium-enhanced head scans and postoperative lumbar spine and cervical spine scans.

A mechanical injector is mandatory for use of injection rates as high as 5 or 6 ml per second and to obtain a sustained, reproducible level of contrast medium enhancement. This usually requires insertion of an 18- or 19-gauge short intravenous needle catheter into a medially directed antecubital vein connected to tubing capable of withstanding the pressures generated in high-flow injections. The major disadvantage of a power injector is the slight risk of extravasation of contrast material into the soft tissues. It therefore is imperative that the patient be able to alert the technologist immediately if a local "burning" sensation occurs so that the injection can be stopped, preventing tissue damage. Most often the injector is loaded with 100 to 180 ml of 60% contrast medium, with injection rates varying from 1 to 6 ml per second depending on the specific indication.

Different delay times are used to match scanning with the arrival of contrast medium at the appropriate vessels and organs. These delays can be set empirically based on experience and published data, or they can be tailored individually through the use of bolus tracking or automated techniques such as "SmartPrep" (General Electric) or "SureStart" (Toshiba). Using helical or spiral volumetric acquisition, a large region (typically 30 cm or more) such as the entire liver can be easily examined in 20 to 30 seconds. The latest generation of scanners, with subsecond and multislice technology, will enhance this capability (Berland and Smith, 1998) by allowing even greater ranges or thinner collimation or both.

With a single bolus injection of contrast medium, the pattern of vascular enhancement during the first circulation and the pattern of vascular and tissue enhancement during recirculation can be studied. This method is useful for studying aortic dissection, in which flow in the false lumen is often delayed, and for evaluation of a possible hemangioma (see Fig. 21-8). In these cases a specific

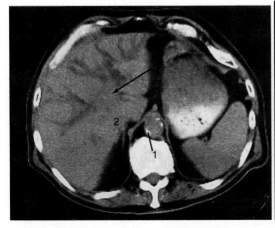 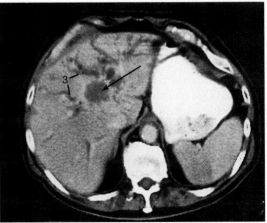

A   B

FIG. 21-26.   Cholangiocarcinoma *(arrow).* **A,** Precontrast scan. **B,** Postcontrast scan. The large mass at the porta hepatis is more evident on the postcontrast scan, which also better differentiates dilated bile ducts from blood vessels. *1,* Aortic calcification; *2,* adrenal gland; *3,* dilated intrahepatic ducts.

area may be examined dynamically and repeatedly over a period of time without table movement.

Other, more specialized techniques include selective catheterization and injection of specific vessels followed by CT scanning such as the proper hepatic artery for CT hepatic arteriography and the superior mesenteric artery or splenic artery for CT arterial portography (Nelson, 1991). These studies are reported to be more sensitive for detecting small liver lesions (less than 2 cm) than either MRI or biphasic CT (Hori et al, 1998).

SCANNING PROTOCOLS

Developing routine protocols is helpful. These protocols serve as general guidelines and can be modified as required, tailoring the examination to a particular patient's clinical problem. In addition to the details specific to a region, scanning protocols should optimize the radiographic technique to maximize lesion detection. This requires careful consideration in choosing the appropriate kV, mA, collimation, reconstruction interval, pitch, range, FOV, reconstruction matrix, field size, reconstruction algorithm, postprocessing filters, and window widths and levels.

Thorax

In most thoracic examinations, scanning begins superiorly from the level of the clavicles and extends to the posterior costophrenic angle. When a neoplasm is suspected, the scans should include the liver and adrenal glands. Because detection of liver metastases is maximized when scans are obtained immediately after administration of a contrast medium, it may be more appropriate to scan in a caudocranial direction through the liver and adrenal glands first and then superiorly through the remainder of the chest, where a high plasma iodine concentration is not as critical (Foley, 1989b).

Scans may be obtained in inspiration or midinspiration. Most important, the patient should try to take the same breath each time to avoid anatomic misregistration. Helical scanning has made this less of a problem because the entire chest can be examined with a single breath (Costello, Anderson, and Blume, 1991). When the posterior lung base is the region of primary concern, prone scans may be helpful to increase aeration to this area. Lateral decubitus scans also are helpful in rare instances in distinguishing between complex pleural and pulmonary pathologic conditions, such as differentiating an empyema from a large lung abscess.

Thoracic CT scans should be viewed with at least two different window width settings (Fig. 21-27). One of these should be optimized for the mediastinum and chest wall and the other for the lungs. If necessary, an additional setting for the bones should be used. The use of higher frequency filters for the lung parenchyma may also be helpful.

Scans of the chest are generally obtained with the patient supine and the arms elevated. The arms should not be so high as to obstruct the flow of IV contrast material, therefore some radiologists prefer to leave the arm with the IV line by the patient's side. especially for high flow rate examinations, even though some artifacts will result.

Some radiologists believe that an IV contrast medium need not be used routinely because the anatomy of the mediastinal structures is not complicated, and they are generally well delineated by the mediastinal fat. Contrast medium is useful, however, for better defining the mediastinum, for determining the relationship of the mass to the mediastinal vessels, or for checking for vascular abnormalities.

CT examination of the thorax usually begins with a digital localizing radiograph (e.g., scout view, topogram, or scanogram), usually in the anteroposterior projection. Scan levels can be prescribed from this image, and the scans obtained can be displayed on it. This can be helpful in correlating the CT images with a plain film abnormality and may be of some value in planning radiation therapy and guiding biopsy. Thicker slices (7 to 10 mm) obtained at 7- to 10-mm slice intervals are routinely used. Thinner sections of 3- to 5-mm collimation with closer slice intervals may be used to improve spatial resolution, particularly in assessing the hila, fissures, and airways. When HRCT is used for assessing diffuse lung disease, 1- to 2-mm thick sections are used, often with a smaller FOV with target reconstruction and a high spatial frequency algorithm to improve spatial resolution (Mayo, 1991) (see Fig. 21-6).

It is impractical to examine the entire chest using contiguous thin slices. The examination therefore is tailored to the particular clinical indication. For the assessment of bronchiectasis and diffuse infiltrative lung disease, 1- to 2-mm thick sections obtained at 10-mm intervals is used most often. Occasionally, selected scans obtained in expiration may be useful for determining the presence or extent of air-trapping. In assessing asbestos-related

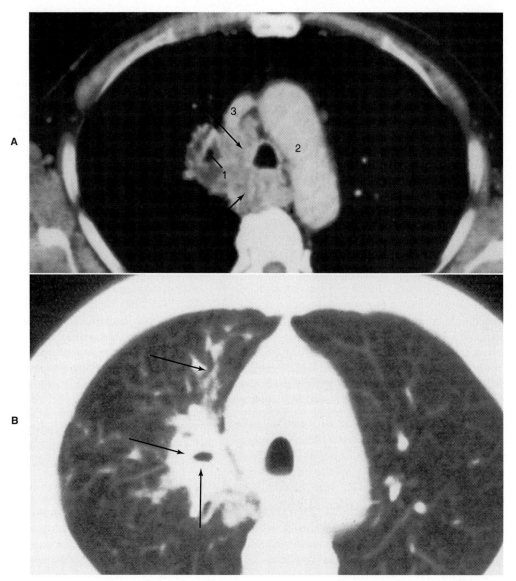

FIG. 21-27. Bronchogenic carcinoma *(arrows)* involving the right hilum with mediastinal invasion and distal obstructive pneumonitis in the right upper lobe. **A,** Mediastinal window. **B,** Lung window. *1,* Right superior segmental bronchus of the right upper lobe; *2,* aortic arch; *3,* superior vena cava.

disease, a more limited examination consisting of five to eight scans spaced throughout the middle and lower thorax usually is sufficient.

Abdomen and Pelvis

Scans are most commonly obtained with the patient supine. Scanning in the prone position may be useful for biopsy of posterior structures, such as the adrenal glands or retroperitoneal lymph nodes.

Thick slices (7 to 10 mm) are most commonly obtained at 7- to 10-mm slice intervals. When the

examination is intended more as a survey, the slices need not be contiguous, and slice intervals of 15 to 20 mm can be used. With helical scanning, pitches of greater than 1 can be selected to quickly cover a longer range, such as in a patient in unstable condition. Newer scanners with dual detectors also permit more extended coverage and quicker examinations. When the adrenal glands or pancreas is the organ of interest, thinner slices of 4- to 5-mm collimation and 4- to 5-mm intervals are necessary. Helical scanning also allows retrospective reconstruction at closer intervals, including

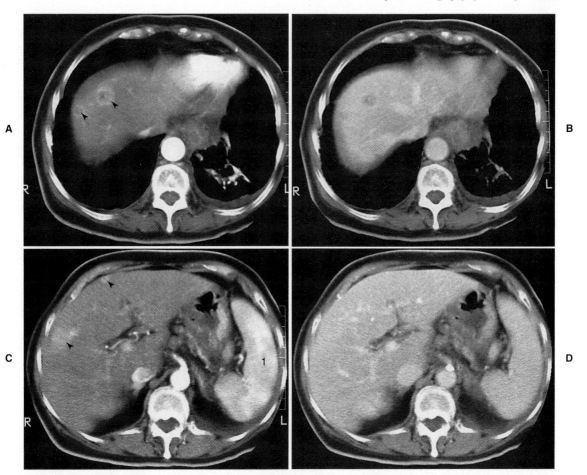

FIG. 21-28. **A** and **C,** Scans obtained within 2 minutes of administration of a contrast medium reveal four hypervascular lesions. **B** and **D,** In "early delayed" scans (i.e., scans obtained approximately 5 minutes after injection of the contrast medium), two of the lesions have "disappeared," and two others are much less conspicuous. *I,* Normal inhomogeneous appearance of the spleen during early enhancement by the contrast medium.

overlapping slices, if the raw data are saved. This may help solve problems of volume averaging and improve multiplanar reformations.

Images obtained without the use of a contrast medium usually are of limited value with the following exceptions: calcific masses or renal calculi, or to localize a hepatic lesion before rapid, contrast medium–enhanced, dynamic scans are obtained at the same level without table movement.

IV contrast medium generally is essential, particularly for evaluating the liver and pancreas. Several factors are important in the detection and differential diagnosis of liver lesions including (1) the liver has a dual blood supply, from the hepatic artery and the portal vein; (2) arterial inflow occurs earlier than portal inflow; and (3) most neoplasms receive their blood primarily from the he-

patic artery, whereas normal hepatocytes primarily receive their blood from the portal vein.

The early "arterial phase" scans with typical scan delays of 20 to 30 seconds best visualize highly vascular lesions, both benign and malignant, such as focal nodular hyperplasia, hepatic adenoma, hepatocellular carcinoma, and hypervascular metastases such as from the kidney, breast, and islet cell tumors (Fig. 21-28). The later "venous phase" scans with scan delays of 60 to 80 seconds are best suited for studying hypovascular lesions such as colonic metastases which, lacking a portal venous supply, enhance much less than normal hepatocytes (Baron, 1994). The trend therefore is to perform these so-called *biphasic examinations* for many hepatic studies. In some cases delayed scans (e.g., 10 minutes) may be helpful in studying cholangiocarcinoma, which may show delayed enhancement. Even very delayed scans (4 to 6 hours) may be useful if at least 60 g of iodine was injected, taking advantage of contrast medium remaining in normal hepatocytes to outline tumors that will appear less dense (Perkerson et al, 1985).

A biphasic protocol for pancreatic scans is also useful. The earlier arterial phase with injection of 150 to 180 ml of contrast medium at a rate of 4 to 5 ml per second, using thin (3 to 5 mm) collimation and a scan delay set to the time of aortic peak plus 5 seconds, optimally enhances the arteries and pancreatic parenchyma, allowing visualization of small hypodense or hyperdense masses (islet cell tumors) and demonstrating any vascular invasion (Hollett, Jorgensen, and Jeffrey, 1995). The later venous phase with a scan delay of 60 seconds and 5- to 7-mm collimation through the liver and pan-

creas delineates the peripancreatic veins, further helping to stage a pancreatic carcinoma; this phase is also best for detecting hepatic metastases from non-islet cell tumors, which tend to be hypovascular.

Renal CT typically is performed to further characterize a renal mass or to stage a tumor. This is best done with a three phase study: examination of the kidneys without a contrast medium (5- to 7-mm collimation) followed by examination after administration of the contrast medium (75 to 100 ml at 2.5 to 4 ml per second) with an early study in the corticomedullary phase (40- to 60-second delay) and by a later scan (3- to 5-minute delay) in the nephrographic or pyelographic phase (Fig. 21-29). The unenhanced scan is useful for detecting stones and fatty tumors (e.g., angiomyolipomas) and for establishing a baseline for determining if a mass is enhancing. Performing

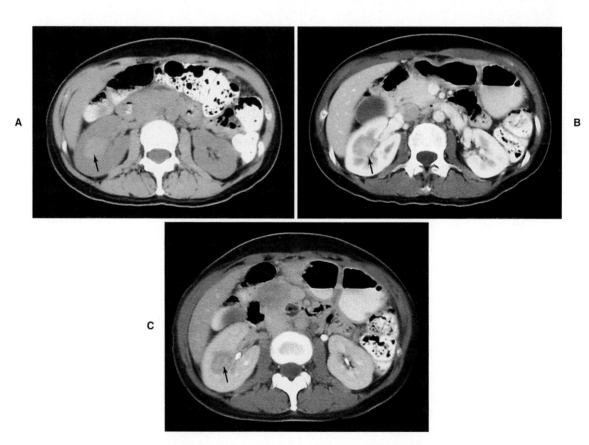

FIG. 21-29.   Renal carcinoma. **A,** Scan obtained before administration of a contrast medium demonstrates a mass of higher density *(arrow)* than renal parenchyma. This is atypical because most renal carcinomas are isodense or hypodense on studies done without use of a contrast medium; the higher density likely indicates recent hemorrhage. **B,** A corticomedullary phase scan demonstrates that the mass *(arrow)* is enhancing, but less than normal renal cortex. **C,** A nephrographic phase scan demonstrates the mass *(arrow)* with greater conspicuity because of the now homogeneous enhancement of the cortex and medulla. Contrast medium is also seen within the collecting system *(arrowhead).*

two studies after administration of the contrast medium improves the detection of masses and provides better characterization and more accurate staging (Kopka et al, 1997).

The protocol for the so-called CT kidney-ureter-bladder examination (CT KUB) is designed specifically to identify renal and ureteral calculi, typically in the acute phase. Neither oral nor IV contrast material is administered. The range scanned extends from the top of the kidneys to the symphysis pubis. Our preferred protocol is to use 3-mm slice collimation, a pitch of 1.5, and overlapping reconstruction every 2.5 mm. The images are transferred to a workstation to be reviewed in cine or movie mode to facilitate interpretation. Only every third image is filmed. The radiation dosage can be significantly diminished by lowering the mA to 80 to 120 since more noisy images are adequate for the purposes of this examination.

For "routine" abdominal scans with less specific indications, an adequate protocol generally is 7- to 10-mm collimated scans, pitch of 1 to 1.5, administration of 150 ml of contrast medium at a rate of 3 ml per second, and a scan delay of 70 seconds.

The use of oral contrast medium has already been emphasized. When examining the pelvis, use of a tampon is an easy means of anatomic localization of the vagina.

Musculoskeletal System

Because the anatomy of the musculoskeletal system varies from one region to another, the technique used for each patient should be tailored to the clinical problem. A computed radiograph is helpful for visualizing any bony abnormalities, to determine the number, location, and range of images needed, and to correlate with plain films.

Precise positioning is important. Whenever possible, the normal extremity should also be examined. The two sides should be symmetrically positioned and displayed to facilitate side-to-side comparison. Slice thickness and interval are determined by the clinical problem. For assessing most tumors and masses, 7- to 10-mm slices are adequate. Smaller lesions require 4- to 5-mm slices, and examination of smaller structures such as the ankle and wrist often requires 1-to 2-mm slices.

Once the images have been obtained, they should always be displayed and viewed at two window settings, soft tissue and bone settings. In some cases reconstruction of the images using higher resolution algorithms and higher spatial frequency filters may be necessary to improve bony detail. Mul-

tiplanar and 3D reconstructions can be helpful with complicated anatomy, particularly in the evaluation of fractures.

When assessing tumors and their relationship to neurovascular structures, bolus injection of IV contrast material is required. Intraarticular injection of a contrast medium or air can be useful when joints are being evaluated.

REFERENCES

Abrams HI et al: Computed tomography versus ultrasound of the adrenal gland: a prospective study, *Radiology* 143:121-128, 1982.

Alpern MB et al: Focal hepatic masses and fatty infiltration detected by enhanced dynamic CT, *Radiology* 158:45-49, 1986.

Androsetti P, Grossholz M, Becker C: Computed tomography in acute left colonic diverticulitis, *Br J Surg* 84(4):532, 1997.

Balthazar EJ: CT of small bowel obstruction, *AJR Am J Roentgenol* 162:255-261, 1994.

Baron RL: Understanding and optimizing use of contrast material for CT of the liver, *AJR Am J Roentgenol* 163:323-331, 1994.

Baron RL et al: A prospective comparison of the evaluation of biliary obstruction using computed tomography and ultrasonography, *Radiology* 145:91-98, 1982.

Berland LL, Smith JK: Multidetector-array CT: once again, technology creates new opportunities, *Radiology* 209:327-329, 1998.

Berry J Jr, Malt RA: Appendicitis near its centenary, *Ann Surg* 200:567-575, 1984.

Boyko OB et al: MR imaging of osteogenic and Ewing's sarcoma, *AJR Am J Roentgenol* 148:317-322, 1987.

Callen PW: Computed tomographic evaluation of abdominal and pelvic abscesses, *Radiology* 131:171-175, 1979.

Castellino RA et al: Computed tomography, lymphography and staging laparotomy: correlations in initial staging of Hodgkin's disease, *AJR Am J Roentgenol* 143:37-41, 1984.

Costello P, Anderson W, Blume D: Pulmonary nodule: evaluation with spiral volumetric CT, *Radiology* 179:875-876, 1991.

Chen MY, Zagoria RJ: Can noncontrast helical computed tomography replace intravenous urography for evaluation of patients with acute urinary tract colic? *J Emerg Med* 17:299-303, 1999.

Davies J et al: Spiral computed tomography and operative staging of gastric carcinoma: a comparison with histopathological staging, *Gut* 41(3):314-319, 1997.

Fenlon HM et al: A comparison of virtual and conventional colonoscopy for the detection of colorectal polyps, *N Engl J Med* 341:1496-1503, 1999.

Ferrucci JT Jr et al: Diagnosis of abdominal malignancy by radiologic fine needle biopsy, *AJR Am J Roentgenol* 134:323-330, 1980.

Fielding JR et al: Unenhanced helical CT of ureteral stones: a replacement for excretory urography in planning treatment, *AJR Am J Roentgenol* 171:1051-1053, 1998.

Foley WD: Dynamic hepatic CT, *Radiology* 170:617-622, 1989b.

Fon GT et al: Computed tomography of the anterior mediastinum in myasthenia gravis, *Radiology* 142:135-141, 1982.

Freeny PC, Marks WM: Hepatic hemangioma: dynamic bolus CT, *AJR Am J Roentgenol* 147:711-719, 1986.

Gamsu G: The mediastinum. In Moss AA, Gamsu G, Genant HK, eds: *Computed tomography of the upper body with magnetic resonance imaging*, ed 2, Philadelphia, 1992, WB Saunders.

Geisinger MA, Zelch MG, Bravo EL: Primary hyperaldosteronism: comparison of CT, adrenal venography, and venous sampling, *AJR Am J Roentgenol* 141:299-302, 1983.

Gerzof SG, Spira R, Robbins AH: Percutaneous abscess drainage, *Semin Roentgenol* 16:62-71, 1981.

Goldman IS et al: Increased hepatic density and phospholipidosis due to amiodarone, *AJR Am J Roentgenol* 144:541-546, 1985.

Gore RM et al: CT features of ulcerative colitis and Crohn's disease, *AJR Am J Roentgenol* 167:3-15, 1996.

Guyer BH et al: Computed tomography of calcaneal fractures: anatomy, pathology, dosimetry, and clinical relevance, *AJR Am J Roentgenol* 145:911-919, 1985.

Halber MD, Daffner RH, Morgan CL: Intraabdominal abscess: current concepts in radiologic evaluation, *AJR Am J Roentgenol* 133:9-13, 1979.

Hara AK et al: Detection of colorectal polyps with CT colography: initial assessment of sensitivity and specificity, *Radiology* 205:59-65, 1997.

Hessel SJ et al: A prospective evaluation of computed tomography and ultrasound of the pancreas, *Radiology* 143:129-133, 1982.

Hollett M, Jorgensen M, Jeffrey R Jr: Quantitative evaluation of pancreatic enhancement during dual-phase helical CT, *Radiology* 195:359-361, 1995.

Hori M et al: Sensitivity in detection of hypervascular hepatocellular carcinoma by helical CT with intraarterial injection of contrast medium and by helical CT and MR imaging with intravenous injection of contrast medium, *Acta Radiol* 39(2):144-151, 1998.

Johnson CD et al: Renal adenocarcinoma: CT staging of 100 tumors, *AJR Am J Roentgenol* 148:59-63, 1987.

Kopka L et al: Dual-phase helical CT of the kidney: value of the corticomedullary and nephrographic phase for evaluation of renal lesions and preoperative staging of renal cell carcinoma, *AJR Am J Roentgenol* 169:1573-1578, 1997.

Korobkin M et al: Differentiation of adrenal adenomas from nonadenomas using CT attenuation values, *AJR Am J Roentgenol* 166:531-536, 1996.

Lane MJ et al: Unenhanced helical CT for suspected acute appendicitis, *AJR Am J Roentgenol* 168:405-409, 1997.

Lange TA, Alter AJ: Evaluation of complex acetabular fractures by computed tomography, *J CAT* 6:849-852, 1980.

Levine E, Grantham JJ: High-density renal cysts in autosomal dominant polycystic kidney disease demonstrated by CT, *Radiology* 154:477-482, 1985.

Manfredi R et al: MAGMA 4:257-262, 1996.

Mayo JR: The high-resolution computed tomography technique, *Semin Roentgenol* 26:104-109, 1991.

Mayo JR et al: Pulmonary embolism: prospective comparison of spiral CT with ventilation-perfusion scintigraphy, *Radiology* 205:447-452, 1997.

Molina PL, Warshauer DM, Lee JK: Computed tomography of thoracoabdominal trauma. In Lee JKT et al, eds: *Computed body tomography with MRI correlation*, ed 3, New York, 1998, Raven Press.

Mucha P Jr: Small intestinal obstruction, *Surg Clin North Am* 67(3):597-620, 1987.

Muhm JR et al: Comparison of whole lung tomography and computed tomography for detecting pulmonary nodules, *AJR Am J Roentgenol* 131:981-984, 1978.

Muller NL: Differential diagnosis of chronic diffuse infiltrative lung disease on high-resolution computed tomography, *Semin Roentgenol* 26:132-142, 1991.

Munk PL, Muller NL, Miller RR: Pulmonary lymphangitic carcinomatosis: CT and pathologic findings, *Radiology* 166:705-709, 1988.

Nelson RC: Techniques for computed tomography of the liver, *Radiol Clin North Am* 29:1199-1212, 1991.

Pang JA, Hamilton-Wood C, Metreweli C: Value of computed tomography in the diagnosis and management of bronchiectasis, *Clin Radiol* 40:40-44, 1989.

Perkerson RB et al: CT densities in delayed iodine hepatic scanning, *Radiology* 155:445-446, 1985.

Petasnick JT et al: Soft tissue masses of the locomotor system: comparison of MR imaging with CT, *Radiology* 160:125-133, 1986.

Pollack HM et al: Computed tomography of renal pelvic filling defects, *Radiology* 138:645-651, 1981.

Posniak HV, Demos TC, Marsan RE: Computed tomography of the normal aorta and thoracic aneurysms, *Semin Roentgenol* 24:7-21, 1989.

Prince MR et al: Breath-hold gadolinium-enhanced MR angiography of the abdominal aorta and its major branches, *Radiology* 197:785-792, 1995.

Rossi P, Baert A, Passariello R: CT of functioning tumours of the pancreas, *AJR Am J Roentgenol* 144:57-60, 1985.

Schaner EG et al: Comparison of computed and conventional whole lung tomography in detecting pulmonary nodules: prospective radiologic-pathologic study, *AJR Am J Roentgenol* 131:51-54, 1978.

Schreiman JS et al: Osteosarcoma: role of CT in limb-sparing treatment, *Radiology* 161:485, 1986.

Siegel CL, Cohan RH: CT of abdominal aortic aneurysms, *AJR Am J Roentgenol* 163:17-29, 1994.

Shuman WP: CT of blunt abdominal trauma in adults, *Radiology* 205(2):297-306, 1997.

Siegelman SS et al: CT of fluid collections associated with pancreatitis, *AJR Am J Roentgenol* 134:1121-1132, 1980.

Smith RC et al: Acute flank pain: comparison of non-contrast-enhanced CT and intravenous urography, *Radiology* 194:789-794, 1995.

Smith RC et al: Acute ureteral obstruction: value of secondary signs on helical unenhanced CT, *AJR Am J Roentgenol* 167:1109-1113, 1996.

Sommer T et al: Aortic dissection: a comparative study of diagnosis with spiral CT, multiplanar transesophageal echocardiography, and MR imaging, *Radiology* 199(2):347-352, 1996.

Stein PD, Henry JW, Relyea B: Untreated patients with pulmonary embolism, *Chest* 107:931-935,1995.

Sundaram M, Wolverson MK, Heiberg E: Utility of CT-guided abdominal aspiration procedures, *AJR Am J Roentgenol* 139:1111-1115, 1982.

Swensen SJ et al: Lung nodule enhancement at CT: prospective findings, *Radiology* 201:447-455, 1996.

Totty WG, McClennan BL, Melson GL: Relative value of computed tomography and ultrasonography in the assessment of renal angiomyolipoma, *J CAT* 5:173-178, 1981.

Weg N, Scheer MR, Gabor MP: Liver lesions: improved detection with dual-detector-array CT and routine 2.5-mm thin collimation, *Radiology* 209:417-426, 1998.

Wing VW et al: The clinical impact of CT for blunt abdominal trauma, *AJR Am J Roentgenol* 145:1191-1194, 1985.

Zerhouni EA et al: CT of the pulmonary nodule: a cooperative study, *Radiology* 160:319-327, 1986.

BIBLIOGRAPHY

Foley WD: Agents in computed tomography. In Skucas J, ed: *Radiographic contrast agents,* ed 2, Rockville, Md, 1989a, Aspen Publishers.

Glazer et al: Adrenal tissue characterization using MR imaging, *Radiology* 158:73, 1986.

Peterson MS et al: Hepatic parenchymal perfusion defects detected with CTAP imaging: pathologic correlation, *Radiology* 185:149, 1992.

The authors would like to thank Marilyn Stuart and Mary Jane Li for their help in typing and preparing the manuscript. They also would like to thank the CT technologists who helped acquire the CT scans.

Pediatric Computed Tomography

JEREMY LYSNE*

* This chapter was originally written by Victoria Bigland, RTR; Gordon Culham, MD, FRCPC; and Kenneth Poskitt, MDCM, of the British Columbia Children's Hospital, Department of Radiology. It has been revised for the second edition by Jeremy Lysne, RT(R)(CT), Department of Radiology, Denver Children's Hospital.

ROLE OF THE CT TECHNOLOGIST

The objective of the pediatric CT examination is to acquire optimum diagnostic images with minimum discomfort and radiation exposure to the patient. To this end, two basic tenets apply: (1) the

PROCEDURE PREPARATION

- Have the patient's radiographic file available for consultation.
- Have a thorough understanding of how the radiologist wishes to conduct the study.
- Register pertinent patient data into the CT system and select the appropriate parameters under which the CT examination is to be conducted.
- Prepare the scanning room and have all necessary accessory equipment (e.g., immobilization devices, monitoring equipment) available for the procedure.
- Prepare the necessary intravenous (IV) contrast media, if required.

technologist should be prepared, and (2) the technologist should be honest. A well-prepared technologist plays an important role in avoiding delays and helps reduce the time the patient must be on the table of the CT scanner. Box 2-1 lists the general duties of the technologist before the patient enters the scanning room.

The CT technologist in a children's hospital should be honest in terms of the exact details of the CT examination. This helps ensure the cooperation of young patients and their parents during the procedure. The results can be successful, especially when the patient and parents are well informed. In most institutions, parents are encouraged to remain in the CT room during the examination.

In addition, a relaxed, nonthreatening environment helps gain the confidence and cooperation of the pediatric patient. Toys, books, and puzzles are a welcome diversion for the child who is waiting for a CT examination. In the CT room, interesting posters (Fig. 22-1) or pictures hung on the walls or ceiling help provide a friendly atmosphere. Young children are encouraged to bring their favorite blanket or cuddly toy with them for

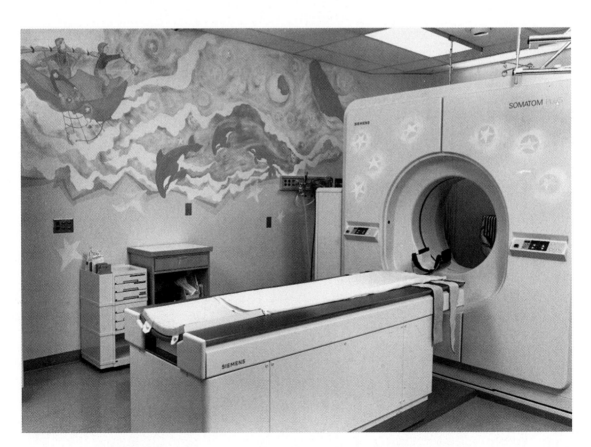

FIG. 22-1. An interesting wall mural helps provide a friendly environment.

reassurance. In addition, a variety of audio tapes for all age groups could be made available.

PATIENT MANAGEMENT
Neonatal Patients

To minimize the risk of infection to the neonatal patient, CT personnel who handle the infant should remove rings and wrist watches, wash hands thoroughly with antibacterial soap, and always wear a cover gown.

During the scanning procedure, it is important to maintain the infant's body temperature. This can be achieved by increasing the temperature in the CT scanning room before the arrival of the patient, wrapping the infant in a warm blanket, and covering the infant's head with a cap or small towel to prevent rapid heat loss. Equally important is placing a heating blanket under the infant that is positioned on the scanning table or focusing a heat lamp on the patient with special attention to the correct distance of the lamp from the patient.

Finally, the patient's vital signs and body temperature throughout the CT examination should be monitored, usually by a nurse who accompanies the patient to the radiology department.

Sedation

The use of sedation is inevitable in pediatric CT scanning. Image degradation from patient motion is still a problem. The introduction of fast, spiral/helical CT scanners have decreased the need for sedation. (For instance, sedation rates at Denver Children's Hospital in Colorado have decreased by 50% compared with a conventional CT scanner.) With scan times as short as 0.5 sec, sedation may not be necessary, although patient motion can still be a problem.

Generally, patients between the ages of 6 months and 5 years are prepared for sedation. This preparation requires patients to ingest nothing by mouth 4 hours for solids and formula and 2 hours for clear liquids including breast milk. The technologist should inform parents of the correct preparation and sedation instructions to help minimize any misunderstanding on the day of the examination.

The sedatives most commonly used in pediatric imaging are oral chloral hydrate and IV pentobarbital sodium. Children younger than 6 months are given chloral hydrate, 50 to 100 mg/kg to a maximum dose of 2000 mg. Patients 6 months and older are given IV pentobarbital sodium, 5 mg/kg to a maximum dose of 200 mg. A dose of 5 mg/kg

is given initially as a slow bolus. If sedation is not achieved, an additional dose of 2 mg/kg is given after 5 minutes.

Children with delayed development delayed are referred to the anesthesia department for sedation. Children under 6 months of age rarely require sedation. Wrapping them in a warm blanket and providing them with a pacifier, as well as using a table restraint system to immobilize them, can be all that is needed for a successful scan. With faster scanners, good patient communication, and the proper use of restraints, sedation can be minimized.

When patients arrive in the radiology department, a careful assessment of their ability to undergo the CT examination without sedation is performed by the CT technologist or the radiology nurse. This assessment includes the following:

1. Consideration of the complexity of the CT study planned. (Is IV contrast required? Will a coronal view be performed?)
2. A brief explanation of the examination to the parents and child.
3. Consideration of the parents' opinion of the child's ability to cooperate.
4. Consideration whether babies seem ready to sleep on their own. With older children, a visit to the scan room to observe another child being scanned may be helpful.

Sedation protocols and standards should be cooperatively established by the departments of radiology and anesthesiology to ensure high-quality care for the sedated patient. At Denver Children's Hospital, most patients are sedated intravenously. Before the examination, an IV line is established by the hospital's IV service and the radiology nurse obtains a patient history. Any syndrome or condition with a respiratory risk that contraindicates sedation is recorded and brought to the attention of the radiologist. The IV sedation is administered by the attending radiologist in the presence of a registered nurse. Immediately following the administration of the drug and during the CT examination, the patient is closely monitored visually and with the pulse oximeter.

Resuscitative supplies are kept in the CT scan room at all times. When the study is completed, the sedated child is moved to the recovery room for monitoring. Patients are discharged when they are easily aroused, have enough muscle tone to hold up their heads, and can drink clear fluids. The parents are given an information sheet about care of the postsedated child that includes a telephone number to call if they have any concerns after their return home.

Use of Intravenous Contrast Media

The use of nonionic contrast media almost eliminates minor reactions such as pain, nausea, vomiting, and urticaria. This is especially important in pediatric CT, and the use of nonionic contrast media is therefore recommended in those examinations requiring contrast media. The removal of these potential reactions and discomforts helps ensure the cooperation of the patient and provides a safer examination for the sedated child.

The dose of contrast material is 2 to 3 ml/kg to a maximum of 150 ml. The use of contrast enhanced studies have become more frequent with spiral/helical CT scanners, in which various vessel and organ enhancement can be evaluated. With spiral/helical CT, larger areas can be covered during optimal enhancement. Until recently, contrast was injected manually, but power injectors are now used in pediatric scanning because they provide a constant rate of injection that allows the more accurate timing of the bolus. The deciding factor for use of a power injector depends on the IV site. Only peripheral IV sites can be obtained on most children. The injection rate is determined by the size of the IV catheter; injection rates of 1 to 3 ml/sec can be used with 22 to 24-gauge catheters. Butterfly-type needles must not be used with power injectors. At the author's institution, the use of smaller catheters have been successful with organ enhancement using slower injection rates.

Several new programs (e.g., Toshiba's Sure Start and General Electric's Smart Prep) facilitate optimum contrast enhancement by allowing the operator to place a region of interest (ROI) on a vessel or organ and track the ROI during enhancement. When the ROI reaches its peak, scanning begins. The disadvantages of these bolus tracking techniques include increased dose to the site where the ROI is set and the loss of the ROI on the target organ if the patient moves.

Regardless of the injection type, it is important to monitor the IV site during injection. If manual injection is used, filling the contrast medium into smaller syringes facilitates injection, compared with the use of a large syringe.

Immobilization

Immobilization of the child is essential to ensure patient safety and to provide images free of motion artifacts. For patients under 5 years old, the immobilizer (Fig. 22-2) is a comfortable device that secures the patient's arms beside the head during body examinations. This device is secured to the patient scanning table with adhesive straps after the patient has been positioned.

Larger children are generally immobilized using other methods such as adhesive straps placed under the mattress and over the patient. After the patient has been immobilized, the CT technologist should still carefully monitor the child by closed-circuit television.

Radiation Protection

Because growing cells are the most sensitive to radiation, and in consideration of the cumulative effect over a lifetime of exposure, radiation exposure has a potentially higher risk for the pediatric patient than for the adult patient. Therefore radiation protection is an integral part of the pediatric CT examination.

With spiral/helical CT, radiation dose can be significantly lower compared with conventional CT. This is mainly because of the improvements in detector technology including the development of multidetector systems. In addition, other variables can be changed to reduce the dose in spiral/helical CT scanning. A pitch of 1.5 can lower the dose by about 25%, whereas a pitch of 2 can reduce the exposure by about 50%. However, as pitch increases, resolution along the z axis decreases.

Radiation dose to the patient can be minimized if the following measures are observed:

1. All CT examination requests should be screened by the radiologist to ensure that CT is the appropriate imaging modality for detection of the clinical problem.

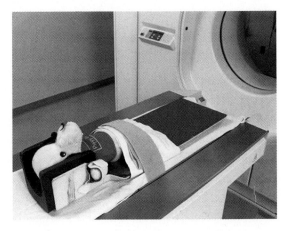

FIG. 22-2.   A patient immobilizer is a comfortable device to secure the pediatric patient.

2. Each study should be tailored to the diagnostic needs of the individual patient.

3. All CT images should be checked by the supervising radiologist before the patient is removed from the CT scanner.

4. Lead shielding should be placed under and over the body regions not being examined.

5. The milliampere (mA) values should be matched appropriately to the size of the patient and the section to be imaged.

6. Low-dose techniques can be employed for certain examinations that do not require optimum spatial resolution. For example, 100 mAs can be used in cranial CT to check for ventricular shunt function only. In addition, 85 mAs can be used to check hip position and postcasting of the patient with congenital hip dislocation.

7. Positioning for routine cranial CT should be done without the aid of prescan localization images (scout view).

8. Axial scans should be done with the gantry angled 20 degrees to the canthomeatal line to avoid exposure to the lens of the eye.

9. Finally, the CT quality assurance program should ensure optimum diagnostic images with minimum radiation dose to the patient.

CT OF THE HEAD AND SPINE

Imaging of the head and spine in children depends on a number of factors including indications for the examination, which determine the imaging modality best suited to the overall assessment of the patient's medical problem. For example, indications for pediatric neuroangiography are limited and are being rapidly replaced by magnetic resonance angiography. The prime remaining indications for neuroangiography are the assessment of arteriovenous malformations, moyamoya disease, aneurysm search, acute idiopathic hemiplegia, and traumatic dissection.

Indications

With a few exceptions, most indications for examination of the central nervous system are best studied by magnetic resonance imaging (MRI). CT remains the primary modality for the assessment of trauma in the acute phase (Fig. 22-3), acute hemorrhage, and the detection of calcification. CT also remains the most sensitive technique for the assessment of hypoxic ischemia damage to the neonatal brain caused by asphyxia at birth (Fig. 22-4) or nonaccidental injury.

CT is also indicated for the following when MRI is not available.

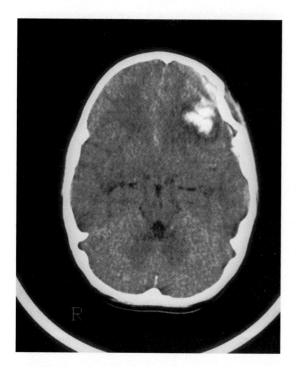

FIG. 22-3. Left frontal depressed skull fracture with associated hematoma and surrounding edema.

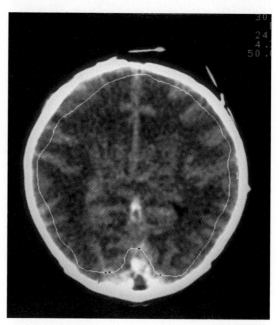

FIG. 22-4. Scan 72 hours after birth shows extensive, low-density changes throughout the white matter with obliteration of much of the overlying cortex. This is typically seen with significant perinatal asphyxia.

Congenital Abnormalities. Abnormalities such as Dandy-Walker syndrome (Fig. 22-5), congenital hydrocephalus, and disorders of migration require attention both to structural relationships and CT technique because the subtle interplay between gray and white matter may be the main diagnostic clue. CT assessment is important for inherited disorders such as neurofibromatosis and tuberous sclerosis (Fig. 22-6) that predispose to future complications such as tumors.

Seizures. A CT examination is included in the assessment of patients with intractable seizures and of those children with seizure types known to have a high association with structural abnormalities.

Vascular Problems. A CT examination is part of the diagnosis and posttreatment evaluation of arteriovenous malformations, infarction, and moyamoya disease.

Inflammation. CT imaging of inflammatory disorders is used primarily to document the complications of infection, rather than to make the initial diagnosis.

Tumors. CT imaging is indicated for the diagnosis and posttreatment evaluation of brain tumors. Brain tumors that occur in the pediatric population differ from those in adults in the areas of location, behavior, and type. Whereas only 5% of adult brain tumors are located in the posterior fossa, over 50% of pediatric brain tumors appear in this location. With the administration of IV contrast, the tumors are frequently enhanced, but this enhancement does not indicate a sinister pathology. Metastatic brain tumors occur less frequently in children than in adults.

The following types of primary brain tumors can be found in children:

- Ependymoma: This can arise in the wall or floor of the fourth ventricle, with possible extension through the fourth ventricle foramina over the medulla and upper cervical cord.
- Cystic astrocytoma: This is the most common posterior fossa tumor, usually centrally located and with cystic and solid components (Fig. 17-7).
- Medulloblastoma: This is usually located midline in the vermis, compressing and displacing the fourth ventricle, and often resulting in hydrocephalus.

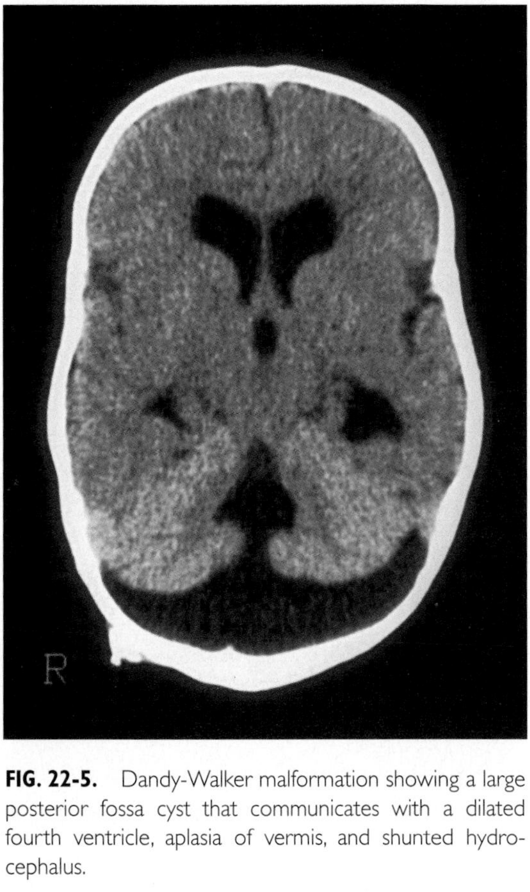

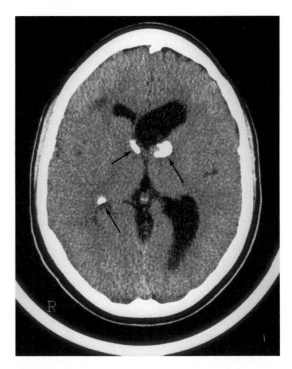

FIG. 22-5. Dandy-Walker malformation showing a large posterior fossa cyst that communicates with a dilated fourth ventricle, aplasia of vermis, and shunted hydrocephalus.

FIG. 22-6. Multiple periventricular cortical calcifications (*arrows*). These represent calcified tubers in patients with tuberous sclerosis.

Spinal cord. CT is indicated for the spinal cord in cases of suspected disk protrusion to assess complex scoliosis and examine the cord following myelography.

Patient Positioning

When positioning the patient, it is essential to have the patient's head geometrically centered in the gantry to ensure artifact-free images. In this respect, the patient's head must be centered accurately from right to left in the head holder and from front to back in the gantry. Multiple small positioning sponges can be used to secure the patient's head in the head holder. For the accurate assessment of midline structures, care must be taken to position the head so that the right and left sides are symmetric and not tilted.

Positioning for axial, coronal, and Water's views are as follows:

- Axial view: Without the aid of a scout view, routine axial scans of the brain are positioned 20 degrees to the canthomeatal line. This position avoids the radiosensitive lens of the eye and includes the complete volume of brain tissue with the least number of scans.

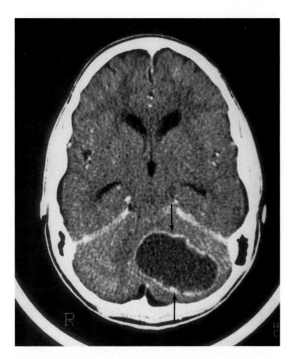

FIG. 22-7. Left cerebellar astrocytoma with enhancing cystic central component (*arrows*).

- Coronal view: In addition to axial scans, direct coronal scans are an essential part of the initial CT assessment of a brain tumor. This view better defines the extent of the tumor into the cerebellar hemispheres and can demonstrate displacement of the fourth ventricle by brain stem or cerebellar tumors. The coronal position is usually comfortable for the pediatric patient and is easily achieved with even sedated children.
- Water's view: Occasionally, a patient cannot tolerate the coronal position. An alternate position is a Water's view, in which the patient's head is extended to maximum tolerance. With the aid of a scout view, the scans are prescribed as close to 90 degrees to the clivus as possible.

Technical Considerations

Pediatric CT examinations of the brain and orbits are first conducted as noncontrast studies and are then reviewed by the radiologist while the patient remains on the scanning table. Based on these unenhanced images, the need for additional views or a contrast study is determined. Routine axial scans of the brain are acquired at a 5-mm slice thickness with 5-mm slice spacing.

Although the kVp value for examinations of head is 120, the mA values should not be too low to cause increased noise, which degrades image quality. Typical mA values are shown in Table 22-1.

In situations in which it is important to reduce minor motion artifacts and interscan tube cooling delays, the multiscan technique is possible on CT scanners with continuously rotating measurement systems. This allows for the measurement of raw data from a series of 1- or 2-second scan rotations

TABLE 22-1

Pediatric Radiographic Technique Factors*

| | TECHNIQUE FACTORS | |
AGE OF PATIENT	kVp	mA
Premature infant	120	180
Term infant to 2 years	120	250
Child 2 to 8 years	120	250
Child more than 8 years	120	300

*All slice thickness = 5 mm.

and for reconstruction of the CT image from the averaged data set. For example, for a head scan, data acquired from four 1-second scan rotations can be averaged to generate a single image that would result in less motion artifact and decreased tube loading compared with an image acquired and reconstructed from one 4-second scan rotation.

In examinations of the posterior fossa, the volume artifact reduction (see Chapter 11) function can be used to reduce streak artifacts caused by partial inclusion of bone structures in the scan. With this technique, the posterior fossa should be scanned with contiguous spiral/helical 2-mm slices at low mA values (250). These 2-mm images are

TABLE 22-2

Pediatric CT Assessment Protocol for Trauma

PARAMETER	RECOMMENDATIONS
Patient position	Supine; scans at 20 to canthomeatal line
Lateral scout view	To include cervical spine
Scan range	From foramen magnum to vertex of skull
Slice thickness	5 mm
Slice spacing	5 mm
Algorithm	Standard; review images to ultrahigh (bone) for evaluation of bony skull and possible fracture
Photography	Brain: W60, C35; bone: W2000, C400; subdural: W150, C50

TABLE 22-3

Pediatric CT Assessment Protocol for Temporal Lobe Seizures

PARAMETER	RECOMMENDATIONS
Patient position	Supine; scans at 20 to canthomeatal line
Scan range	Contiguous 5-mm scans through temporal lobes with 5-mm scans of rest of brain volume
Plus-patient position	Supine; scans at −20 to canthomeatal line

LATERAL SCOUT VIEW

Slice thickness	5 mm
Slice spacing	5 mm
Scan range	Entire temporal lobes

TABLE 22-4

Pediatric CT Assessment Protocol for Seizure Disorder, Hydrocephalus*, Migraine, and Congenital Malformations†

PARAMETER	RECOMMENDATIONS
Patient position	Supine; scans at 20 degrees to canthomeatal line
Scout view	No
Scan range	From foramen magnum to vertex of skull
Slice thickness	5 mm
Slice spacing	5 mm

*Determine possible cause.
†The radiologist views the images while the patient is on the scan table and determines whether a contrast study is required.

TABLE 22-5

Pediatric CT Assessment Protocol for Hydrocephalus, Periventricular Leukomalacia, and Tuberous Sclerosis

PARAMETER	RECOMMENDATIONS
Hydrocephalus	Shunt dysfunction (?)
Patient position	Supine; scans at 20 degrees to canthomeatal line
Slice thickness	10 mm
Slice spacing	10 mm
Mas	150
Scan time	1 second

PVL (PERIVENTRICULAR LEUKOMALACIA)

Tuberous sclerosis

Patient position	Supine; scans at 20 degrees to canthomeatal line
Slice thickness	Contiguous 5-mm scans through the lateral ventricles
Slice spacing	5-mm scans every 5 mm above and below the lateral ventricles

then summed to create 4-mm images with superior spatial resolution. If this technique is to be effective, the patient must be fully cooperative and must not move during acquisition of the 2-mm images.

Scanning Protocols

Scanning protocols are usually established to include information such as patient position, prescan localization (scout view) scan range, slice thickness and spacing, algorithm, and mA values. These are intended to assist the technologist performing the CT examination and generally help increase the overall efficiency of the examination. Tables 22-2 through 22-9 are examples of protocols of the head orbit and spine used in our department. In addition, Figs. 22-3 through 22-11 illustrate

other important clinical problems demonstrated by CT.

Spiral/Helical Scanning

Spiral/helical scanning offers several advantages compared with conventional single-slice CT scanning in pediatrics. For example, faster scanning times decrease the need for sedation and allow the performance of examinations during peak contrast enhancement. Volume data acquisition allows for retrospective data reconstruction, which facilitates further evaluation of pathology without the need to scan additional slices. The data can be reconstructed in overlapping slice intervals. Volume data acquisition also improves the quality of MPR images and 3D images. Additionally, with in-

TABLE 22-6

Pediatric CT Assessment Protocol for Tumors

PARAMETER	RECOMMENDATIONS
Patient position	Supine; scans at 20 degrees to canthomeatal line
PRECONTRAST	
Scan range	From just below to just above tumor site
Slice thickness	5 mm
Slice spacing	5 mm
POSTCONTRAST	
Lateral scout view	
Posterior fossa tumor (volume artifact reduction technique)	2-mm contiguous scans summed to 4-mm images from the foramen magnum to just above the tumor site; alternate: 5-mm contiguous scans
SUPRATENTORIAL TUMOR	
Slice thickness	5 mm
Slice spacing	5 mm
Scan range	From just below to just above the tumor site
REMAINDER OF BRAIN VOLUME ABOVE AND BELOW SITE OF PATHOLOGY	
Slice thickness	5 mm
Slice spacing	5 mm
PLUS	
Patient position:	Coronal view or −20 degrees to the canthomeatal line (for temporal lobe tumor)
LATERAL SCOUT VIEW	
Slice thickness	5 mm
Slice spacing	5 mm
Scan range	From just below to just above tumor site

TABLE 22-7

Pediatric CT Assessment Protocol for the Internal Auditory Meatus*

PARAMETER	RECOMMENDATIONS
Patient position 1	0-degree axials
Patient position 2	Coronals or reverse coronals to image cochlea
LATERAL SCOUT VIEW	
Slice thickness	2 mm
Slice spacing	2 mm
Scan range	Petrous bones
Algorithm	Ultrahigh (bone)
Postscan review	Using raw data saved during image acquisition, scans are targeted to right and then left sides, magnified ×8
Reverse coronal	Patient supine; head view flexed as much as possible; gantry angled so that scans are 70 degrees to axial scans

*Maximum cooperation of the patient is required for this study; therefore children under the age of 5 years are usually sedated.

TABLE 22-8

Pediatric CT Assessment Protocol for the Orbits

PARAMETER	RECOMMENDATIONS
Patient position	Supine; scans at −10 degrees to canthomeatal line
LATERAL SCOUT VIEW PRECONTRAST	
Scan range	From inferior orbital margin to superior orbital margin
Slice thickness	3 mm
Slice spacing	3 mm
Magnify	×3
Algorithm	Standard; review images to ultrahigh (bone) algorithm for assessment of bony involvement
Postcontrast	Same as for precontrast; for malignant orbital lesions, routine axial scans of brain 20 degrees to canthomeatal line for possible metastases

TABLE 22-9

Pediatric CT Assessment Protocol for Spinal Fracture, Dislocation, and Disk Protrusion

PARAMETER	RECOMMENDATIONS
PATIENT POSITION	
Cervical spine	Supine; arms down with shoulders down as much as possible
Thoracolumbar spine	Supine; arms raised
Scout view	Lateral and/or AP
Slice thickness	3 or 5 mm
Slice spacing	3 or 5 mm
Scan range	Specific to pathology
Algorithm	Ultrahigh (bone); review images to standard for soft tissue detail

creased pitch in pediatric imaging, the dose to the patient can be reduced.

CT OF THE BODY

Indications

Trauma. CT is the modality of choice for examination of the abdomen following blunt injury or high-speed trauma to evaluate possible laceration of liver, spleen, pancreas, or kidney (Fig. 22-12). Abdominal CT is used to evaluate for kidney stones and acute appendicitis in children. CT also provides useful information in the assessment of complex fractures of the pelvis, ankle, and foot (Fig. 22-13).

Tumors. Bony lesions (e.g., Ewing's sarcoma and osteogenic sarcoma) are best imaged with MRI. When MRI is not available, CT is the appropriate imaging modality (Fig. 22-14). CT is an integral

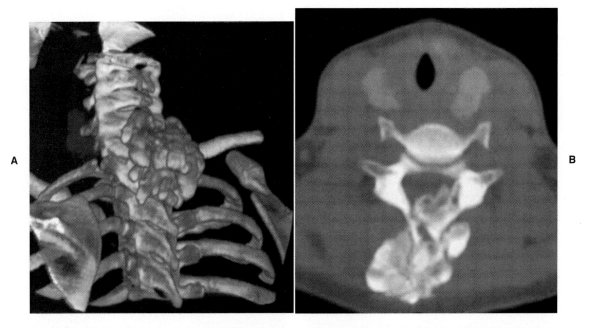

FIG. 22-8. Osteochondroma. The 3D image shows a large calcified mass of the thoracic spine (**A**), which is also demonstrated on the unenhanced axial image (**B**).

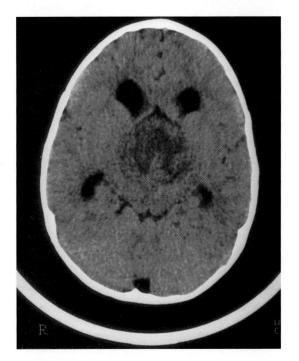

FIG. 22-9. Unenhanced axial image reveals large suprasellar mass with no calcification and obstructed ventricle system.

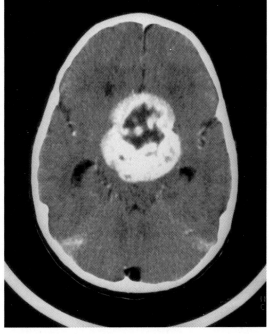

FIG. 22-10. Postcontrast axial image shows marked tumor enhancement.

part of the diagnostic workup and posttreatment assessment of pediatric solid tumors including lymphoma (e.g., Burkitt's or Hodgkins), and abdominal tumors (e.g., Wilms' tumor of the kidney, neuroblastoma, rhabdomyosarcoma, and hepato-

blastoma) (Figs. 22-15, 22-16). The investigation of these oncologic diseases generally includes a noncontrast chest CT to look for lung metastases. Chest CT for mediastinal disease includes a contrast examination.

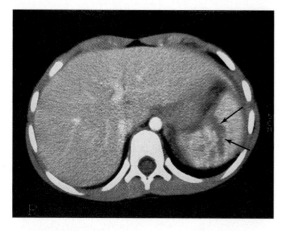

FIG. 22-11. Postcontrast coronal image. This defines superior and inferior tumor margins and aids surgical or radiation treatment planning.

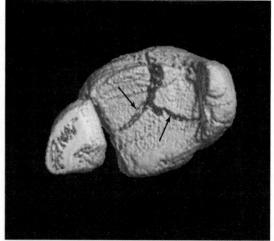

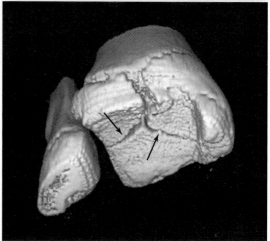

FIG. 22-13. 3D reconstruction following computer disarticulation of ankle joint showing extensive tibial fractures (*arrows*). **A,** Looking from below and in front. **B,** Looking directly up the tibial epiphyseal surface.

FIG. 22-12. Postcontrast axial CT scan in a child struck by a car. A laceration and a contusion (*arrows*) are present in the spleen.

the ability of patients to hold their breath for the scan, the use of this technology may be limited in pediatrics.

Chronic Pulmonary Disease. High-resolution CT is sometimes performed on the pediatric patient for the assessment of parenchymal lung disease such as cystic fibrosis or bronchiectasis (Fig. 22-17).

Orthopedic Disorders. CT digital radiography is used to produce an accurate assessment of leg length discrepancy. A CT scout view technique for measuring limb length has the following advantages:

    1. Speed: Both limbs are imaged simultaneously with less chance of patient motion.

Spiral/helical CT of the chest is used to evaluate central and peripheral airways, pulmonary nodules, vascular anatomy, and lung parenchyma. CT is also used to evaluate the trachea for stenosis, malacia, and atresia with virtual endoscopy. Because these evaluations are limited by

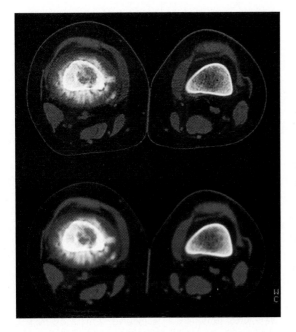

FIG. 22-14. Axial unenhanced images through distal femur on bone (*top*) and soft tissue (*bottom*) algorithms. A large bone tumor is spreading out of the femur with a soft tissue mass and spicules of new bone.

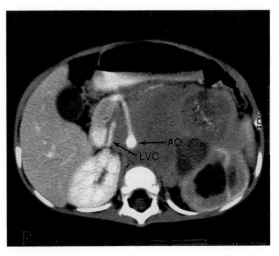

FIG. 22-16. Retroperitoneal neuroblastoma causing obstructive hydronephrosis of the left kidney, displacement of the aorta (AO), and compression of the inferior vena cava. Note the calcifications within the mass.

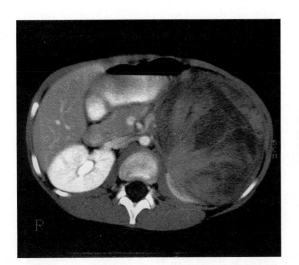

FIG. 22-15. Large Wilms' tumor of the left kidney with focal areas of low attenuation caused by hemorrhage or necrosis.

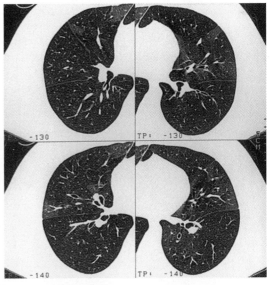

FIG. 22-17. High-resolution, 1-mm images reveal bronchiectasis, extensive areas of low attenuation caused by bronchiolitis obliterans, and patchy dense areas, which represent overperfusion of the normal lung. The chest x-ray (not shown) was normal.

2. Accuracy: Comparison studies between conventional and CT leg length examinations have confirmed the accuracy of the CT examination.

3. Less radiation: The radiation dose of the CT examination is three to six times less than that of conventional radiography, which may be of special significance to the pediatric population.

The rotational deformities of long bones that cause gait problems are accurately measured with a CT examination to assess tibial torsion, femoral anteversion, or acetabular anteversion. A CT examination of the hindfoot provides essential data for the evaluation of tarsal coalition.

Patient Positioning

Patients are positioned feet-first in the gantry. The young patient finds this a less intimidating experience, and the IV lines can be more easily managed.

Geometric centering of the patient in the gantry is essential to achieve artifact-free images from which accurate measurements can be derived. This objective is easily achieved with a child immobilizer or a second mattress placed on the patient couch.

Respiration

For children 8 years and younger, shallow breathing on chest and abdomen examinations works well with helical CT scanning. This reduces the chance of misregistration when compared with instructing them to hold their breath. For children more than 8 years old, a little coaching and practice can generally help them to hold their breath for the required scan time.

Technique

Several parameters need to be considered before scanning the pediatric patient. These include the kVp, mA, table speed, collimation, reconstruction interval, and pitch.

TABLE 22-10

Pediatric CT Assessment Protocol for Lymphoma, Thyroid Tumor, and Neuroblastoma

PARAMETER	RECOMMENDATIONS
Patient position	Supine; arms down
LATERAL SCOUT VIEW	
Spiral CT	Pre- and post-IV contrast
Slice thickness	5 mm
Table feed	5 mm
Reconstructions	3-mm standard algorithm for soft tissue detail; 3-mm ultrahigh (bone) algorithm to evaluate bony involvement

A 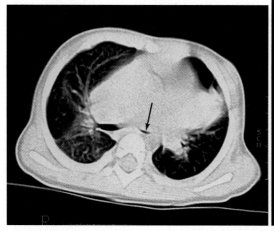 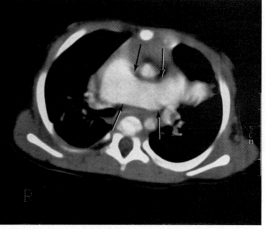 B

FIG. 22-18. Giant pulmonary artery aneurysm. **A,** Unenhanced 5-mm image showing obstructed left bronchus (*arrow*), decreased blood flow to the left lung, and increased blood flow to the right lung. **B,** Postcontrast, dynamic, 5-mm image showing aneurysmal dilatation of main pulmonary artery (*arrows*) compared with normal ascending aorta.

The radiologist is responsible for selecting the pitch for each examination. For CT scanning of the lungs, a 1 to 1 pitch is preferred because of the increase in nodule detection when reconstructed with overlapping slices. For the abdomen, a 1.5 to 1 pitch can be used to decrease radiation exposure to the patient. Studies are underway to determine the optimum pitch selections for different body parts.

Scanning Protocols

Neck and Chest. The scanning protocol for the neck and chest are given in Tables 22-10 and 22-11, respectively. Fig. 22-18 shows a giant pulmonary artery aneurysm.

The young child is prepared for sedation as previously mentioned. If IV contrast is to be administered to an older child, IV access is established and the child is given nothing orally for 2 hours before examination.

Abdomen. The protocol for CT of the pediatric abdomen is given in Table 22-12. To prepare the patient, nothing is given by mouth 4 hours before examination. IV access is established before examination, and oral contrast is administered to opacify the small bowel.

The nonsedated patient is given an oral contrast drink (Table 22-13) to be consumed slowly during the 1 hour before examination. Oral hypaque has a salt concentration of 40%. If using oral gastrografin, which has a salt concentration of 76%, the solution proportions should be adjusted accordingly.

No bowel preparation is required for the abdominal study of the acute trauma patient.

To ensure that inpatients are correctly prepared for their abdominal scan, a detailed instruction sheet should be delivered to the ward with the oral contrast medium.

Pelvis. An example of the protocol for the pelvis is shown in Table 22-14. Preparation of the patient is the same as for the nonsedated and sedated abdomen with one exception: the oral contrast is consumed 2 hours before examination. Also, after viewing the precontrast pelvic scans,

TABLE 22-11

Pediatric CT Assessment Protocol for the Chest

PARAMETER	RECOMMENDATIONS
Lung metastases and tumors	Scan range from superior lung apices to inferior aspect of costophrenic angles
KVp	120 kVp
mA	Newborn to 18 months: 150 mA
	18 months to 3 years: 200 mA
	3 to 10 years: 230 mA
	10 years and older: 250 to 300 mA
Collimation (Helical protocol)	5-mm slice on children 2 years and under
	10-mm slice on children 3 years and older
Reconstruction interval	Every 5 mm on children 2 years and under
	Every 5 mm on children 3 years and older (no overlapping of slices on routine chests)
Pitch	1 to 1 pitch is recommended on chests
Algorithm	Ultrahigh and soft tissue for mediastinum
Intravenous contrast	
Power injector	1.5 ml/sec scan after 75% is injected
Hand injector	Scan after 75% of contrast is injected
Chronic lung disease (high resolution)	
Collimation	2-mm slice on children 2 years and younger
	1-mm slice on children 2 years and older (2-mm slice helps decrease respiratory motion)
Slice spacing	5 mm on children 2 years and younger
	10 mm on children 3 years and older
Algorithm	Ultrahigh detail
Scan time	1 second or faster

TABLE 22-12

Pediatric CT Assessment Protocol for the Abdomen

PARAMETER	RECOMMENDATIONS
Routine abdomen	Scan from dome of diaphragm to symphysis pubis
kVp	120 kVp
mA	Newborn to 18 months: 150 mA
	18 months to 3 years: 200 mA
	3 to 10 years: 230 mA
	10 years and older: 250 to 350 mA
Collimation (Helical protocol)	5-mm slice on children 2 years and under
	10-mm slice on children 3 years and older
Pitch	1 to 2 (use a higher pitch on routine screening of abdomen to reduce patient dose)
Algorithm	Soft tissue
Intravenous contrast	
Power injector	1 to 2 ml/sec (depends on patient size and catheter size); scan 45 to 60 seconds after injection begins
Hand injection	Scan 60 seconds after injection begins
Nephrolithiasis	Scan from top of kidneys through the bladder. No oral or IV contrast required.
Collimation (helical)	5-mm slices
Reconstruction interval	Through kidneys every 3 mm
Pitch	1 to 1
Appendicitis	Scan from umbilicus through symphysis; rectal and IV contrast required
Collimation (helical)	5-mm slices
Reconstruction interval	Every 3 mm
Pitch	1 to 1

TABLE 22-13

Oral Contrast Amounts for Abdominal CT

AGE	AMOUNT GIVEN FOR THE SCAN	MIXTURE RATIO
Newborn to 3 months	50 to 100ml	3-cc G : 100-cc J or P
4 months to 1 year	175 ml	5-cc G : 175-cc J or P
1 to 5 years	250 ml	8-cc G : 250-cc J or P
6 to 10 years	500 ml	16-cc G : 500-cc J or P
11 to 15 years	750 ml	24-cc G : 750-cc J or P
16 years to adult	1000 ml	32-cc G : 1000-cc J or P

G, Oral gastrografin.
J, Juice.
P, Powered drink mix (e.g., Kool-Aid).

the radiologist may decide to administer rectal contrast.

Extremities. The extremity protocol is given in Table 22-15. Tables 22-16 and 22-17 list the protocols for joints and leg length studies, respectively. CT scanning can be used to detect bone le-sions of the upper or lower limb when MRI is not available.

The young child is prepared for sedation as pre-viously mentioned. If IV contrast is to be adminis-tered to the older child, IV access is established and the child is given nothing orally 2 hours before examination.

TABLE 22-14

Pediatric CT Assessment Protocol for the Pelvis

PARAMETER	RECOMMENDATIONS
Patient position	Supine; arms raised
AP scout view	
Precontrast	Scan range to include from iliac crest to symphysis pubis
Slice thickness	Contiguous 5 or 10 mm, depending on patient size and size of lesion
Algorithm	Standard: to image soft tissue structures; postscan review: to ultrahigh (bone) algorithm to assess any bone involvement
Scan time	0.7 second
Postcontrast	During rapid bolus hand injection, contiguous 5-mm or 10-mm 1-second dynamic scans are acquired to visualize major blood vessels, vascularity of lesion, and urinary tract

From Hooper KD: CT bronchoscopy, *Semin Ultrasound CT MRI* 20(1):10-15, 1999.

TABLE 22-15

Pediatric CT Assessment Protocol for the Extremity

PARAMETER	RECOMMENDATIONS
Patient position	Supine
AP scout view	
Precontrast	Scan range to include above and below lesion and both extremities for bone marrow comparison
Algorithm	Ultrahigh
Slice thickness	5 mm
Slice spacing	5 mm
Postscan review	Images targeted to site of pathology and magnified 2.5 to 4.0 × on standard algorithm for soft tissue detail and on ultrahigh for bone detail
Postcontrast algorithm	Standard; during rapid bolus hand injection, contiguous 5-mm, 1-second dynamic scans targeted and magnified to site of pathology are acquired to image vascularity of lesion and surrounding soft tissue structures

From Hooper KD: CT bronchoscopy, *Semin Ultrasound CT MRI* 20(1):10-15, 1999.

TABLE 22-16

Pediatric CT Assessment Protocol for the Ankle and Subtalar Joints

PARAMETER	RECOMMENDATIONS
Patient position	Supine with feet positioned as symmetrically as possible: (1) coronal view, feet flat, knees flexed to limit of gantry opening; (2) axial view, ankles flexed.
Lateral scout view	Right and left ankles and feet will be superimposed
Slice thickness	5 × 5 mm—possible dislocation
Slice spacing	3 × 3 mm—possible subtalar coalition, fracture
Algorithm	Ultrahigh (bone)
mA	Low values, 85 to 125 mA; right and left sides imaged for comparison

From Hooper KD: CT bronchoscopy, *Semin Ultrasound CT MRI* 20(1):10-15, 1999.

XENON CT

Diagnostically useful data about cerebral tissue function that is not obtainable from angiography or conventional CT can be acquired during a xenon-CT cerebral blood flow study. Diseases such as infarction, edema, neoplasm, and focal epilepsy can cause altered local cerebral blood flow values. The xenon-CT cerebral blood flow study is a non-invasive technique used to quantify cerebral tissue perfusion.

The patient is positioned so that scans are acquired in a plane 20 degrees to the canthomeatal line. Baseline scans at three levels of interest are acquired. A closed xenon gas delivery circuit delivers 28% xenon gas to the patient through a breathing mask for 4 minutes. Sequential scans at 1-minute intervals are acquired at each level during xenon gas inhalation, the wash-in phase, and the wash-out phase following inhalation. Throughout the wash-in and wash-out phases, expired xenon and CO_2 concentrations are recorded for use in the blood flow calculations.

After inhalation, xenon gas rapidly diffuses from the lungs into the arterial blood and freely crosses the blood-brain barrier. Xenon induces regional changes in CT density (measured in Hounsfield units). Because stable xenon is radiodense, tissues that are perfused with xenon appear white on CT images and tissues that have low xenon perfusion appear black (Fig. 22-19).

Data evaluation is performed using a subtraction technique, in which the baseline images are

TABLE 22-17

*Pediatric CT Assessment Protocol for Leg Length**

PARAMETER	RECOMMENDATIONS
Patient position	Supine; geometric centering at level of the greater trochanter is essential for accurate measurements
AP scout view†	(1) To include both hip joints; (2) to include both knee joints; and (3) to include both ankle joints

*Gonadal shielding is always used for both male and female patients; minimum mA values produce diagnostic images.
†Using the scout view evaluation program, accurate measurements of each femur and tibial length are made and the total lengths of each leg are compared.

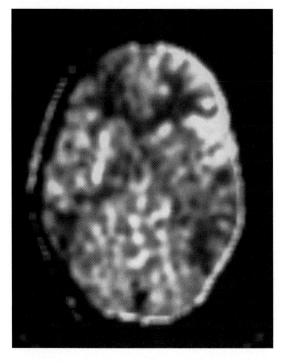

FIG. 22-19. Tissues perfused with xenon gas appear white on xenon-CT flow images, whereas tissues with low xenon perfusion appear black.

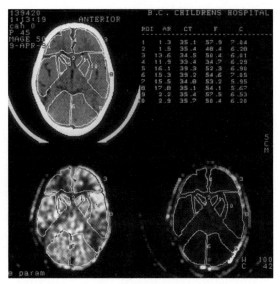

FIG. 22-20. Blood flow maps. Multiple regions of interest are defined and a statistical analysis is displayed.

subtracted from the xenon-enhanced images. Special software for functional image calculations defines each image voxel by a series of enhancement values as a function of time. Blood flow maps that have exact anatomic correlation to the baseline CT images are constructed and displayed. The radiologist then defines multiple regions of interest for quantitative analysis (Fig. 22-20) and uses the statistical and visual analyses of the images to interpret the study.

BIBLIOGRAPHY

Aitken GF et al: Leg length determination by CT digital radiograph, *Am J Roentgenol* 144:613-615, 1985.

Daneman A: *Pediatric body CT*, New York, 1987, Springer-Verlag.

Flodmark O et al: Periventricular leukomalacia radiologic diagnosis, *Radiology* 162:119-124, 1987.

Frush D et al: Challenges of pediatric spiral CT, *Radiographics* 17:939-959, 1997.

Frush D, Donnelly LF: Helical CT in children: technical considerations and body applications, *Radiology* 209:37-48, 1998.

Fuchs WA, ed: *Advances in CT*, New York, 1990, Springer-Verlag.

Huda W et al: An approach for the estimation of effective radiation dose at CT in pediatric patients, *Radiology* 203:417-422, 1997.

Jacob RP et al: Tibial torsion calculated by computerized tomography, *J Bone Joint Surg* 62B:238-242, 1980.

Jacquenier M et al: Acetabular anteversion in children, *J Pediatr Orthop* 12:373-375, 1992.

Keeter S et al: Sedation in pediatric CT: national survey of current practice, *Radiology* 175:745-752, 1990.

Lee SH, Rao KCVG: *Cranial computed tomography*, New York, 1983, McGraw-Hill.

Mettler FA, Moseley RD: *Medical effects of ionizing radiation*, Orlando, 1985, Grune & Stratton.

Ozonoff MB: *Pediatric orthopedic radiology*, ed 2, Philadelphia, 1992, WB Saunders.

Wilmot DM, Sharko GA, eds: *Pediatric imaging for the technologist*, New York, 1987, Springer-Verlag.

23

Quality Control
for Computed
Tomography Scanners

ROBERT CACAK

WHAT IS QUALITY CONTROL?

What is quality control (QC), and how does it relate to CT scanners? For CT scanners, QC may be defined as a program that periodically tests the performance of a CT scanner and compares its performance with some standard. If the scanner is performing suboptimally, then steps must be initiated to correct the problem. The goal of a QC program is to ensure that every image created by the CT scanner is a quality image. High-quality images provide the radiologist maximum information, improve the chances for correct diagnosis, and ultimately contribute to quality patient care.

The definition of QC consists of two parts. Quality assurance requires a measurement of the CT scanner's performance to ensure the scanner is operating at some acceptable level. Unfortunately, quality assurance does not prescribe what to do if the standards are not met. Quality control carries the concept of quality assurance one step further—if the quality is inadequate, then steps are taken to correct the problem.

This simple definition does not attempt to describe how such a program might work or how to apply QC to a CT scanner. However, the remainder of this chapter describes aspects of a QC program for CT scanners and includes descriptions of some tests that have proven useful in QC testing. Descriptions of the testing instruments, an outline of necessary measurements, and hints on interpretation of the results are presented.

This chapter describes a generic QC program that can be adapted to almost any CT scanner system. As part of the purchase package, CT manufacturers often prescribe a daily QC program for use on their CT system. Sometimes their QC program includes a specially furnished phantom or test object to be imaged with selected techniques. In some cases, internal software is used to interpret the measurements and to notify the operator of unsatisfactory results.

Unfortunately, manufacturers' tests are often restricted to images from one or two scans. The amount of information that can be gained from the images is limited. The tests described later in this chapter can be used to augment or to replace the manufacturers' tests. The information gained from these augmentation tests may prove useful in the assessment of additional aspects of the scanner's performance.

Many tests are based on QC tests published in the literature (Cacak and Hendee, 1979; Cacak, 1985; Burkhart et al, 1987) and described in Report 99 of the National Council on Radiation Protection and Measurement (1988). More complex physics tests are outlined in Report 39 of the American Association of Physics in Medicine (1993). Although the tests are similar to those described in these references, the types and frequency of the QC tests may vary somewhat to reflect advances in CT scanner technology. One recent and significant advance of CT scanner technology has been the introduction of spiral/helical CT scanners. The "wind-up" cables that connect the moving and stationary parts of the CT scanner are eliminated through a series of sliding electrical contacts, or slip rings. Because no cables follow the moving part of the scanner, it is no longer necessary to stop and unwind the twisting cables after every scan. Consequently, the heavy motors, brakes, and clutches can be made lighter and the moving sections can be rotated faster, which allows for shorter scan times. These scanners can make a complete revolution of an x-ray tube (and sometimes detectors) in 0.5 second or less. Some CT scanners have two or more banks of detectors, which allows them to acquire data for several scan planes simultaneously. With this multidetector system, many images can be acquired very quickly. For example, if a CT scanner has four sets of detectors and can complete one revolution in 0.5 second, then eight images can be acquired in 1 second. This is incredibly fast compared to the CT scanners from only a few years ago.

Because of their sliding electrical contacts, continuously rotating x-ray tube and detectors do not need to stop at the end of each scan. If necessary, the x-ray tube can merely stop the production of x-rays while the bed advances to the next scan location. In fact, most CT scanners do not stop x-ray production to move the bed, but instead allow the bed and patient to move continuously as the x-ray tube continues to rotate and data are collected. The pattern of the x-ray beam as it winds around the patient in a screw-like fashion is sometimes called *spiral/helical scanning*. Most of the QC tests described here are applicable to both spiral/helical CT scanners and more conventional scan-and-stop scanners. However, when tests involve a phantom, the alignment of the phantom to the x-ray beam is much easier if these QC tests are performed in the stationary bed, single-scan mode. For most tests, the measurements performed in the stationary bed mode closely resemble measurements performed in the spiral/helical mode.

Generally, some absolute standard of imaging performance exists that should be exceeded by the

CT scanner. For example, the CT scanner may be required to always resolve a certain size (presumably small) object in a clinical image. Therefore the QC program sets up an internal standard for high-contrast resolution capabilities of the scanner (e.g., the CT scanner must be able to image high-contrast objects at least as small as 0.75 mm). If the performance is below this standard (i.e., it cannot resolve small objects), then the scanner must be adjusted or repaired.

Some tests are too complex and require too much time for routine use. Depending on the skill, comfort level, and available time, the QC technician can select the tests to be performed and their frequency. A majority of the tests described in this chapter are designed to be performed by radiation technologists. For more complex tests, help can be sought from a medical physicist.

Experience has shown that if a QC program is to be effective, the tests must be objective, quantitative, easy, and quick. If the test results determine that the scanner is working at an acceptable level, then the results are merely recorded. If the results demonstrate that the scanner is not functioning well, alternative corrective procedures should be followed. The tests in this chapter suggest some alternative procedures to follow when acceptable limits are exceeded.

WHY QUALITY CONTROL?

The answer to the question, "Is a QC program needed for the CT scanner?" is usually "yes." Progressive hospitals and clinics that operate CT scanners and other complex instruments have long recognized the value of QC programs to maintain high performance standards for their patients. In addition, regulatory agencies increasingly demand that some standard of quality be maintained on x-ray units and other equipment that can potentially harm patients if the units are not performing optimally. These agencies frequently require that institutions using CT scanners verify the scanner's performance periodically (e.g., daily, monthly, annually) and often prescribe alternative measures if the performance standards are not met. To meet these regulatory requirements, a quality control program must be operational.

In the case of CT scanners, the engineering is exceedingly complex. With so many mechanical and electronic parts involved in the creation of the images, there are many opportunities for the quality of the images to subtly and unnoticeably degrade. The mechanical parts of these complex, heavy instruments can wear slowly. Electronic parts can change characteristics and drift out of optimal adjustment. When this occurs, the CT scanner may no longer yield the same quality images as it did when it was in proper adjustment. Often, this wear and drift can be repaired or compensated, but the suboptimal imaging problems must first be recognized. Comparing modern QC data with past data can demonstrate that the scanner is not performing as well as in the past.

A quality control program can be an important ally in many aspects of CT scanner service. For example, if the QC data are used to define the problem and its extent, the service person will be better able to correct a subtle image quality problem. If a measurable change can be quantitatively demonstrated to the service person, the necessity of repair will be more apparent, and the degree to which it should be repaired can be specified (i.e., "we want it to perform like new" or "as good as last August.").

Often a QC program can result in reduced downtime. A good QC program may recognize weakened or marginally performing parts before complete failure, and unscheduled service may be avoided.

PRINCIPLES OF QUALITY CONTROL

Three basic tenets of quality control are as follows:
1. The QC must be performed on a regular, periodic basis. Ideally, these tests might be performed between each patient exam. At this testing frequency, there would be maximal insurance that the CT scanner was always operating correctly. However, in reality, this very frequent QC attention is too costly in terms of the time taken from patient examinations. Some compromises must be made for the sake of time and effort.

It does seem prudent to perform certain quick tests on a daily basis. Less important or more time-consuming tests might be performed less frequently (e.g., monthly), and the most complex tests might be performed semiannually or yearly. The institution's philosophy and its willingness to devote time to periodic QC tests often dictate which tests are performed and how often. To an administrator watching the revenues generated by a CT scanner, QC has a double affliction of requiring labor, which must be paid, and reducing the availability of the CT scanner for patients, which reduces revenue. A compromise must be reached that balances the effort and expense of a QC program with the expected benefits, such as better images, consistent images, reduced downtime, and legal and regulatory requirements.

2. The second tenet is prompt interpretation of the measurements. Data usually show that the CT scanner is operating within specified guidelines. But on those occasions when it is not, this fact must be recognized and some remedial action must be taken. This action may be as simple as notifying the physicist, service person, or radiologist, or it may be as aggressive as taking the unit out of service until it is repaired. But to institute this facet of the QC program, the person making the test must be able to recognize that the results are outside of acceptable limits. Some mechanism should be in place that alerts the QC technician to errant behavior of the scanner. For example, on the data form for a particular test, acceptable limits of the data may be stated. From an inspection of the measured results, the QC technician can recognize immediately that the results are out of tolerance. Another method is to enter data into a computer, then instruct the computer to issue an appropriate alert when limits are exceeded. In the latter case, the temptation to sit on data for a few days or weeks before they are entered into the computer must be avoided. If a computer is to be relied upon to make the necessary comparisons and if the program is to be effective, the data must be entered promptly.

3. The third tenet of good QC is faithful bookkeeping. If time and effort are to be expended to perform the tests, then the results should be recorded. These results should be maintained in a logbook, data form, or computer for a reasonable period, usually as long as the CT scanner is active (i.e., for its lifetime). Keeping good records is not just a tedious exercise. These results will prove invaluable if the unit appears to be malfunctioning some time in the future. A comparison of past measurements with current results can easily demonstrate a change in performance (usually degradation). These data can also prove important to defend a lawsuit that might arise because of a reading of a CT image. For example, if litigation arises that is dependent on an interpretation (or misinterpretation) of a CT image and data can be produced from the QC logbook to demonstrate that the CT scanner was functioning satisfactorily at the time of interpretation, then the CT scanner is removed as a source of blame for the interpretation.

QUALITY CONTROL TESTS FOR CT SCANNERS

The methods described in the remainder of this chapter provide some details of the testing procedure, the equipment required, interpretation of the results, some suggestions for acceptable limits, and how often the test should be performed. The tests are listed in approximate order of importance, with some weighting of the tests according to the ability perform the test quickly and easily.

Choosing a Technique for QC Measurements

The selection of technique for the QC tests depends on the type of CT scanner and the test being performed. Many variables can be selected for each test, including kVp, mA, scan time, slice width, type of algorithm, x-ray filter type, and focal spot size. The number of possible combinations of techniques is usually overwhelming, and the best that can be done is to select one or two representative techniques. In general, the technique should remain the same for a specific test from day to day. However, the technique for one test does not have to be the same as the technique for other tests. A good rule of thumb is to use a technique that matches a frequently used clinical technique. One method to select a QC technique is to choose the most frequently used head or body technique and use it for the tests. As many tests as possible should be performed with this technique, with the understanding that deviations may be required for some tests.

Test Frequency

It is usually necessary to limit the more complex tests to annual surveys, those occasions when the CT scanner is being initially tested for acceptance, and subsequent occasions when the deterioration of image quality is suspected. It is good practice to repeat appropriate tests after replacement of a major component such as an x-ray tube or after the performance of extensive service or adjustments. If data from CT scanner images are used quantitatively or if the precision of an image is used for accurately localizing tissue (e.g., to perform biopsies or plan radiation therapy treatment), the frequency of appropriate tests should be increased.

Limits of a "Passing" Test

What are acceptable limits? How big should the window of acceptable values be for each test described here before the CT scanner is considered "out of tolerance"? These complex questions depend on the technology of the unit being tested, the type of test instrument being used, and the imaging technique.

Perhaps more important than the actual value of the measured variable is a change in the variable between measurements. A CT scanner that is operating the same today as it did yesterday should produce nearly the same results when the test is repeated. After acceptable limits are established, a quick inspection of the measurements can identify deviant values. Past history can provide good insight into what the values have been. A range that includes most values when the unit was operating optimally can be easily determined from an inspection of past values. Of course, it is never absolutely certain that the CT scanner was operating optimally in the past when these supposedly "good" readings were taken. But if the readings were taken when the unit was new or believed to be functioning well, then they can be presumed to be "good" readings and used as a standard. Some generic limits are suggested in the following sections.

QC Tests

QC tests are proposed in this section. Suggestions are given regarding the following: phantom or equipment, expected results, acceptance limits, possible causes of failure, and frequency of tests.

TEST I Average CT Number of Water (CT Number Calibration)

PHANTOM OR EQUIPMENT: A simple water-filled cylindric plastic container about 20 cm in diameter. Commercial phantoms are available for this test, but some institutions have used 1-gallon plastic

containers from liquid laundry bleach. The bleach, of course, is replaced with water.

MEASUREMENT: Take a scan through the water phantom at the usual technique. Reconstruct the image of the water phantom. Examine the region of interest (ROI) feature available on the imaging monitor of most scanners to verify that the scanner can measure the average of the CT numbers of the pixels inside the ROI. Enlarge the ROI area to include an area of about 2 to 3 square centimeters (i.e., about 200 to 300 pixels). Position the ROI near the center of the phantom image and measure the average CT number (Fig. 23-1).

Two media that serve as calibration points for CT numbers are water and air. Occasionally (e.g., once a month), move the ROI outside the phantom into the region of the image that is known to contain air. Check the average CT number of air. It should be −1000 if the CT scanner is calibrated properly.

EXPECTED RESULTS: The average CT number of water should be very close to zero.

ACCEPTANCE LIMITS: If the average CT number of water is more than 3 CT numbers away from 0 (i.e., outside the range −3 to +3), the CT scanner fails the test. The CT number of air should be −1000 ±5.

POSSIBLE CAUSES OF FAILURE: Miscalibration of the algorithm that generates the CT number. If a recalibration does not help, notify the service person. Usually the

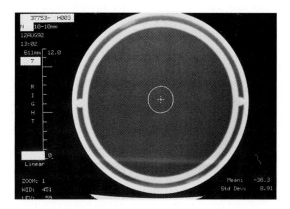

FIG. 23-1. CT scanner image of an uniform water phantom. The region of interest (ROI) is placed in the center of the water-filled phantom to measure the average CT number and the standard deviation of the CT numbers inside the ROI. In this case, the average or "mean" CT number measures −36.3, which is not acceptable.

manufacturer provides a procedure to recalibrate the CT number scale.

FREQUENCY: This should be performed daily.

TEST 2 Standard Deviation of CT Number in Water

PHANTOM OR EQUIPMENT: A simple water-filled cylindric plastic container about 20 cm in diameter (the same phantom used in Test 1).

MEASUREMENT: Use the same image as for Test 1 (see Fig. 23-1). Use the ROI feature available on the CRT monitor of most scanners. Ensure that the scanner's ROI can measure the standard deviation of the numbers inside the ROI. Enlarge the ROI area to include an area of about 2 to 3 square centimeters (i.e., about 200 to 300 pixels). Position the ROI near the center of the phantom image and measure the standard deviation of the CT number.

EXPECTED RESULTS: Typical values are in the range of 2 to 7 CT numbers. The actual value will depend on the dose at the location of the ROI, which depends on the kVp, mA, duration of the scan, slice width, and phantom size, and the type of reconstruction algorithm. The standard deviation of the CT number also depends on the position of the ROI. For example, the standard deviation may be slightly smaller at the edge of the phantom image than in the center. Ensure that the technique is the same each day and that the standard deviation is measured at the same place each day (e.g., the center of the phantom).

ACCEPTANCE LIMITS: Ideally, the standard deviation should be very small. The actual acceptance limits must be determined by examination of past measurements that were presumably performed when the performance of the CT scanner was good. The technique must stay the same for this measurement from day to day. If the standard deviation starts to increase, this indicates a "noisier" image with more variation in pixel-to-pixel CT numbers and poorer low contrast resolution.

POSSIBLE CAUSES OF FAILURE: Something is causing a noisier image, such as decreased dose (x-ray tube output) or increased electronic noise of the x-ray detectors, amplifiers, or A/D converters. Notify the service person.

FREQUENCY: This should be performed daily.

TEST 3 High Contrast Resolution

PHANTOM OR EQUIPMENT: High contrast (contrast difference of 10% or greater) resolution pattern in an imaging phantom. Although a variety of patterns are available to perform high-contrast tests, including patterns for generating modulation transfer function (MTF) measurements, a quick and easy test pattern is most suitable for QC tests. One such pattern consists of a series of rows of holes drilled in plastic (Fig. 23-2). Each row contains a set of holes (usually five) of constant diameter with the centers of the holes 2 diameters apart. The holes decrease in size from one row to the next. If the holes are drilled in acrylic and filled with water, the contrast is about 20%. If the holes are filled with air, the contrast is about 100%. Either filling is satisfactory.

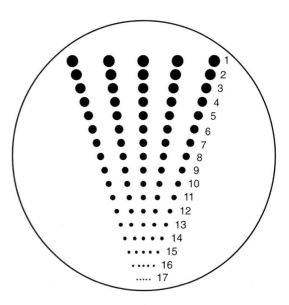

FIG. 23-2. Hole pattern for a high-contrast phantom test object. The test pattern consists of rows of holes of various sizes drilled in plastic. Each row contains five holes of the same diameter. In a row of constant sizes, the holes are separated by two diameters from center to center.

MEASUREMENT: On the CT image (Fig. 23-3), determine the smallest row of holes in which all holes can be clearly seen. The smaller the holes that can be clearly seen, the better the performance of the CT scanner. Be certain that all holes can be seen in the image. Sometimes it appears that one fewer hole is seen in the row than is actually in the phantom. This is usually a phase reversal phenomenon and should not be counted as a complete set of holes.

EXPECTED RESULTS: Most modern CT scanners have a high-contrast resolving power slightly smaller than 1 mm by using a typical head image technique. Therefore they will be able to visualize a complete set of holes in some of the rows in the range of 0.75 to 1.0 mm. With the highest resolution technique available to a particular scanner, some CT scanner manufacturers claim to be able to visualize holes as small as 0.25 mm.

ACCEPTANCE LIMITS: This baseline number should be established when the CT scanner is working well by scanning the phantom and noting the smallest set of holes that can be seen. This initial measurement becomes the baseline for future tests. Subsequent tests can be compared with this baseline. Alternatively, the manufacturer's specifications for this test can

be used to verify that the performance of the CT scanner is at least as good as the specifications.

POSSIBLE CAUSES OF FAILURE: Enlarged focal spot in the x-ray tube, excessive mechanical wear in the motion of the gantry, mechanical misalignments or poor registration of electromechanical components, vibrations, or detector failures. If the resolution has degraded from the baseline, inform the service person.

FREQUENCY: This should be performed monthly.

TEST 4 Low Contrast Resolution

PHANTOM OR EQUIPMENT: Low contrast resolution pattern in imaging phantom. A quick and easy test pattern of low-contrast test objects consists of a series of holes (2 to 8 mm diameter) drilled in polystrene. The holes are filled with liquid (often water) to which has been added a small amount some other material (usually methanol or sucrose) to bring the liquid's CT number close (about 0.5% different) to that of the plastic itself. One such pattern (Fig. 23-4) consists of a series of rows of holes drilled in relatively thick plastic. Each row contains holes of a constant diameter. The holes decrease in size from one row to the next. In a CT image, the holes appear to have a density similar to their surround (i.e., the holes have low contrast).

Another technique is to use partial voluming by making the plastic very thin (e.g., a plastic membrane). Low contrast in the image is achieved by a different principle than the solid plastic type of low-contrast phantom. The membrane type of phantom consists of a thin membrane containing a pattern of holes (the same pattern shown in Fig. 23-4). The membrane is stretched across a plane of the phantom and is then immersed in water. The CT x-ray beam, as visualized from its edge (Fig. 23-5) strikes mostly water. But a small fraction of the beam is absorbed by the plastic, forming a faint (low-contrast) image of the hole pattern. By varying the thickness of the plastic relative to the width of the x-ray beam, the contrast can be varied.

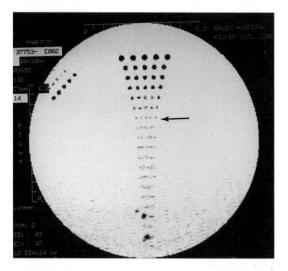

FIG. 23-3. CT image of the high-contrast test pattern shown in Fig. 23-2. The CT scanner is judged by the smallest row in which all five holes can be seen (*arrow*).

In both techniques, the contrast of the object is difficult to calculate. In QC testing, it is sufficient that the contrast be constant between tests. The contrast should be selected so that the standard test image shows about 50% of the holes. At that level of hole imaging, a decrease in low contrast imaging performance will result in the visualization of fewer rows of holes.

MEASUREMENT: On the CT image, determine the smallest row of holes in which all holes can be clearly seen. The smaller the holes that can be seen at a particular technique, the better the performance of the CT scanner. A sample of a "low noise" (high dose) image and a "high noise" (low dose) image are seen in Fig. 23-6. In the low noise image, more sets of smaller objects can be seen.

EXPECTED RESULTS: The smallest holes that can be imaged by modern CT scanners should be 4 to 5 mm in diameter or smaller for 0.5% contrast objects. Perhaps more importantly, the minimum size of holes visualized should not increase over the life of the scanner.

ACCEPTANCE LIMITS: The number of holes that can be visualized varies widely between techniques. For example, if a partial volume phantom is used, the apparent contrast of the object depends on the thickness of the membrane and the slice width of the image. In addition, an increase in mA value of the scan technique will usually reduce the noise in the image and will permit smaller holes to be visualized. Therefore a baseline scan at a chosen technique (usually a commonly used head technique) performed when the scanner is functioning well can serve as baseline against which future images can be compared. This technique, once chosen, should not be changed from day to day.

A smoothing algorithm filter can also reduce the apparent statistical fluctuations be-

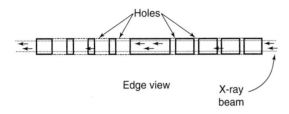

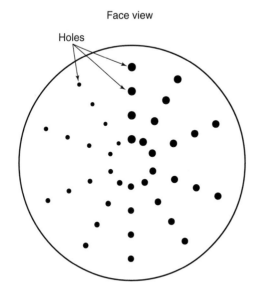

FIG. 23-4. "Solid plastic" type of low-contrast phantom test object that consists of a pattern of holes (face view) drilled in a piece of plastic with the holes filled with liquid. The low-contrast aspect of this test object is achieved by adjusting the absorption characteristics of the water solution to nearly match (about 0.5% difference) the absorption of the plastic.

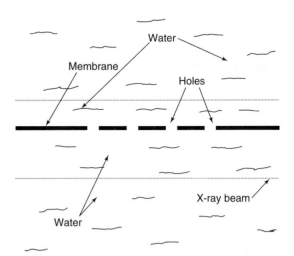

FIG. 23-5. Edge view of a membrane of partial-volume type of low-contrast test object. The presence of the thin membrane alters the absorption characteristics very slightly wherever there is membrane. Where the membrane is not present (i.e., in the holes), the absorption is that of just water. The slight difference in absorption characteristics between the water and the water-plus-membrane combination produce a low-contrast test pattern that appears as the hole pattern in the membrane.

tween pixels. These algorithms produce images with smaller standard deviations and usually permit visualization of smaller low-contrast objects by sacrificing some high-contrast resolution. Therefore it is important to always use the same reconstruction algorithm to compare repeated results from this test.

POSSIBLE CAUSES OF FAILURE: A higher noise level in the image usually causes reduced low-contrast resolution. Some possible sources of increased noise are decreased dose, decreased mA values, or any other factor that will reduce the x-ray tube output, such as a tungsten coating build-up on the inside of older x-ray tubes. Increased electronic noise is also possible and may arise from noise in the x-ray detectors, amplifiers, or A/D converters. The service person should be informed of decreasing low-contrast resolution and asked to perform further diagnosis.

FREQUENCY: This should be performed monthly.

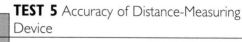

TEST 5 Accuracy of Distance-Measuring Device

PHANTOM OR EQUIPMENT: An object with two or more small objects that have a precisely known spatial relationship (i.e., the distance between them is precisely known). One such object is a large "+" pattern of small holes in a plastic phantom (Fig. 23-7). The holes are precisely 1 cm apart, and the size of the "+" is large enough to fill most of the image.

Some institutions have used an image of a regular square grid that covers most of the field of view. One source of square grids is a type of fluorescent light fixture that uses square grid light diffusers made of plastic with a

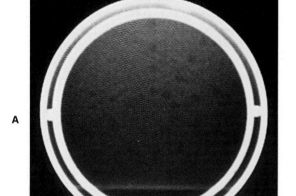

A

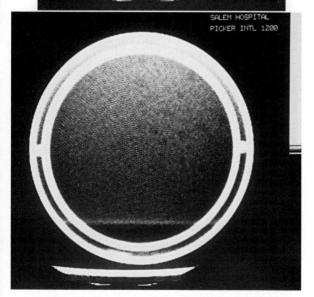

FIG. 23-6. Low-noise (**A**) and high-noise (**B**) low-contrast images produced with a membrane-type low-contrast test object obtained from a high-dose (low noise) CT scan and a low-dose (high noise) type of scan.

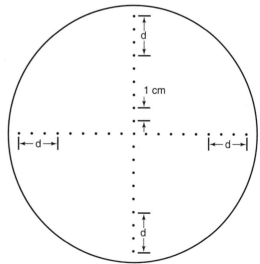

FIG. 23-7. A pattern of holes to measure image distortion. The pattern consists of a series of holes arranged in a "+" pattern that spans the diameter of the phantom. The holes are exactly 1 cm apart.

square spacing of about 0.5 inch (12 mm). With a moderate amount of effort, the grids can be cut to fit inside a phantom or scanned in air (no phantom).

MEASUREMENT: Using the distance-measuring feature available on the video monitors of most scanners, measure the distance between two well-visualized holes near the periphery of the phantom, one near the top, and one near the bottom (Fig. 23-8). Repeat the measurement between two holes, moving right to left. If required, a diagonal measurement between two holes can be made and the true distance can be calculated using the Pythagorean theorem.

EXPECTED RESULTS: The distance indicated by the CT scanner should agree with the true distance as determined by counting the spaces between the two holes.

ACCEPTANCE LIMITS: Disagreement of 1 mm or less is good. Disagreement of greater than 2 mm should be corrected.

POSSIBLE CAUSES OF FAILURE: Reconstruction algorithm may be improperly calibrated. If the manufacturer has not provided the user with a means to recalibrate the algorithm, a service person should be notified.

FREQUENCY: This should be performed annually.

TEST 6 Distortion of Video Monitor

PHANTOM OR EQUIPMENT: Any object with a precisely spaced and regular geometric pattern. One such object is a large "+" pattern of small holes in a plastic phantom described in Test 5.

MEASUREMENT: Using a ruler pressed lightly against the screen of the video monitor (Fig. 23-9), measure the distance between n holes (*n* = 3 to 5) at the top, bottom, and right and left sides of the image as shown on the video monitor being tested.

EXPECTED RESULTS: An equivalent size object (or equivalent distances between sets of holes) should produce an image of the same size at any location on the monitor.

ACCEPTANCE LIMITS: The true distance between holes as measured on the monitor is not very important, but equivalent distances should measure the same at all points on the monitor. For example, a 30-mm object near the top of the phantom measures 17 mm on the monitor, which is fine, assuming that the magnification from the object to the image is 17/30. But if a similar 30-mm object measures 12 mm on

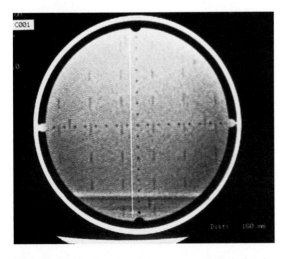

FIG. 23-8. Testing the distance-measuring device by measuring the distance between two holes separated by a precisely known distance. In this case the measured distance (*Dist*) between two holes spaced 16 cm apart is 160 mm (perfect).

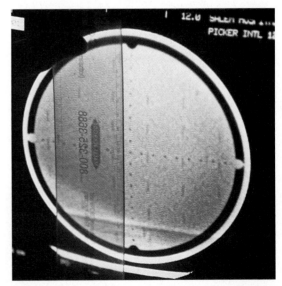

FIG. 23-9. Measuring distortion of a video monitor. A ruler pressed lightly against the screen of the video monitor is used to measure the distance between two holes at various locations on the video screen. Equal distances on the object (e.g., the separation between two easily visualized holes) should measure the same at all locations on the screen.

the monitor at the bottom of the image, the magnification is not constant and there is distortion in the monitor from top to bottom. From just two measurements, it is difficult to determine which measurement is correct; additional equivalent lengths should be measured at the right and left parts of the monitor to determine which (if any) of the four measurements is different. The maximal difference between any of the four measured values should be less than 1% of the diameter of the phantom as measured on the monitor. For example, if the phantom diameter is 170 mm on the monitor image, the maximum allowable difference between any of the four measured values would be 170 mm × 1% = 1.7 mm. This requirement may be relaxed slightly at the edge of the video monitor screen, where distortion is typically more severe.

POSSIBLE CAUSES OF FAILURE: Usually these types of distortions are produced in the video monitor itself. Many types of distortion can occur in video monitors. Usually these are caused by improper voltages or nonlinearities in voltages that sweep the electrons across the phosphor screen of the monitor. Often, a service person can adjust these voltages to values in which the distortion is small enough to be acceptable.

FREQUENCY: This should be performed monthly.

TEST 7 Distortion of Film Image or Other Hard Copy Output

PHANTOM OR EQUIPMENT: The same "+" pattern of holes described in Tests 5 and 6.

MEASUREMENT: Put an image of this phantom on film. On the film image, measure with a caliper (a fine-ruled ruler will work if necessary) the distance between n (n = 3 to 5) holes near the top, the bottom, and both sides of the image for a total of four measurements. The true distance between holes as measured on the film is not so important, but equivalent distances should measure the same at all points on the film. This measurement is the film equivalent of the measurement of video monitor distortion (Test 6).

EXPECTED RESULTS: Distances between two equally spaced holes anywhere in the phantom should appear as equal distances on the film image.

ACCEPTANCE LIMITS: The maximum difference between any of the four measured values should be less than 1% of the diameter of the phantom as measured on the film. For example, if the phantom diameter is 50 mm on the film image, the maximum allowable difference between any of the four measured values would be 50 mm × 1% = 0.5 mm.

This test is particularly important if the film images are to be used to locate tissues very precisely. For example, if the CT images are used to develop radiation therapy treatment plans, the acceptable limits of distortion may be somewhat smaller.

POSSIBLE CAUSES OF FAILURE: Misalignments or maladjustments of the optical system of the film camera or hard copy output device. Photographing a video monitor creates some film images, and these monitors are subject to the same types of distortions as the video monitors previously described. Nonlinearities in the camera electronics may also cause these types of distortions. Usually, the service person can adjust these devices relatively easily to reduce distortions.

FREQUENCY: This should be performed monthly.

TEST 8 Flatness of CT Number

PHANTOM OR EQUIPMENT: A simple cylindric plastic container about 20 cm in diameter (the same phantom used for Test 1).

MEASUREMENT: Using the ROI feature available on most CT scanners, measure the CT number of water near the top, bottom, right, and left of the phantom (Fig. 23-10). Use a ROI large enough to cover an area of 200 to 300 pixels. Compare with the measurement in Test 1.

EXPECTED RESULTS: Ideally, the CT number of water will be zero at all points in the phantom.

ACCEPTANCE LIMITS: If the CT number anywhere in the phantom differs by more

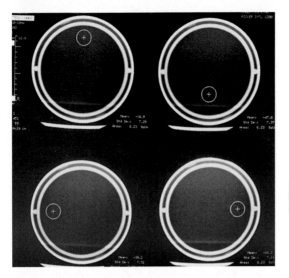

FIG. 23-10. Use several regions of interest (ROI) to measure flatness. In a homogenous water phantom, the CT number should measure zero at any location in the phantom. In these images, the CT number at the top measures −16.9 and the rest of the image has values in the range of −37 to −47. This image is unacceptable because it is not "flat."

than 5 CT numbers from the average CT number collected from all measurements, then the CT image does not have a *flat* image. If the CT number is high in the center and low near the perimeter of the phantom, the image exhibits *capping*. A low value in the center relative to the edges exhibits *cupping*.

POSSIBLE CAUSES OF FAILURE: Often capping and cupping are the result of the hardening of the x-ray beam as it penetrates the phantom. Near the edges of the phantom, the x-ray beam does not penetrate as much phantom material, and the beam is softer (i.e., it has a lower average energy). To arrive at the center, the x-rays must penetrate more phantom material and are harder near the center of the phantom. Because the effective energy of the x-rays determines the absorption characteristics of the x-rays, the absorption characteristics of water change slightly from center to edge in the phantom. Because the CT number is calculated from the number of x-rays absorbed, slight differences in CT number may indicate differences of the average energy of the x-ray beam at various points in the phantom. Some CT scanners

have software corrections built into the algorithm that compensate for these x-ray beam hardening effects, and these corrections sometimes overcompensate or undercompensate for the beam hardening. The service person may be able to adjust the algorithm to compensate for an unflat image.

FREQUENCY: This should be performed annually.

TEST 9 Hard Copy Output

PHANTOM OR EQUIPMENT: A stepped gray-scale image generated by the computer or by some other means and a film densitometer. Scanning a stairstep wedge constructed of plastic can generate a gray scale. Each step of the wedge fills the width of the x-ray beam with a larger fraction of plastic than the thinner step adjacent to it, and therefore it absorbs more x rays. The greater absorption produces a slightly higher CT number at that step and a slightly lighter shade of gray in the image. After a satisfactory image has been generated, it should be saved and used as a standard against which future tests can be compared.

MEASUREMENT: Generate an image on film of the gray-scale image. Using a film densitometer, measure the density in the center of each step of the stepped gray-scale image. One of the points of measurement is marked on the third step of the image (Fig. 23-11).

EXPECTED RESULTS: The same image should be reproduced with the hard copy device each time the image is recorded. The levels of gray as measured by the densitometer should be unchanged between images.

ACCEPTANCE LIMITS: If the measured density steps differ by more than 0.12 optical density (OD) from the accepted standard image, then the drift should be investigated and corrected.

POSSIBLE CAUSES OF FAILURE: Most frequently, drifts in the optical density of films from the camera can be traced to problems in the film processing. However, if the processor has been eliminated as a source of the problem, then the camera must be assumed to be the errant instrument. Some-

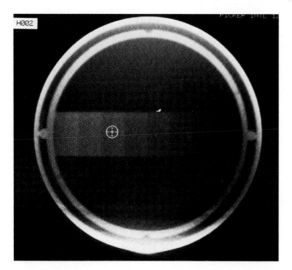

FIG. 23-11. Gray-scale test wedge for checking hard copy output. A film image of this gray-scale pattern is processed and the optical density is measured on each step and recorded.

times the video monitor, laser, or other light device used to expose the film has changed its output. In this case a service person should be called for repairs.

FREQUENCY: This should be performed monthly.

TEST 10 Accuracy of Localization Device

PHANTOM OR EQUIPMENT: A test object with a target that can be aimed for in the localization image, and a gauge that indicates how far the resulting CT images falls from the target. One example of this phantom is a set of two small holes drilled in plastic that are perpendicular to each other but at 45 degrees to the plane of the image. A cross-sectional drawing of the device is shown in Fig. 23-12. The two holes are offset slightly and do not intersect. The localization target is centered on the point where the two holes appear to intersect in the localization image, and a scan is performed. After the CT image is reconstructed, the holes should appear directly opposite each other with perfect alignment between the holes. If there is offset in the holes, the scan is not being performed where the localization image shows it to be.

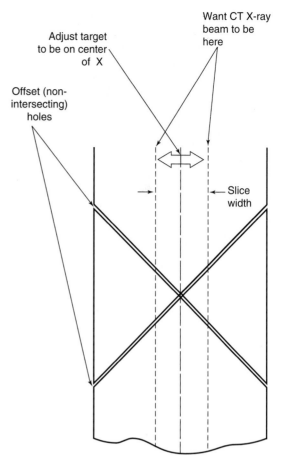

FIG. 23-12. Target pattern to test localization device. After this section is imaged with the localization image, the CT image is targeted directly on the spot where the two holes tilted 45 degrees to the scan plane appear to cross. Then a scan is performed and an image at the targeted location is reconstructed. In the image, the relative location of the two slanted holes indicates the position of the scan relative to the target.

MEASUREMENT: Image the phantom using the localization device (sometimes called a *scout* or *targeting* image). Using this localization image, set up the scanner to make a single scan at a certain thickness, such that the center of the scan is directly on the intersection of the holes. Make a scan and reconstruct the image. At the very least, both holes should appear in the CT image. If they do not, then the localization device is so poorly adjusted that the width of the x-ray beam does not intersect the plastic section in which the holes are drilled. If the localization device is working properly, the image of the two holes should appear exactly side by side (Fig. 23-13). If the holes are not aligned, then the center of the slice is off target. The distance that the center of the CT image is located from its targeted position (the intersection of the holes) can be quantified by measuring the amount of offset of the two holes in the image. Using the distance measuring device on the video monitor (the measurement can be made with a ruler on the video monitor or on the hard copy image if there is no distortion in these devices and if appropriate compensation for the magnification of the image is made), measure the distance from the tip of one hole to the tip of the other hole (Fig. 23-14). The distance that the center of the CT slice is from the targeted location is equal to the length L.

Repeat the test at other slice widths.

Note that the lengths of the holes on the image, measured from end to end, are a direct measurement of the width of the CT slice. See Test 14 for a more thorough description of why this is so.

EXPECTED RESULTS: In the ideal case, the holes should be exactly aligned.

ACCEPTANCE LIMITS: If the measured value of L is 3 mm or greater, the localization device is out of adjustment and a service person should be called.

POSSIBLE CAUSES OF FAILURE: Miscalibration of the patient bed positioning mechanisms is usually the cause, although a software problem is also possible.

FREQUENCY: This should be performed monthly.

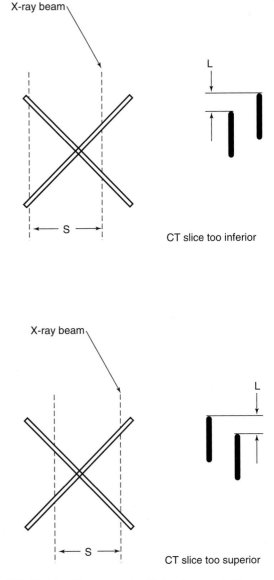

CT slice too inferior

CT slice too superior

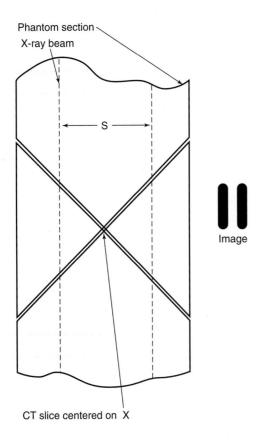

CT slice centered on X

FIG. 23-13. Example of CT slice centered on the spot where the holes appear to cross. If the two holes are aligned as shown, the localization feature is on target.

FIG. 23-14. Measurement of L for slice localization accuracy. If the two holes appear offset in the image, the error in the localization feature can be determined by measuring the offset of the lines L.

TEST 11 Bed Indexing

PHANTOM OR EQUIPMENT: A single piece of x-ray film. A 10 × 12-inch "Ready-pak" film (Kodak) works particularly well.

MEASUREMENT: The x-ray film is taped to the patient table; the length of the film is parallel to the length of the table. The scanner is programmed to perform a series of 10 to 12 scans; each scan is 10 mm from the preceding scan with the slice width set to the smallest width available (less than 5 mm). The bed is loaded with at least 100 lb (50 kg) of material to simulate the weight of a patient. When the scan is initiated, the x-ray beam exposes a series of narrow bands on the film (Fig. 23-15). With a ruler, measure the distance between the bands to determine how much the film (and bed) has moved between each scan.

EXPECTED RESULTS: The distance from center to center of the exposed bands on the film is expected to be 10 mm, or whatever the scan spacing was chosen to be.

ACCEPTANCE LIMITS: A series of 10 scans (9 interscan spacings) should create a series of exposed bands exactly 90 mm from the first to the last band. If the measured length of this band distance differs by more than 1 mm, the bed movement is not accurate and a service person should be notified.

POSSIBLE CAUSES OF FAILURE: Excessive slippage in the bed drive mechanism or miscalibration of the bed position indicators. Notify a service person.

FREQUENCY: This should be performed annually.

TEST 12 Bed Backlash

PHANTOM OR EQUIPMENT: Two small lengths of masking tape, a pencil, and a ruler.

MEASUREMENT: The patient bed is loaded with at least 100 lb (50 kg) of material to simulate the weight of a patient. The bed is moved to a convenient location to serve as a zero point. Two strips of masking tape are placed adjacent to each other, one on the edge of the moveable part of the bed, the other on a part of the bed that does not move (Fig. 23-16). A pencil mark is placed on each piece of tape so that the two marks are exactly opposite each other. The CT

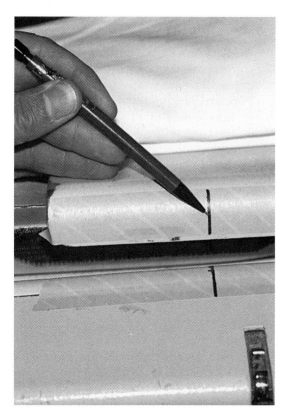

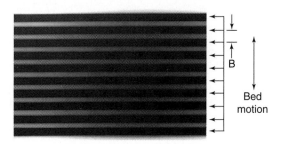

FIG. 23-15. Measurement of bed indexing from an exposed x-ray film. The series of dark lines on the film are produced by several scans through a piece of x-ray film, moving the bed after each scan. The distance between the lines (*B*) is a measure of the distance that the patient bed has moved between scans.

FIG. 23-16. Two strips of tape on the bed to determine bed backlash for both the moveable and stationary parts of the bed. The two pencil marks opposite each other define the starting or zero location of the bed.

scanner is programmed to move the bed automatically about 150 to 200 mm in 10- or 20-mm increments in one direction (for example, bed into scanner), and then return to its original (zero) starting location. After all the motions, the mark on the moving bed should return to its original position opposite the stationary mark. A measurement of the distance between the two marks indicates if there are mechanical discrepancies ("backlash") in the patient bed.

This measurement should be repeated driving the bed in the opposite direction as the first test.

If there is a position readout on the bed, the readout should be tested by driving the bed in and out about 200 to 300 mm and then returning the bed to its original position, as determined by the readout. Again, the marks on the tape should align if there is no backlash.

EXPECTED RESULTS: The marks on the two pieces of tape should always align when the bed is returned to its starting (zero) location.

ACCEPTANCE LIMITS: If the bed does not return to its starting position within 1 mm, then a service person should be notified.

POSSIBLE CAUSES OF FAILURE: Various types of mechanical backlash in the gears, belts, and pulleys driving the table, or slippage of the sensors that indicate the position of the bed. A service person can usually adjust the bed drive mechanism to eliminate this problem.

FREQUENCY: This should be performed annually.

TEST 13 Light Field Accuracy

PHANTOM OR EQUIPMENT: A piece of x-ray film. The same piece of film used for Test 11 can be used for this test.

MEASUREMENT: Tape a sheet of "Ready-pak" film to the patient bed. Raise the patient bed so that the film is approximately centered (vertically) in the gantry opening. Turn on the external or internal light field (some CT scanners use a laser beam) that indicates the location of the first scan. Using a needle or other sharp object (e.g., a penknife), poke two very small holes

through the paper wrapper of the film and into the film (Fig. 23-17). The two holes should be exactly on top of the light field, with one hole near the left edge of the film and the other on the right edge. These holes, which will be visible after the film is processed, will indicate the location of the light field.

If an external light field was used, move the bed into position for the first scan. Make a medium-technique scan with the slice width set to the minimal width. The radiation should produce a narrow dark band on the film that indicates where the radiation struck the film. Process the film and examine the location of the dark band relative to the two pinholes.

EXPECTED RESULTS: If the light field is correctly centered on the radiation field, which is also the position of the image, the dark exposed band caused by the radiation should be centered on both pinholes.

ACCEPTANCE LIMITS: The light field should be coincident with (i.e., on top of) the radiation field to within 2 mm.

POSSIBLE CAUSES OF FAILURE: Often the optical field light system is out of alignment. Less frequently, the x-ray tube may have been installed off center. Notify your service person.

FREQUENCY: This should be performed annually.

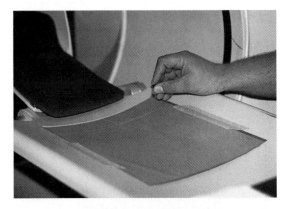

FIG. 23-17. Marking the light field position on film with a needle. Two small holes are poked into the film at the center of the light field. The film is then scanned (exposed) with a narrow beam slice to produce a darkened stripe of the film where the radiation field hit the beam. The needle marks indicate the location of the light field. The position of the light field and the radiation field should coincide.

TEST 14 Slice Width
(Nonspiral/Nonhelical Scanner)

PHANTOM OR EQUIPMENT: A phantom with a thin wire or a hole oriented at a 45-degree angle to the scan plane. The test object described in Test 10 will work.

Do not rely on the measurement of the width of the radiation bands on film to determine the slice width.

MEASUREMENT: A series of at least three scans are performed through the 45-degree hole. The scans should include a selection of possible beam widths available on the CT scanner. A selection of three slice thicknesses—narrow, medium, and wide—is usually sufficient. Using the distance-measuring device on the reconstructed image, measure the length of the hole visible on the image. When the hole is oriented at 45 degrees to the incoming radiation beam, the projection of the hole onto the CT image is the same length as the width of the x-ray beam that strikes the detectors (Fig. 23-18).

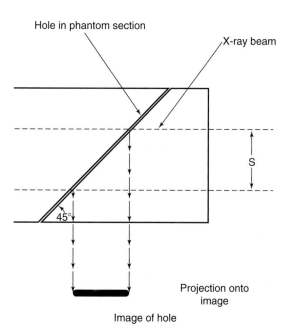

Hole in phantom section

X-ray beam

S

45°

Projection onto image

Image of hole

FIG. 23-18. X-ray beam intersecting a hole angled at 45 degrees through a thick plastic plate. As a radiation beam with a certain actual width strikes a hole or wire oriented at 45 degrees to the radiation beam, the beam intersects a certain width of that hole. When that width of hole is projected onto an image, the length of the hole in the image is exactly the same as the width of the radiation beam.

EXPECTED RESULTS: The beam width measured from the image should agree with the set (i.e., nominal) beam width.

ACCEPTANCE LIMITS: For slice widths 7 mm and greater, the measured slice width should agree with the nominal slice width to within 2 mm or less. Unfortunately, at narrower slice widths, the discrepancy between nominal and measured slice widths often becomes greater. For example, at nominal slice widths of 2 to 3 mm, the measured beam width may be twice the nominal slice width.

POSSIBLE CAUSES OF FAILURE: Miscalibration of the mechanism (e.g., shutters or collimators) that collimates that portion of the x-ray beam that reaches the detectors. Notify a service person.

FREQUENCY: This should be performed annually.

TEST 15 Pitch and Slice Width
(Spiral/Helical Scanner)

NOTE: A single test may be used to determine both the slice width and pitch of spiral/helical CT scanners. For a CT scanner with a single array of detectors, the *pitch* is defined as the ratio of bed movement (mm) that occurs during one complete revolution to the slice width (mm). For CT scanners with a single array of detectors, the slice width is determined by collimator spacing.

In the case of CT scanners with several (e.g., four) arrays of detectors that enable several slices of data to be acquired simultaneously, the definition of pitch must be clarified. In these multiarray cases, the slice width is usually determined by the size of the detectors, not by the collimator. Using a logical extension, the new definition of *pitch* is still the ratio of the distance the bed moves (mm) during one complete revolution to the slice width (mm). But it should be realized the detector size is determining the slice width, and it is not unusual to see pitch settings of 4 to 8 on these multiarray units.

PHANTOM OR EQUIPMENT: A phantom with a small diameter wire, several centimeters long, placed in the center of the scan plane at 45 degrees to the scan plane.

This test involves several adjacent scans, which may be either single scans separated by bed indexing between scans, or if the scanner is capable of spiral/helical scanning, several revolutions of the x-ray tube while the bed moves several centimeters.

Do not rely on the measurement of the width of the radiation bands on film to determine the slice width.

MEASUREMENT: For an axial scanner, set up the scanner to perform a series of 5 or 6 single scans with a constant bed indexing between the scans. Analysis of this test is easier if the slice width is selected to be the same as the bed indexing (e.g., set the bed indexing = slice width = 10 mm). For spiral/helical scans from a single array CT scanner, set the bed index the same as the slice width (pitch = 1). For a multiarray CT scanner, set the bed indexing equal to the slice width multiplied by the number of detector arrays used. Perform the scans of the wire and reconstruct the images. For spiral/helical scans, make sure that the data from the same 360-degree arc is used to reconstruct each image. To measure the slice width, use the distance-measuring device on the reconstructed image. Measure the length of the wire visible on the image. When the wire is oriented at 45 degrees to the incoming radiation beam, the projection of the wire onto the CT image is the same length as the width of the x-ray beam that strikes the wire (Fig. 23-19, A).

From this same set of images, the slice overlap or gap may be determined. To do this, overlay any two adjacent images, electronically if possible. If the images cannot be added electronically (some scanners do not have this feature), then make a film copy of the two images. Cut the adjacent images from the hard copy film, and manually overlay them on a viewbox.

EXPECTED RESULTS: First, the beam width measured from the image should agree with the set or nominal beam width using a technique similar to that described in Test 14. Next, examine the images for correct pitch by looking at the overlaid images. The image of the wires (inclined at 45 degrees) should appear in different positions in the two images. If the bed indexing is exactly the same as the slice width, the images of the wire segments should just touch

at the two ends of the wire that are closest to each other. If the ends of the wire seem to overlap as shown in Fig. 23-19, B, this indicates that the adjacent slices also overlap. If the two images of the wires do not touch at the ends as shown at the bottom of Fig. 23-19, C, the adjacent slices also have a gap between them. Ideally, the ends of the wires will just touch. Either overlap or a gap indicates that the bed indexing is not the same as the slice width. If the bed indexing test (Test 11) verifies the bed indexing accuracy, then the slice width is usually at fault.

ACCEPTANCE LIMITS: For slice widths 7 mm and greater, the measured slice width should agree with the nominal slice width to within 2 mm or less. The gap or overlap between adjacent slices should be less than 3 mm. Unfortunately, at narrower slice widths and bed index settings, the discrepancy between nominal and measured often becomes greater and these values may be relaxed somewhat.

POSSIBLE CAUSES OF FAILURE: Errors in beam width are usually caused by miscalibration of the mechanism (e.g., shutters or collimators) that collimates the portion of the x-ray beam reaching the detectors. Overlap or gaps in adjacent images or improper pitch settings may be caused by inaccuracies in the bed indexing (see Test 11) or more frequently, inaccuracy in the slice width setting. In either case, notify a service person.

FREQUENCY: This should be performed annually.

TEST 16 CT Number versus Patient Position

PHANTOM OR EQUIPMENT: A simple cylindric plastic container about 20 cm in diameter (the same phantom used for Test 1).

MEASUREMENT: At least five scans of the same phantom at the same technique are performed. However, the position of the phantom in the gantry should be changed for each scan. Place the phantom near the center of the gantry (use this image as the "standard"), top, bottom, and right and left

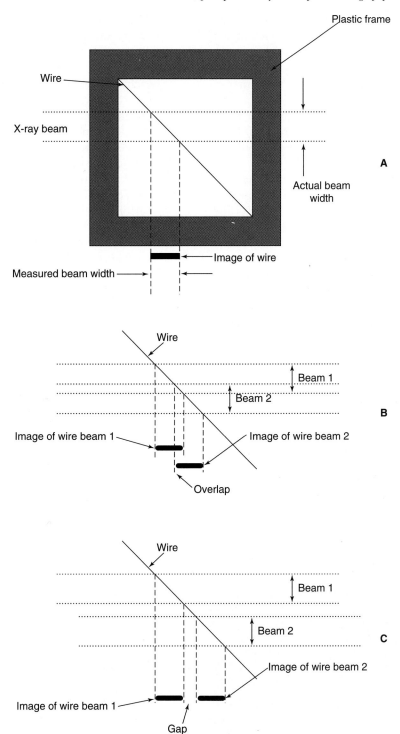

FIG. 23-19. **A,** A several centimeter-long (e.g., 10 cm) piece of wire stretched 45 degrees diagonally across a plastic frame serves as an object that projects the beam width directly to the CT scanner image. **B,** Overlaying the images from adjacent slices allows a comparison of the relative location of the adjacent slices. If adjacent slices overlap, the ends of the wire on the overlaid images will also overlap. **C,** If the adjacent slices are too far apart, a gap will appear in the overlaid images.

sides. Set the ROI feature available on the video monitor to about 200 to 300 square millimeters (or 200 to 300 pixels) and measure the average CT number of water at the center of the phantom (not the center of the image) in each image.

EXPECTED RESULTS: The average CT number of water should always be zero, independent of the position of the phantom in the CT scanner.

ACCEPTANCE LIMITS: If the average CT number varies by more than 5 CT numbers from the CT number at the center of the CT scanner, there may be a problem with the symmetry of the CT scanner.

POSSIBLE CAUSES OF FAILURE: Various asymmetries in the CT scanner system. Consult a service person.

FREQUENCY: This should be performed annually

TEST 17 CT Number versus Patient Size

PHANTOM OR EQUIPMENT: Three or four water filled phantoms, each of different diameters (Fig. 23-20). Typical diameters are 30 cm (body), 20 cm (adult head), and 15 cm (pediatric head). Fig. 23-20 also shows a very small phantom (8 cm in diameter) that models extremities.

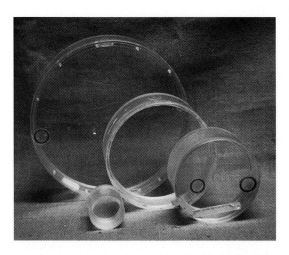

FIG. 23-20. Water phantoms of several diameters. A selection of water phantom sizes is used to test whether the CT number of water changes as the phantom (patient) size changes.

MEASUREMENT: A scan of each phantom size at the same technique is performed. The size of the phantoms should cover the sizes of the anatomy used clinically. For each CT scan, set the CT scanner field of view just large enough to view the entire phantom. Set the ROI feature available on the video monitor to about 200 to 300 square millimeters (or 200 to 300 pixels) and measure the average CT number of water at the center of each phantom image.

EXPECTED RESULTS: The average CT number of water should always be zero, independent of the size of the phantom.

ACCEPTANCE LIMITS: The average CT number of water should vary no more than 20 CT numbers from the smallest to the largest phantom.

POSSIBLE CAUSES OF FAILURE: Some CT scanners have electronic circuitry that compensates for the wide range of x-ray intensities that activate the detectors. The intensity of the x-ray signal depends on the amount of tissue that the x rays penetrate before they strike the detector. Improper compensation for the number of x-rays that reach the detector may cause the calibration of CT for water and other materials to shift from the ideal value. A service person is usually required to trace the problem.

FREQUENCY: This should be performed annually

TEST 18 CT Number versus Algorithm

PHANTOM OR EQUIPMENT: A simple cylindric plastic container about 20 cm in diameter (the same phantom used for Test 1).

MEASUREMENT: Perform a single scan of the phantom. If possible, use the same raw data to construct the image several times, each time using a different reconstruction algorithm or filter. If it is not possible to use the same data for several reconstructions, rescan the phantom using a different algorithm for each image.

EXPECTED RESULTS: The average CT number of water should always be zero, independent of the type of algorithm used to reconstruct the image.

ACCEPTANCE LIMITS: The average CT number should vary no more than three CT numbers from one algorithm to the next.

POSSIBLE CAUSES OF FAILURE: Miscalibration of the algorithm. If a recalibration of the CT scanner does not remedy the problem, a service person should be notified.

FREQUENCY: This should be performed annually.

TEST 19 CT Number versus Slice Width

PHANTOM OR EQUIPMENT: A simple cylindric plastic container about 20 cm in diameter (the same phantom used for Test 1).

MEASUREMENT: A few scans of the water phantom are performed at the same technique; however, the nominal slice width is changed between each scan. The slice widths used should cover the sizes of slice widths used clinically. Set the ROI feature available on the video monitor to about 200 to 300 square millimeters (or 200 to 300 pixels) and measure the average CT number of water at the center of each phantom image.

EXPECTED RESULTS: The average CT number of water should always be zero, independent of the slice width.

ACCEPTANCE LIMITS: The average CT number should vary no more than three CT numbers from one slice width to the next.

POSSIBLE CAUSES OF FAILURE: Miscalibration of the electronic detection circuitry or algorithm, especially the part that compensates for changes in x-ray intensity striking the detectors. Notify the service person.

FREQUENCY: This should be performed annually.

TEST 20 Noise Characteristics

PHANTOM OR EQUIPMENT: A simple cylindric plastic container about 20 cm in diameter (the same phantom used for Test 1).

MEASUREMENT: A few scans of the water phantom are performed at different mAs and different slice widths, with all other parameters constant. The settings should start at the smallest mA value available and fast scans (low mAs) and increase to the highest mAs value and slow scans (high mAs). Set the ROI feature available on the video monitor to about 200 to 300 square millimeters (or 200 to 300 pixels) and measure the standard deviation (not the average) of the CT number of water at the center of each phantom image.

EXPECTED RESULTS: The noise in the image is proportional to the standard deviation of the CT number measured in a homogeneous medium (water). Generally, the standard deviation of the CT numbers in the ROI (σ) should decrease as the mAs values and slice width are increased, keeping all other parameters constant (Brooks and Di Chiro, 1976). At lower mAs values, the dependence is $\sigma \propto (mAs \cdot Slice\ width)^{-1/2}$

The low mAs region is called the *photon noise region* and is statistical in nature. On a sheet of graph paper, plot the standard deviation versus $(mAs \times slice\ width)^{-1/2}$ (Fig. 23-21). As the mAs value is increased, the standard deviation will decrease; eventually the image noise will not be lim-

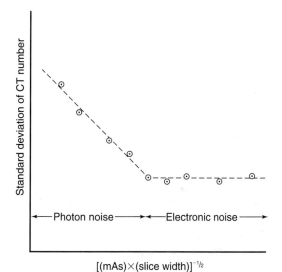

$[(mAs)\times(slice\ width)]^{-1/2}$

FIG. 23-21. Standard deviation of CT number (*noise versus mAs* × *slice width*)$^{-1/2}$. The noise decreases gradually in the photon noise (low-dose) region and assumes an approximately constant value at high-dose levels. In the high-dose region, the noise is mostly inherent electronic noise that cannot be easily reduced.

ited by the number of photons. At that point, the noise will become more or less constant and characteristic of the inherent electronic noise of the CT scanner.

ACCEPTANCE LIMITS: The noise curve that was obtained when the CT scanner was new should not change appreciably with age. Be especially sensitive to increased standard deviation as the CT scanner ages in the high-mA portion of the curve, in which the noise is dominated by electronic components.

POSSIBLE CAUSES OF FAILURE: Anything that can cause the noise of the system to change, such as changed sensitivity of the detectors, increased noise in the detector amplification circuits, or reduced photon output per mA. Notify the service person.

FREQUENCY: This should be performed annually.

TEST 21 Radiation Scatter and Leakage

PHANTOM OR EQUIPMENT: An integrating or total exposure/dose survey meter (Geiger counter) or large volume ion chamber and a head-size water phantom. An integrating exposure meter is essential for these measurements. A simple dose-rate meter is not very satisfactory because of the wide variation in dose received as the CT gantry rotates.

MEASUREMENT: Insert the head phantom into the scan plane to provide radiation scatter for the measurements. Put on a lead apron normally used for fluoroscopic procedures. Position the radiation detector at the location where the radiation measurement will be performed, and initiate a scan. It may be helpful to have a colleague initiate the scan during these measurements. Measure the total radiation emitted at that location per one complete scan. Repeat the measurements for several locations, paying particular attention to locations where attending personnel might stand during a scan. To determine an attendant's total radiation dose, simply multiply the number of attending scans by the dose per scan at the attendant's location during the scans.

EXPECTED RESULTS: The results will vary according to location and distance from the scanner. Usually, the highest exposure

rate will be next to the patient and close to the scanner (Fig. 23-22).

ACCEPTANCE LIMITS: None.

POSSIBLE CAUSES OF FAILURE: If the exposure rate is exceedingly high (>25 mR/scan), there may be a problem with the collimation system or the x-ray tube shielding. In that case, notify the service person.

FREQUENCY: This should be performed annually.

TEST 22 kVp Waveform

PHANTOM OR EQUIPMENT: There are several methods to measure the kVp of the CT scanner. The most invasive method, which is falling into more disfavor, is to install a high-voltage divider in the high-voltage cables between the x-ray generator and x-ray tube, and connect the divider to a storage-type oscilloscope. This carries a potential hazard to the technician (from high voltage) and the equipment (from failure to keep the cable clean or failure to make good electrical contact during reinsertion of the cables into their respective connectors).

Some manufacturers of testing equipment offer a noninvasive kVp meter that measures the emitted radiation to infer the shape of the kVp waveform. These devices offer consid-

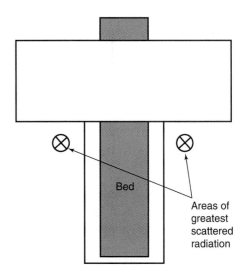

FIG. 23-22. Top view of a CT scanner suite showing areas of highest radiation intensity near a CT scanner (⊗).

erable savings in time and reduction of risk to the operator and the equipment. One of these devices, connected to a storage-type oscilloscope, can provide a kVp waveform of the CT scanner without disassembling the scanner. This latter technique is recommended.

MEASUREMENT: Select a clinically used kVp and perform a scan with the noninvasive kVp meter (or a high-voltage divider) and a storage oscilloscope. Measure the kVp from the oscilloscope trace.

EXPECTED RESULTS: The measured kVp should agree with the nominal or set kVp. The kVp waveform should be "well-behaved"; that is, it should not have excessive spikes or anomalous shapes, and it should not change kV over the duration of the scan.

ACCEPTANCE LIMITS: The measured kVp should agree with the nominal kVp to within 2 kVp.

POSSIBLE CAUSES OF FAILURE: Miscalibration of the x-ray generator. The service person can usually adjust the x-ray generator to within acceptable tolerances.

FREQUENCY: This should be performed annually

REFERENCES

American Association of Physics in Medicine: *Specifications and acceptance testing of computed tomographic scanners*, Report 39, 1993.

Brooks RA, Di Chiro G: Statistical limitations in x-ray reconstructive tomography, *Med Phys* 3:237-240, 1976.

Burkhart RL, McCrohan JL, Shuman FG: CT quality assurance in the mid-1980s, *Appl Radiol* 25-37, 1987.

Cacak RK, Design of a quality assurance program. In Hendee WR, ed: *The selection and performance of radiographic equipment*, Baltimore, 1985, Williams & Wilkins.

Cacak RK, Hendee WR: Performance evaluation of a fourth-generation computed tomography (CT) scanner, *Proc Soc Photo-optic Instr Eng* 173:194-207, 1979.

National Council on Radiation Protection and Measurements: *Quality Assurance for Diagnostic Imaging*, Report 99, pp 120-124, 1988.

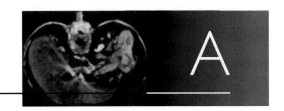

Spiral versus *Helical*

SPIRAL OR HELICAL CT: RIGHT OR WRONG?

From:
Willi A. Kalender, PhD
Siemens Medical Systems
Henkestrasse 127, D-91050 Erlangen, Germany

Editor:

The term spiral computed tomography (CT) was first made public at the 1989 RSNA scientific assembly (1). Peter Vock, MD, from Switzerland and myself, not native speakers of the English language, had had some trouble in deciding on the name for the technique. Both spiral and helical appeared to be acceptable to us—helical was possibly more precise (which is very important to the Swiss), and spiral was more readily understandable. Authoritative dictionaries of the English language told us that both terms were correct. Having walked up and down spiral staircases with spiral binders under our arms without any problems, we believed that the term spiral might be more readily understood and accepted intuitively. Indeed, the term was accepted. However, in several of our communications, we stressed that spiral and helical can be considered as synonyms (2).

Apparently, a controversy arose in the past 1–2 years, as documented by letters to editors of scientific journals (3,4). The authors made very intelligent and acceptable statements voting for either one of the terms. I think that the discussion is unnecessary. There is no right or wrong term; both terms should be kept as synonyms.

Last, but not least, for yet another reason I recommend that the scientific community and their journals stay away from deciding that one term is right and the other one is wrong. There are some commercial implications and interests connected to the terms, and any decision might be misinterpreted. For what I hope are understandable reasons, I will continue to use the original term spiral CT in my communications; however, it shall not imply a decision about which term is right and which term is wrong.

References

1. Kalender WA, Seissler W, Vock P. Single-breathhold spiral volumetric CT by continuous patient translation and scanner rotation (abstr). Radiology 1989; 173(P):414.
2. Kalender WA. Technical foundations of spiral CT. Semin Ultrasound CT MR 1994; 15:81–89.
3. Towers MJ. Spiral or helical CT? (letter) AJR 1993; 161:901.
4. Mintz RD. Spiral vs helical: a matter of precision (letter). AJR 1994; 162:1507.

Editor's note.—We concur; hereafter, *Radiology* will accept either term.

Stanley S. Siegelman, MD
Editor, *Radiology*

Letter to editor, *Radiology* 171:20, 1990.

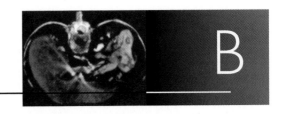

Equipment Specifications for Three Computed Tomography Scanners

PICKER PQ-6000 CT IMAGING SYSTEM

Scan time	0.6 (230 degrees), 1, 1.5, 2, 3, and 4 sec
Slice thickness	1, 1.5, 2, 3, 4, 5, 8, and 10 mm
Scan angle	230, 360, 379 degrees
Scan plane	Gantry tilt range of ±30 degrees
Image processing	1024 samples per view
	512 × 512 image matrix
	1024 × 1,024 image display
	Pixel size: 0.04 to 0.47-mm standard scanning
	CT number range: −2048 to +6143
	Hounsfield units
Reconstruction times	Axial and spiral: 3 sec
Pilot scan	Half field: 2 sec (25 cm) 512 matrix
	2 sec (51 cm) 512 matrix
	Full field: 3 sec (51 cm) 1024 matrix
	5 sec (102 cm) 1024 matrix
Image-to-image display	
Cycle time	3 sec (axial and spiral)
Spatial resolution	21.5 Lp/cm
Low-contrast resolution	2.0 mm at 0.35%
	(1-sec scan, 6-in CatPhan phantom) and 4 mm at 0.35% with 2.5 rads
	(1-sec scan, 8-in CatPhan phantom)
Noise	0.14% (2-sec scan, 6-¼-in water phantom) or 0.21% (1-sec scan, 8-in water phantom)
X-ray tube	Duplex graphite anode
	Dual focal spot:
	Small: 0.4 mm × 0.5 mm length (nominal)
	Large: 0.6 mm × 0.9 mm length (nominal)

CT imaging system. (Courtesy Picker International; Cleveland, Ohio.)

Continued

X-ray tube—cont'd	10,000 RPM
	Anode heat storage capacity: 5.0 MHU
	Anode cooling rate: 830 kHU/min
	Continuous anode cooling rate: 600 kHU/min
	Housing heat storage: 4.0 MHU
	Housing heat dissipation rate: 550 kHU min
Generator	High-frequency inverter generator mounted on a rotating scan frame
	50 kW maximum
	mA selections: 30, 50, 60, 100, 125, 150, 175, 200, 225, 250, 300, 325, 350, 375, and 400 kV selections: 80, 100, 110, 120, 130, 140
	Output specifications (480 VAC 10%, 3-phase rated output) mA accuracy ±6% or 3 mA (whichever is greater)
	kV accuracy ± 6%
	Efficiency: > 75%
	Reproducibility:
	Long term: less than 0.25% during 24-hour period
	Short term: 0.1% in 1-hour line
	Frequency ripple: less than 0.02%
Detectors	CSD (continuous spiral detectors)
	Cadmium tungstate, active-response detectors
	Cadmium tungstate crystal–99% photon conversion efficiency
	Continuous calibration
	Performs both angular and ray sampling
	Dynamic range: > 1,000,000 : 1
Gantry	Length: 34 in (86 cm)
	Width: 89 in (226 cm)
	Height: 77 in (196 cm)
	Weight: 3550 lbs (1,610 kg)
	The gantry will fit through a standard door way for easy installation
	±30 degree gantry angulation
	70 cm aperture
	Sagittal, coronal, and z-axis laser positioning lights
	Controls for gantry tilt, patient support system, and laser lights are located on both sides of the gantry
	Digital readout of gantry angle, patient support height, and horizontal position

PICKER Mx-8000 MULTISLICE CT IMAGING SYSTEM

Scan time	0.3 (240 degrees), 0.5, 0.75, 1, 1.5, and 2 sec
Spiral ontime	Up to 100 sec continuous
Spiral pitches	Q-0.25 to Q-2.0 in 4-slice modes
	D-0.5 to D-2.0 in 2-slice modes
Slice thickness	0.5, 1.0, 2.5, 5, 8, and 10 mm
Scan angle	240, 360, 420 degrees
Scan plane	Gantry tilt range of ±30 degrees
Surview	Up to 1000 mm scan length, 500 mm scan width
Image processing	2320 views/revolution/element
	Reconstruction matrices of 340^2, 512^2, 768^2, and 1024^2
System color monitor	20-inch, 1280 × 1024, high resolution
CT number range	−1024 to +3072 Hounsfield units
Computer	Silicon Graphics RISC host computer with UNIX multitasking graphic interface, SGI R5000 RISC processor at 200 MHz
	Hard drive: 4 GByte SCSI, optional EOD with 1.2 GByte or 2.3 GByte EOD cartridges
Reconstruction time	1.5 to 2 sec for 512^2 image
Spatial resolution	24.0 Lp/cm in ultrahigh mode, 22.0 Lp/cm at 0.3%
Low contrast resolution	4.0 mm at 0.3% with 27 mGy (20 cm CATPHAN phantom)
Noise	0.30%, 27 mGy as measured on a 21.6-cm water equivalent phantom
Generator	60 kW maximum mA selections: from 28 to 500 in 1 mA increments
	kV selections: 90, 120, and 140
X-ray tube	Dynamic focal spot rotating graphite composite anode; continuous operation during scan
	Maximum heat anode storage: 6.5 MHU
	Maximum anode cooling rate: 730 kHU/min
	Dual focal spot: 1.2 mm × 1.5 mm and 0.7 mm × 1.0 mm
Detectors	Asymmetrix: Picker-patented variable wide area detector arranged in an array consisting of 5376 elements in eight distinct arcs
Dynamic range	1,000,000:1
Field of view	50-cm field of view inside 70-cm aperture
DICOM	DICOM 3.0 hierarchical model in a DICOM 3.0 image format. Advanced database type sorting of patients and images enables fast and easy manipulation of files.
Gantry	70-cm aperture
	Controls for gantry tilt, table elevation, stroke, and swivel are conveniently located on both sides of the gantry and on the operator console
Patient support	1570-mm scannable range
	200 kg (440 lbs) capacity with ± 0.25-mm accuracy
Data processing computer	1.9 GIPS (giga instructions per sec)
	512 MByte (expandable to 1 GByte*) plus an 18 GByte fast disk array for scan data

(Courtesy Picker International; Cleveland, Ohio.)

TOSHIBA AQUILLION MULTISLICE CT SCANNER

SCAN PARAMETERS

Scan regions	Whole body, including head
Scan system	360-degree continuous rotate/rotate
Scan time	
CT scan	0.32 sec (229°) sec, 0.5, 0.75, 1, 1.5, 2 and 3 sec (360°)
Scanoscope	Arbitrary up to 14 sec depending on the length of the scan field along the patient axis.

Scan cycle time (for 0.5-sec scan)

SCAN & VIEW mode	1.5 sec
SCAN & SCAN mode	1.5 sec (rapid sequence)

NOTE: Scan cycle time refers to the time between one scan initiation and the next.
SCAN & VIEW mode permits immediate viewing of images upon completion of each individual slice.

Scan field	
CT scan	ø180 mm (SS)
	ø240 mm (S)
	ø320 mm (M)
	ø400 mm (L)
	ø500 mm (LL)
Scanoscope	

LATERAL DIRECTION	AXIAL DIRECTION
240 mm (S)	Arbitrary from 200 mm
400 mm (L)	to 1390 mm
500 mm (LL)	

Slice thickness	0.8, 1, 2, 3, 5, 7, and 10 mm
Number of slices	1 slice/scan
Gantry tilting angle	From forward 30 degrees to backward 30 degrees (in increments of 0.5 degrees)
	Remote control from the console is possible.
Tube position for scanoscope	0 degrees, 90 degrees, 180 degrees, and 270 degrees
	Any arbitrary angle can be specified (in 5 degrees increments)
Gantry aperture	720-mm diameter

PATIENT COUCH

Vertical movement system	Hydraulically driven
Speed of vertical movement	16 to 30 mm/sec
Stroke	Approx. 650 mm
Minimum couchtop height	Approx. 300 mm
	Remote control from the console is possible.

NOTE: This function allows the user to check the image on the console and adjust the couchtop without leaving the console. Adjustment can be made in 10-mm increments at the console.

Couchtop movement	
System	Motor driven or manual
Speed of movement	100 mm/sec (fast)
	10 mm/sec (slow)
Stroke	1820 mm
Scannable range	1440 mm (with head rest)
Step feed pitch	0.5 to 200 mm in 0.5-mm unit
Reproducibility	± 0.25 mm
	Repeatable to within ± 0.25 mm after 600 mm of movement

Remote control from the console is possible.

Couchtop width	470 mm
Load limitation	
Maximum allowable load	205 kg (450 lb)

VOICE-RECORDED INSTRUCTION AND SCAN SYSTEM (VOICELINK)

Vocal instructions to the patient can be recorded electronically by the operator and replayed during scan sequences automatically as a part of the eXam Plan.

Available number of messages	Maximum of 32
Available number of seconds	Maximum of 128 sec for a total of 32 messages
Delay time setting	Time between the end of reproduction and scan start can be set up to 10 sec in increments of 1 sec.

HELICAL SCAN

X-ray tube rotation speed	0.5, 0.75, 1, 1.5 sec/ 360 degrees
Maximum helical scan time	100 sec
Scan start time delay	Min. 1 sec
	Setting is possible in steps of 0.1
Scan field in axial direction	Maximum 1390 mm/scan
	Up to 10 scan plans are programmable in one eXam Plan. (Multiple and/or Multidirectional Helical)

Continued

HELICAL SCAN—cont'd

Couch feed speed — This can be specified arbitrarily within the range of 0.5 to 40 mm/sec (in steps of 0.1 mm/sec).

Image reconstruction time — 1.5 sec

Real-time helical reconstruction time — 8 images/sec (12 images/sec option)

SureStart

Max continuous scan time — 100 sec

Region of interest (ROI) — Maximum 3 ROIs

CT number measurement interval — 0.25 sec

Specification of reconstruction position — By entering the couchtop position, or on the scanogram (in minimum units of 0.1 mm)

Reconstruction method — No interpolation
360-degree interpolation
Opposite beam interpolation
Stack reconstruction

DYNAMIC SCAN

Scan time — 0.5, 0.75, 1, 1.5 sec/ 360 degree

Programmable time — Maximum 1 hour
This refers to the maximum time within which a series of scans are performed following a predetermined eXam Plan.

Number of programmable scans — Maximum 100 scans
This refers to the maximum number of scans possible as a series of dynamic scanning data.
Maximum time of one continuous scan is 100 sec.

Scan plan

Scan interval — Minimum interval is 1 sec.
Setting is possible in steps of 0.1 sec in scan interval more than 1 sec.

NOTE: When a scanning mode with patient couch movement is used, the minimum scan interval is limited by the time for the movement.

Scan plan programming — Up to 360 different Sequences can be preprogrammed.

Scan start time delay — Minimum 0.5 sec
Setting is possible in steps of 0.1 sec.

Maximum scan rate — Maximum 200 scans/100 sec (0.5-sec scan, 200 rotations)

Image reconstruction

Full image — 1 image/scan

Partial image — Reconstruction is possible in steps of 0.1 sec.

Reconstruction time — 1.5 sec

Real-time reconstruction time — 8 images/sec (12 images/sec: option)

Rapid sequence scan: — Minimum scan cycle time
Approx. 1.5 sec at 10 mm pitch with 0.5 sec scan

Multislice dynamic scan: — Maximum number of 8 positions

X-RAY GENERATION

X-ray beam shape — Fan shaped, fan angle 49.2 degrees

X-ray exposure — Continuous

X-ray tube voltage — 80, 100, 120, and 135 kV

X-ray tube current — 10 to 500 mA (in increments of 10 mA)

X-ray tube heat capacity — 7.5 MHU

X-ray tube cooling rate — 1386 kHU/min (maximum)
1008 kHU/min (actual)

Focal spot size

IEC standard, nominal — 0.9 × 0.8 mm (small)
1.6 × 1.4 mm (large)

X-RAY DETECTION

Detection system — Solid state detectors

Main detector — 896 channels

Reference detector — 1 set

Viewing rate — 1800 views/s (maximum)

DATA PROCESSING

Reconstruction matrix 512 × 512

Picture element (pixel) size

CT IMAGE				UNIT: MM	
Scan field	**SS**	**S**	**M**	**L**	**LL**
Pixel size	*to	*to	*to	*to	*to
	0.35	0.47	0.63	0.78	0.98

(*: depending on Vari-Area or Zoom factors)

Continued

DATA PROCESSING—cont'd

SCANOGRAM UNIT: MM

Enlargement

Ratio (area)	Standard	2×	4×	8×	16×
	2.00 (LL)	1.41	1.0	0.71	0.50
Pixel size	1.00 (L)	0.71	0.50	—	—
	0.50 (S)	—	—	—	—

Reconstruction filter functions — Total of 99 available filter functions

	REGION
From FC01	Abdomen with BHC
From FC10	Abdomen without BHC
From FC20	Brain with BHC
From FC30	Inner ear and bone
From FC40	Brain without BHC
From FC50	Lung
FC70	Maintenance
From FC80	Super resolution mode for inner ear, bone and lung
FC90	Maintenance

Image reconstruction time
  CT scan — 1 sec (for 0.5-sec scan)
  Scanoscope — Reconstructed and displayed simultaneously with scanning (real-time reconstruction)

Data processor
  Central processing unit — 64-bit microprocessors
  Magnetic disk unit: — Storage capacity, 12 Gbytes
  Magnetooptical disk unit — 5-inch type, 2.4 Gbytes (double sided)

DATA STORAGE

System
  Raw data — 2000 (maximum)
  Image data — 8000 (maximum)
Magnetooptical disk: — Approximately 9600 images or 2400 raw image data per cassette (2.4 Gbyte)

IMAGE DISPLAY

Display matrix — 1024 × 1024 (maximum)
CT number display range — From −1024 to +8191
Window width — Continuously variable (adjustable at variable speed)
Window level — Continuously variable (adjustable at variable speed)

Preset window — 3 kinds of window settings may be preset for each image.
Window types — Linear, nonlinear (6 user-programmable), and double windows.
Image retrieval
  Method — On-screen menus and keyboard
  Mode — Image, series and patient
Image display monitor — 21-in color display
Autoview function — Software control, function key
Multiframe display — ROI processing
  Inset scanogram display
  Selective related information display
  Cine display
    Number of frames — Up to 128
    Image display speed — The display speed can be varied up to a maximum of 20 frames/sec.
    Display image: — All images in the magnetic disk can be selected.

IMAGE PROCESSING

Scanogram processing
  Slice position display (display of planned slice, preset slice, and last scanned slice)
  Anatomic scale (display of relative position, taking any point selected as standard as 0)
  Slice position setting
  Enlargement (2×, 4× for L and LL size; 8×, 16× for LL size)
  Target tracking
CT image processing
  ROI setting and processing
    ROI shape — Point, rectangular, polygonal elliptical, irregular
    ROI processing — Mean value, standard deviation, area, number of pixels
    ROI display — 3 ROIs can be displayed on an image
    ROI control — Size, position, rotation
  Measurement of distance and angle between two points
  Profile (oblique profile also available)
  Histogram
  CT number display
  Mark display (grid display, scale display)
  Volume calculation
  Enlargement (2×, 4×, and arbitrary size)
  Addition/subtraction between images

Continued

IMAGE PROCESSING—cont'd

Band display (nonlinear windowing)

Comment and arrow insertion

Top/bottom, right/left, black/white reversal of image

Image filtering

Screen save

High-speed axial interpolation

Raw data processing

Multizooming (processing of raw data for 4 ROIs and multiple images)

Stack reconstruction

System management

Warm-up

Calibration data

Picture retouching

Scanogram/CT image switching

CLINICAL APPLICATION

Dynamic study*

A mathematical function is fitted to the time curve generated for the designated ROI within an image, and the functional parameters are displayed.

ROI shape: Rectangular, polygonal, elliptical, irregular

Fitting function: Gamma function (perform least squares approximation)

NOTE: The above parameters may be modified or additional parameters may be provided to upgrade the system.

Functional image*

In addition to processing images, Aquilion can create functional images or image maps as well. Parameters which can be used to generate a functional image

Peak height

Peak time

Appearance time

Area under curve

Mean transit time

Second moment

Transit time

NOTE: These parameters may be modified or additional parameters may be provided to upgrade the system.

Size of the calcu-   1 × 1 to 10 × 10 pixels, lation area   variable

Area to be   By specifying a rectangular calculated   ROI, the ROI is divided into elements of the size above and parameters for each element are calculated.

Resultant file   Filed as a 512 × 512 matrix image.

*Works in progress

3D COLOR IMAGE PROCESSING

High-quality 3D images can be obtained very quickly with easy operation.

3D surface rendering

Clipping, texture or non-texture

3D volume rendering

Maximum intensity projection (Max-IP)

Minimum intensity projection (Min-IP)

X-ray volume rendering

Intensity volume rendering

Shaded volume rendering (opacity curve can be set freely)

Display/processing function

Zooming, panning, measurement (distance, angle), annotation, cutting, drilling

Cine display

Segmentation

Partial extraction can be performed

MPR

3 orthogonal planes/oblique image

Curved MPR

IMAGE TRANSFER

DICOM3 storage SCU

AUTO FILMING

Ethernet network

IMAGE QUALITY

Noise

Standard deviation Less than 0.35%

Scan parameters

Tube voltage   120 kV

Tube current   300 mA

Scan time   1 sec

Function type   FC41

Slice thickness 10 mm

Scan field   S

Water phantom   ø240 mm

Spatial resolution 1   14.5 lp/cm at MTF 2%

18 lp/cm at Cut off

Scan parameter

Tube voltage   120 kV

Tube current   200 mA

Scan time   1 sec

Slice thickness 2 mm

Scan field   S

Function type   FC90

Phantom   IRIS QA*

*ø160 mm CATPHAN

Continued

IMAGE QUALITY

		Low contrast resolution		
Spatial resolution 2			2.5 mm	
Super resolution	0.35 mm ± 0.05 mm		at 0.25%	
mode (FC90)			or 2 mm	4 mm
Standard mode	0.55 mm ± 0.05 mm		at 0.3%	at 0.3%
(FC30)		Scan parameters		
Scan parameters		Tube voltage	120 kV	120 kV
Tube voltage	120 kV	Tube current	500 mA	300 mA
Tube current	300 mA	Scan time	0.5 sec	0.5 sec
Scan time	0.5 sec	Function type	FC41	FC41
Slice thickness	2 mm	Slice thickness	10 mm	10 mm
Scan field	S	Scan field	S	S
Phantom	Toshiba standard	Phantom	IRIS QA*	IRIS QA*

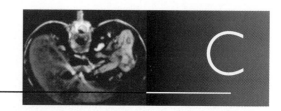

OmniPro 2 Visualization and Multislice CT Workstation

OMNIPRO 2

DESCRIPTION
Picker's OmniPro2™ is an independent, multimodality, advanced visualization workstation. It provides quick processing, analysis, manipulation, display, filming, storage and retrieval of images from different modalities. OmniPRO2 is based on a Silicon Graphics© platform and powerful UNIX multitasking system for optimum speed and response.

OmniPro2's speed and power make it the perfect workstation for multislice CT systems that require the ability to manipulate datasets with hundreds of images. Large image sets are efficiently and quickly reviewed and displayed with real-time 2D, multiplanar reformation (MPR), and 3D volume rendering.

OmniPro2's mouse-driven graphical user interface (GUI) makes learning and using the system both fast and easy. Beyond its basic functions and features, OmniPro2's modular design allows the addition of the most advanced image processing applications.

FEATURES
Volume rendering. Picker's exclusive 4D Angio™ volume rendering package provides simultaneous viewing of vasculature, soft tissue and bone. 4D Angio provides real-time interactive control over opacity and transparency values, which permits viewing through and beyond surrounding structures such as metallic stents and arterial calcification.

4D Angio virtually eliminates the need for organ segmentation by displaying the entire dynamic range of Hounsfield units in a single image. CT angiography (CTA) studies can be completed rapidly with minimal operator effort for improved throughput and efficiency.

Virtual endoscopy. Voyager™ is a real-time CT endoscopy tool that renders spiral CT data to provide fly-through images within and around hollow organs. Possible uses are virtual colonoscopy, bronchoscopy, angioscopy and more. Interactive exploration of the patient anatomy from inside or automatic replay of a previously traversed path are available.

Advancement direction, traversed path and field-of-view are displayed on-line on MPR and 3D reference images for guidance in the endoscopic space.

Rotation of point-of-view enables looking at the anatomy from any angle and not necessarily in the direction of movement. Image graphics enable distance and angle measurements in 3D space and annotations with arrows and text.

Multitissue 3D. Fast reformatting of three-dimensional images of up to 15 different tissues or organs provides easy to understand presentation of complex anatomy. To enhance the display, light source placement can be changed interactively.

Real-time manipulation of 3D images includes zoom, pan, rotation around any axis, and cutting of the organs with a user-defined viewing aperture to expose underlying tissues. Making a tissue transparent enables viewing of underlying organs.

CT or MR values can be displayed on the cutting aperture surfaces, and the 3D image can be correlated with the original images. Cine of up to 30 frames/second may be displayed. 3D volumes, distances and angles can be measured.

To define tissues and organs, a variety of segmentation tools are available: thresholding level adjustment, seed planting region growing and morphological methods (e.g. erosion, dilation, etc).

Maximum and minimum intensity projection (MIP). MIP images from a volumetric set of images can be quickly reformatted to demonstrate enhanced vascular structures. The projection images can be interactively generated in any arbitrary viewing angle, and can be windowed, zoomed and panned in realtime.

Easy-to-use tools to define a volume-of-interest for the projection and to extract unwanted tissues (e.g., bones) are available. The projection can also be correlated with the original images.

With the MasterCut™ feature, MPR curved cuts along vascular structures can be defined on the MIP image to display panoramic and cross-sectional views. A series of cross-sectional cuts with 2.5 mm spacing can be saved for full evaluation of changes across the vessels. Cine of up to 30 frames/second may be displayed.

In addition to the standard MIP, minimum intensity projection for visualization of airways is available. This display mode is especially helpful for determining and localizing bronchial stenosis in adults and children.

Multiplanar reformations (MPR). Volumetric datasets may be quickly reformatted into any user-defined plane (axial, sagittal, coronal, oblique) or curved planes in realtime. Interactive and easy manipulation is provided, including plane thickness, position and orientation, number of displayed planes and spacing between planes.

Other manipulations such as zoom, pan, windowing and leafing through images are also available. Flexible display formats include multiplanar oblique display (with reference images), orthogonal planes display, or single image with reference acquired slice.

Continued

Graphic aids may be used to annotate and measure on MPR cuts. User-defined series of cuts may be archived and filmed for full coverage of the interesting region in any orientation.

Combiner™. OmniPro2 provides the ability to combine multiple images and display them as a single, thick-slice image. This is especially useful for viewing and filming multislice CT datasets that have as many as 800 or more images, making review and filming of every slice impractical.

Thin-slice (0.5 mm or 1.0 mm) images can be combined to limit the number of images displayed, drastically shortening filming and interpretation time. Select, original thin-slice images can be reviewed when necessary.

In addition, this feature also permits weighted subtraction of images for better visualization of contrast uptake by subtracting pre-contrast images from the corresponding images after contrast.

MasterMatch image fusion. MasterMatch™ allows for the three-dimensional co-registration of studies acquired in different modalities (CT and MR), or in the same modality at different times or with different scan conditions. Some of the uses are:

- Analysis of pathological change over time
- Complimenting the data from one modality with data from another

DentaCT. The DentaCT™ application is used to perform imaging of the mandible or maxilla for assisting oral surgeons in planning implantation of prostheses. The patient is scanned on the CT scanner using a specially tailored DentaCT procedure and the scanned images are then used as input in the DentaCT application. The program allows real-time generation and display of panoramic views and cross-sectional cuts, and true-size printing on film.

Image viewing. OmniPro2's interactive image viewer is designed for fast, efficient and simple image review and film preparation. Multiple series of images are chosen by the user and called up for rapid display in the viewer window. Several series containing images from different modalities can be displayed concurrently. Images can be manipulated individually or in user-selected groups. Image viewing features include:

- Zoom and pan
- Random image placement on the viewer
- Image enhancement filters
- Scrolling
- Cine
- Flip and rotate images
- Display image parameters in-frame or separately
- Predefined and mouse-driven window and level

Image graphics. A variety of graphic aids may be individually positioned and manipulated with the mouse to assist in the interpretation of clinical images. They include:

- Text annotation anywhere on the image
- Cursors for pixel value measurement
- Regions of interest
- Lines, grid, and scales for distance measurements
- Arrows for pointing to features
- Angle measurements
- Histogram of pixel values
- Profile of the pixel values along any line
- Grid with adjustable spacing for distance assessment

COMMUNICATIONS AND NETWORKING

OmniPro2's full implementation of the DICOM v3.0 communications protocol allows connectivity to Picker and other vendors DICOM v3.0-compliant scanners and workstations

In addition, OmniPro2 can retrieve and return images directly from Picker CT scanners and OmniView consoles. The OmniPro2 can function both as a server and a client.

The OmniPro2 can communicate with the following DICOM compliant modalities:

- Computed tomography (CT)
- Magnetic resonance imaging (MRI)
- Nuclear medicine (NM)
- Computed Radiography (CR)
- Radio-fluoroscopy (RF)
- Secondary-capture images (for display only)

InterView-OP. InterView-OP™ is used for sharing images by multiple users, irrespective of where they are located. Images stored on the OmniPro2 are viewed and manipulated locally on the end-user PC. In-site users will be connected to the site LAN which ensures fast response. Users outside the site may use modem and ISDN lines or can be connected via the Internet. They operate the service from their standard PCs using the familiar web browser interface.

The Java technology used in this product obviates the need to install any software on their Pcs as all modules (applets) are downloaded automatically from the server.

IMAGE MANAGEMENT AND ARCHIVING

Images in the OmniPro2 archive are organized according to the DICOM v3.0 hirarchical model. Images can reside on local devices such as the workstation fixed disc, on optional removable EOD (erasable optical disk), or on remote devices connected via LAN (e.g., Mx8000™, MxTwin™).

Continued

Archive Capacity (typical number of images)

MATRIX	DISK		EOD
	4 GBytes	1.2 GBytes	2.3 GBytes
512^2	16000	6000	11000
340^2	29000	11000	21000
256^2	48000	18000	34000

COMPUTER AND DISPLAY

System computer. Silicon Graphics workstation based on the R5000SC RISC microprocessor at 200 Mhz with 4 Gbytes hard disk.

Main memory. 128 Mbytes RAM (up to 1 Gbyte optional)

Operating system. Unix system V5. Mouse-driven graphic user interface, OSF/Motif-compliant.

Display monitor. 1280 × 1024
120 MHz bandwidth
17-in color high resolution
21-in and magnetically shielded
20-in color monitors are optional

Gray levels and colors. 256 gray levels and up to a total of 4096 colors simultaneously on screen.

OPTIONS

Special applications packages

3D-OP-2. Multitissue 3D image reformations, manipulation, and display package.

4D Angio. New advanced 3D volume rendering algorithms to reproduce whole tissue and organs for display.

Angio+MIP-OP-2. Maximum and minimum intensity projection (MIP) reformation and manipulation. MasterCut panoramic and cross-sectional views option.

Voyager virtual endoscopy. Virtual endoscopy package providing a noninvasive method to fly-through and fly-around hollow anatomic organs such as the colon, bronchus and vessels.

M-Match. Image fusion for 3D coregistration of studies taken at different times or by different modalities.

Dent-3. Dental package for producing panoramic and cross-sectional cuts through the mandible or maxilla.

DICOM-NM. Viewing and transferring of images in DICOM v3.0 protocol./format. Images can be stored in archives or retrieved for viewing and filming and also windowed, zoomed, panned, and rotated.

DICOM-CR. Viewing and transferring of CR (computed radiography) images in DICOM v3.0 protocol/format. Images can be stored in archives or retrieved for viewing and filming and also windowed, zoomed, panned, and rotated.

DICOM-RF. Viewing and transferring of RF (radiofluoroscopy) images in DICOM v3.0 protocol/format. Images can be stored in archives or retrieved for viewing and filming and also windowed, zoomed, panned, and rotated.

InterView-OP. A package to access and view medical images by up to five users on their standard PC computers. Users are connected via LAN, WAN or through the Internet (not included).

SYSTEM EXPANSIONS

MEM-4, MEM-5. Memory expansion to a total RAM of 192 and 256 Mbytes respectively.

MEM-6, MEM-7. Memory modules of 128 and 256 Mbytes respectively. Total memory is limited to 1 Gbyte.

CMD-1. 21-in. high-resolution color display in lieu of the standard 17-in monitor.

ECL-4. 180 meters of path-cable in lieu of the 60 meters of path-cable included in OmniPro2.

PHYSICAL SPECIFICATIONS

- Power requirements: 115 VAC/2.5A
- Heat dissipation: 1000 BTU/hr
- Operating temperature: 13° to 35° C
                               (56° to 95° F)
- Relative humidity: 10% to 80%
                               noncondensing

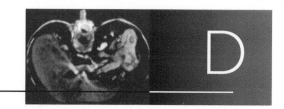

Historical Look at Specific Features of CT Scanners, 1973 to 1983

YEAR	DEVELOPMENTS
1973	EMI is sole manufacturer and delivers 60-head computer tomographs with 6.5-min scan time.
1974	Siemens brings similar unit SIRETOM to clinical use as first x-ray company; Ledley presents his whole-body ACTA scanner, which is built by Pfizer in the following year; Ohio Nuclear announces the whole-body DELTA-Scan 50 with 2.5-min scan time; Artronix announces a rotation system for a 9-sec computer tomograph with water-compensating body.
1975	EMI presents the 60-sec head unit CT 1010 and the 20-sec whole-body computer tomograph 5005; GE presents a 10-sec mamma unit CT/M with rotation system as pilot project, announces the 5-sec whole-body unit CT/T and sells the 270-sec head unit CT/N of the Neuroscan Company; Siemens takes the DELTA-Scan 50 into the worldwide sales program (apart from United States and Canada) and afterward the following DELTA-Scan types as well, up to 1977.
1976	Ohio Nuclear introduces the 18.8-sec DELTA-Scan 50 FS, Pfizer the 20-sec computer tomograph 0200 FS, and Philips the 20-sec TOMOSCAN, and thus follow the EMI unit CT 5005; Syntex shows a 12-sec whole-body computer tomograph with translation-rotation system that is, however, dropped in the following year; Eiscint introduces the 10-sec whole-body computer tomograph SCANEX (also with translation-rotation); AS & E presents the ring detector system for 5-sec scan time; Siemens introduces the SOMATOM with crystal semiconductor detector and instant image.
1977	Ohio Nuclear comes in the spring with the DELTA-Scan 2000 series and thus "shoots down" the DELTA-Scan 50 FS prematurely; three manufacturers announce at the RSNA Meeting at the end of the year ring detector systems without showing image results: EMI, Picker, and Artronix; Philips announces the 5-sec whole-body TOMOSCAN 300 and thus makes the just-available TOMOSCAN 200 into a special offer unit; Syntex 60 is added to the Philips sales program as neurocomputer tomograph TOMOSCAN 100; Syntex drops out of the computed tomography field in the following year; CGR takes over the sale of the Pfizer units and afterward those of the Varian scanner and brings their own 20-sec head unit ND 8000 onto the market.
1978	Syntex, AS & E, Searle "bail out"; Pfizer takes over technology and production of the AS & E scanner; EMI distributes Searle computer tomographs because their own CT 7070 is not yet ready; Eiscint exploits the translation-rotation system up to a minimum scan time of 5.8 sec.
1979	CGR announces its own whole-body unit CE 10,000 with 1024 xenon detectors, of which the first head scans were shown only 2 years later; Siemens is successful in breaking through to the American market with the SOMATOM 2; all x-ray firms except for Picker prefer the rotation system with the traveling detector.
1980	EMI drops out of the computer tomography field; GE takes over the service, apart from in the United States and Canada, where Omnimedical takes over servicing and finally continues in the following year with the CT 7070 modified as QUAD 1; Eiscint brings a hybrid computer tomograph onto the market with the EXEL 1002 with translation-rotation for high resolution and 1.9-sec rotation with only 280 detectors; Pfizer shows CT images from its new ring detector with 2400 elements and a resolution of 0.4 mm.
1981	Pfizer "bails out"; Picker is taken over by the British GEC; GE and Siemens present at the RSNA Meeting the CT 9800 and the SOMATOM DR, with minimum scan times of 1.3 sec and 1.4 sec, respectively.
1981 to 1983	Eight manufacturers still represented with worldwide activities; among these, GE has the peak position in the United States, Siemens in Europe, and Toshiba in Japan.

From Dümmling K: 10 years' computed tomography: a retrospective view, *Electromedica* 52:13-28, 1984.

Index